Readings in Family Nursing

Readings
in Family Nursing

Edited by

GAIL D. WEGNER, RN, MS
Associate Professor
Department of Nursing
Purdue University Calumet
Hammond, Indiana

RINDA J. ALEXANDER, RN, PhD
Professor
Department of Nursing
Purdue University Calumet
Hammond, Indiana

J. B. LIPPINCOTT COMPANY   Philadelphia

Acquiring Editor: Barbara Nelson Cullen
Coordinating Editorial Assistant: Jennifer E. Brogan
Indexer: Barbara S. Littlewood
Interior Designer: Publishers' WorkGroup
Cover Designer: Thomas Jackson
Production Manager: Lori J. Bainbridge
Compositor: Publication Services, Inc.
Printer/Binder: R.R. Donnelley & Sons
Cover Printer: New England Book Components

6 5 4 3 2 1

Library of Congress Cataloging-in-Publication Data
Readings in family nursing / edited by Gail D. Wegner, Rinda J.
   Alexander.
       p.   cm.
   Includes bibliographical references and index.
   ISBN 0-397-55033-2
   1. Family nursing.   I. Wegner, Gail D.   II. Alexander, Rinda J.
   RT120.F34R4   1993
   610.73'6—dc20   92-42193
                                                            CIP

Any procedure or practice described in this book should be applied by the health-care practitioner under appropriate supervision in accordance with professional standards of care used with regard to the unique circumstances that apply in each practice situation. Care has been taken to confirm the accuracy of information presented and to describe generally accepted practices. However, the authors, editors, and publisher cannot accept any responsibility for errors or omissions or for any consequences from application of the information in this book and make no warranty express or implied, with respect to the contents of the book.

Every effort has been made to ensure drug selections and dosages are in accordance with current recommendations and practice. Because of ongoing research, changes in government regulations and the constant flow of information on drug therapy, reactions and interactions, the reader is cautioned to check the package insert for each drug for indications, dosages, warnings and precautions, particularly if the drug is new or infrequently used.

Contributors

David E. Balk, PhD, MC
Assistant Professor
Department of Human Development and
  Family Studies
Kansas State University
Manhattan, Kansas

Janice M. Bell, RN, PhD
Associate Professor
Faculty of Nursing
Research Coordinator
Family Nursing Unit
The University of Calgary
Calgary, Alberta, Canada

Andrea S. Berne, MPH, CPNP
Associate Staff Analyst
Office of Child Health Planning
New York City Department of Health
New York, New York

Nancy J. Briggs, MS, RN
Consultant
Quality Assurance and Case Management
Kansas City, Kansas

Tess L. Briones, MSN, RN
Department of Surgical Nursing
Surgical Intensive Care Unit
University of Michigan Medical Center
Ann Arbor, Michigan

Kathleen C. Buckwalter, PhD, RN
Professor, College of Nursing
The University of Iowa
Iowa City, Iowa

Angeline Bushy, PhD, RN
Assistant Professor
College of Nursing
University of Utah
Salt Lake City, Utah

Mary Jo Butler, RN, MS
West Virginia University–School of
   Nursing
Charleston, West Virginia

Patricia H. Byers, PhD, RN
Associate Chief of the Nursing Service for
   Research
Veterans' Administration Medical Center
Bay Pines, Florida

Mary Woods Byrne, PhD, RN
Division of Nursing
Lehman College
The City University of New York
Bronx, New York

Doris W. Campbell, RN, PhD
Associate Professor of Nursing
College of Nursing
University of Florida–Gainesville
Gainesville, Florida

Constance Captain, PhD, RN
Nurse Researcher
Nursing Service
Audie Murphy Memorial Veterans
   Hospital
San Antonio, Texas

Karen I. Chalmers, MSc(A)
Assistant Professor
School of Nursing
University of Manitoba
Winnipeg, Manitoba, Canada

Donelle Cusack, MS, RN
Clinical Instructor
Veterans Administration Medical Center
Knoxville, Iowa

Candy Dato, RN, CS, MS
Administrative Coordinator
St. Luke's–Roosevelt Hospital Center
New York, New York

Carrie Dawson, BSN, RN
Department of Surgical Nursing
Surgical Intensive Care Unit
University of Michigan Medical Center
Ann Arbor, Michigan

Carol Ann Diemert, RN, MS
Community Health Faculty
School of Nursing
University of Minnesota
Minneapolis, Minnesota

Mildred A. Dietz-Omar, PhD, RN
Michigan State University
College of Nursing
East Lansing, Michigan

Eileen Donnelly, RN, PhD
Assistant Professor
Graduate Program
Community Health Nursing Department
Boston College School of Nursing
Chestnut Hill, Massachusetts

Cheryl Drongowski, BSN, RN
Department of Surgical Nursing
Surgical Intensive Care Unit
University of Michigan
Ann Arbor, Michigan

Mary E. Duffy, RN, PhD
Assistant Professor
Department of Mental Health
Community and Administrative Nursing
University of California
San Francisco, California

Ruth Enestvedt, RN, MS
Community Health Faculty
School of Nursing
University of Minnesota
Minneapolis, Minnesota

Jacqueline Fawcett, RN, PhD, FAAN, Upsilon and Xi
Associate Professor and Division
    Chairperson
Science and Role Development
University of Pennsylvania
School of Nursing
Philadelphia, Pennsylvania

Marie-Luise Friedemann, RN, PhD
Assistant Professor
Department of Psychiatric–Mental Health
    Nursing
College of Nursing
Wayne State University
Detroit, Michigan

Catherine L. Gilliss, RN, C, DNSc, FAAN, Alpha Eta
Associate Professor & Director
Family Nurse Practitioner Program
University of California-San Francisco
San Francisco, California

Lynne Goodykoontz, PhD, RN, CNA
Dean of Nursing
University of North Carolina
Greensboro, North Carolina

Rebecca Graner, RNC
Supervisor
Department of Obstetrics and
    Gynecology
Coordinator, Planning Pregnancy Class
Medcenter One
Bismarck, North Dakota

Diana N. Gurley, PhD
Postdoctoral Fellow in Psychiatric
    Epidemiology
Columbia University
New York, New York

Lynne A. Hall, DrPH, RN
Associate Professor
College of Nursing
Department of Behavioral Science
College of Medicine
University of Kentucky
Lexington, Kentucky

Sue P. Heiney, MN, RN, CS
Mental Health Clinical Nurse Specialist
Center for Cancer and Blood Disorders
Children's Hospital at Richland Memorial
Columbia, South Carolina

Charlotte A. Herrick, PhD, RN, CS
University of South Alabama
College of Nursing
Department of Community Mental
    Health Nursing
Mobile, Alabama

Nancy S. Hogan, PhD, RN
Associate Professor
School of Nursing
University of Miami
Miami, Florida

Susan R. Jacob, MSN, RN
Assistant Professor
Loewenberg School of Nursing
Memphis State University
Memphis, Tennessee

Susan J. Kelley, PhD, RN
Assistant Professor
Maternal Child Health Graduate Program
School of Nursing
Boston College
Chestnut Hill, Massachusetts

Linda J. Kristjanson, MN
Assistant Professor
School of Nursing
University of Manitoba
Winnipeg, Manitoba, Canada

Thomas Kruckeberg, MS
Systems Programmer
College of Nursing
The University of Iowa
Iowa City, Iowa

Richard J. Kryscio, PhD
Professor and Chair
Department of Statistics
Director of Statistics Consulting
    Laboratory and Biostatistics Consulting
    Unit
University of Kentucky
Lexington, Kentucky

Barbara J. Kupferschmid, MSN, RN
Department of Surgical Nursing
Surgical Intensive Care Unit
University of Michigan Medical Center
Ann Arbor, Michigan

Cheryl Ann Lapp, RN, MPH, MA
Community Health Faculty
School of Nursing
University of Minnesota
Minneapolis, Minnesota

Maureen Leahey, RN, PhD
Adjunct Associate Professor, University of
    Calgary
Team Director, Mental Health Services
    Director,
Family Therapy Institute, Holy Cross
    Hospital
Calgary, Canada

Nancy W. Kline Leidy, PhD, RN
Assistant Professor
College of Nursing
The University of Arizona
Tucson, Arizona

Helen Lerner, EdD, RN
Division of Nursing
Lehman College
The City University of New York
Bronx, New York

Carol J. Loveland-Cherry, PhD, RN
Assistant Professor
School of Nursing
The University of Michigan
Ann Arbor, Michigan

**Debra J. Lynn-McHale, MSN, RN, CS,
    CCRN**
Surgical Cardiac Care Unit
Surgical Intensive Care Unit
Thomas Jefferson University Hospital
Philadelphia, Pennsylvania

**Donna J. MacLachlan, BSN, RN,
    COHN**
Staff Nurse
AT&T Bell Laboratories
Lincroft, New Jersey

Diana J. Mason, RNC, PhD, Upsilon
Assistant Professor
Henry Rutgers Research Fellow
College of Nursing
Rutgers–The State University of
    New Jersey
Newark, New Jersey

Shelby F. Merkel, BSN, RN
Staff Nurse
AT&T Bell Laboratories
Indian Hill
Naperville, Illinois

Janice M. Morse, RN, PhD, Gamma Rho
Professor
Faculty of Nursing
University of Alberta
Alberta, Canada

Dorothea C. Pfohl, BS, RN
Clinical Research Coordinator
Cerebrovascular Research Center
School of Medicine
University of Pennsylvania
Philadelphia, Pennsylvania

Margaret Rafferty, RN, MA, MPH
Instructor
Long Island College Hospital
School of Nursing
Brooklyn, New York

Sharon R. Reeves, RN, MPH, MS
Vice President Patient Care Services
Community Nursing Services of DuPage
    County
Lombard, Illinois

Marlene M. Rosenkoetter, PhD, RN, FAAN
Dean and Professor
School of Nursing
University of North Carolina at
    Wilmington
Wilmington, North Carolina

Sister Callista Roy, RN, PhD, FAAN
University of California–San Francisco
San Francisco, California

Barbara Sachs, PhD, RN, FAAN
Associate Professor
College of Nursing
University of Kentucky
Lexington, Kentucky

Harry J. Satariano, MSW, LSCSW
Family Psychotherapist
Critten Outpatient Clinic–Johnson
    County
Overland Park, Kansas

Margaret Schmelzer, RN, MSPH
Director of Public Health Nursing
Madison Department of Public Health
Madison, Wisconsin

Amy Shoemaker, BSN
Staff Nurse
The University of Iowa Hospitals and
    Clinics
Iowa City, Iowa

Mary Cipriano Silva, PhD, RN, FAAN
School of Nursing
George Mason University
Fairfax, Virginia

Ann Smith, MSN, RN, CCRN
Surgical Cardiac Care Unit
Surgical Intensive Care Unit
Thomas Jefferson University Hospital
Philadelphia, Pennsylvania

Ora L. Strickland, PhD, RN, FAAN
Professor
School of Nursing
University of Maryland
Baltimore, Maryland

Susan G. Taylor, RN, PhD
University of Missouri–Columbia School
    of Nursing
Columbia, Missouri

Rosanne Trost, RN, MPH
Coordinator of Clinical Studies
Division of Education
Baylor College of Medicine
Houston, Texas

Constance R. Uphold, MS, PhD, RN
Assistant Professor
College of Nursing
University of Florida
Gainesville, Florida

**Rosemary K. Vahldieck, RN, MPH,
    MS**
Public Health Nursing Consultant
Wisconsin Division of Health
Madison, Wisconsin

Ann L. Whall, PhD, FAAN
Professor
Department of Psychiatric Mental Health
    Nursing
University of Michigan School of Nursing
Ann Arbor, Michigan

Fay W. Whitney, PhD, CRNP
Assistant Professor
Primary Care Graduate Program
School of Nursing
University of Pennsylvania
Philadelphia, Pennsylvania

Holly Skodol Wilson, PhD, FAAN
Professor
Department of Mental Health,
Community and Administrative Nursing
School of Nursing
University of California
San Francisco, California

Nancy L. Wilson, MA
Instructor and Coordinator of Academic
    Affairs
Department of Medicine
Geriatric Program
Baylor College of Medicine
Houston, Texas

Sharon Wilson, RN, MEd, MN
Professor
School of Nursing
Ryerson Polytechnical Institute
Toronto, Canada

Lorraine M. Wright, RN, PhD
Director, Family Nursing Unit
Professor, Faculty of Nursing
University of Calgary, Calgary
Calgary, Alberta, Canada

JoAnne M. Youngblut, PhD, RN
Assistant Professor
Frances Payne Bolton School of Nursing
Case Western Reserve University
Cleveland, Ohio

Preface

Over the last ten years, family nursing has emerged as a subspecialty in nursing. A body of knowledge now exists that addresses family nursing as a relevant domain within nursing science. Currently family nursing literature on issues in theory development, research, clinical practice, and education is scattered in various nursing journals and books; however, there is no one source that brings together, under one cover, past and present insights on the issues that shape family nursing. This book, composed of selected reprinted articles from journals, fills this void.

This anthology provides those interested and involved in family nursing a framework for practice. Issues in theory development, research, and education are included because we strongly believe that practice is based on the knowledge and understanding gathered through theory, research, and education.

Although this text is extensive, it is not comprehensive. We selected those articles that share the most current developments in family nursing. The majority of the reprinted articles from nursing journals appeared in 1989, 1990, and 1991. Some articles written prior to these years are included because they contribute a richness to the family nursing discussion and add dimensions that are not found elsewhere. There are a variety of formats found in these articles. They include case studies evolved from theory-based clinical practice; and nursing research testing nursing theory or exploring clinical questions or nursing interventions. All copies include a reference list.

This text is unique because it is useful in baccalaureate, master's, and doctoral nursing programs, as well as in family nurse practitioner programs. For a core course or elective course in family nursing, on any level, this book can be a required textbook.

Additionally, there is a focus in baccalaureate programs on community health nursing, in which the client is the family. Thus this book could be used in a community health course as supplemental or recommended reading. And it can be used as supplemental or recommended reading in a graduate program in community health/adult nursing. It should certainly be a required textbook in family nurse practitioner programs. Also, it is an excellent resource for doctoral students in nursing and for postdoctoral nurse researchers interested in expanding the knowledge base in family nursing.

Besides being useful in undergraduate and graduate programs in family nursing, community health nursing, and family nurse practitioners, this book can add to the knowledge base of practicing health professionals. Because family nursing is practiced in a variety of settings, we hope all nurses will be challenged to incorporate some of this knowledge into their practice. Other nurses who will find the book especially informative are nurses who practice maternal-child nursing, psychiatric nursing, and advanced medical surgical nursing in hospitals; nurses who work in schools, in community health centers, and home health agencies; and nurses who are family nurse practitioners.

Our intent with this book is to reach all nurses regardless of educational preparation who are interested in current developments in family nursing theory, research, clinical practice, and education. Our hope is that the articles in this book will provide a forum from which to improve family health.

Acknowledgments

We would like to acknowledge and thank the following people:

- —Those who authored the articles and the publishers who gave us permission to reprint them;
- —Our editor, Barbara Nelson Cullen, for her encouragement and editorial contributions;
- —Our typist, Cecilia Weimer, whose painstaking care helped us go through this process more easily;
- —And, to each of our families, and particularly to Irene C. Wegner and David Alexander, for their support and patience.

Contents

UNIT 2
Family Health Nursing Research

UNIT 3
Family Health Nursing Clinical Practice

UNIT 4
Family Health Nursing Education

Readings in Family Nursing

UNIT 1

FAMILY HEALTH NURSING THEORY DEVELOPMENT

As a consequence of the renewed interest in family nursing, a major goal of family nurses is to elaborate and substantiate the knowledge base to create a science of family nursing through theory development. There are several areas within family nursing that need theoretical development. One is the further explication of concepts such as "family" and "family health" in present nursing paradigms. Another is the development of middle-range nursing theories in family health. The articles collected for this section are examples of such work. They serve as a sound theoretical foundation for the nurse who is engaged in family health nursing, regardless of the clinical area.

CHAPTER 1

The Family as the Unit of Care in Nursing: A Historical Review

Ann L. Whall

ABSTRACT

Current discussions of nursing theory identify the metaparadigm of nursing as focused upon person, environment, health, and nursing. Literature was reviewed to determine if historical and current sources supported the understanding that the family as recipient of care was a continuing nursing focus. The review supported the contention that the family unit has been an early, continuing, and ever increasing focus of nursing care. Public health nursing was the first clinical area to emphasize service to families, and this continuing emphasis is evident for this practice area. The conclusion is drawn that if the family is now deemphasized as a unit of analysis and care, an historically important focus will be abandoned.

Current discussions of theory in nursing make reference to the metaparadigm of nursing as being focused upon person, environment, health, and nursing (Fawcett, 1983). Not explicit is the understanding that the family as well as individuals may be recipients of care. A review of the literature was conducted to determine the emphasis on the family as the recipient of care. The review covered representative historical documents pertaining to standards of care as represented by Nightingale's comments, journal articles, historical texts, curriculum guides, standards of practice, and nursing

From *Public Health Nursing, Vol. 3* (No. 4), 1986, pp. 240–249. Reprinted by permission of Blackwell Scientific Publications, Inc.

models. Nursing research was not covered explicitly, as the focus upon family in this body of knowledge is documented elsewhere by Feetham (1984).

Knowledge of the early discussions of family in nursing led to the observation that the term family was implied rather than explicit in the very early literature, that is, terms of family position such as mother and child were used rather than the term family. It was also observed that later discussions came to regard the family as a single entity, and this made possible the consideration of family as a unit of care.

DEFINITIONS

Present definitions of family were identified and compared with the historical evolution of the concept. In this first step, a portion of the concept analysis discussions of Walker and Avant (1983) was followed. The two definitions examined were "family" and "family unit."

Reisner (1980, p. 8) defined the family as a relational group that consists of two or more individuals who are associated with each other and whose association is characterized by such terms as parent, mother, father, sister, brother, and grandparent. In Logan's (1979, p. 9) definition, the family is a "social system" and "a set of components interacting with each other"; the sense of a whole is both implied and explicit. In this perspective, the family member is responsive to the larger whole or family system, and changes in patterns between persons result in changes in the entire system. Gillis (1983) defined the family as a complex unit with attributes of its own, but containing component parts that are significant as individual units. According to Roberts (1983), there are several ways in which to define a family but all have some negative features. For example, definitions based on bloodlines and law exclude groups that consider themselves to be a family but who are not related by bloodlines or law (p. 8).

Examination of discussions of the family and family unit in major reviews led to several conclusions. The family is a self-identified group of two or more individuals whose association is characterized by special terms, who may or may not be related by bloodlines or law, but who function in such a way that they consider themselves to be a family. A unitary approach is one in which the wholeness of the unit is recognized. With these definitions in mind, the literature was reviewed to identify important instances in which the family unit was discussed as a focus of care. After the time of Nightingale, the nursing literature was grouped into 20-year time frames to facilitate coverage of the material. No historical evidence was identified that suggested another chronologic grouping.

NIGHTINGALE

A biography of Florence Nightingale (Tooley, 1905, p. 153) was one of the earliest texts examined. Tooley stated, "Miss Nightingale found the wives of soldiers, respectable women, without decent clothing, living in three or four rooms of the damp basement of a hospital. There by light of rushlight, measures were taken, the sick attended, and their babies born and nourished." In all, 22 babies were born to this group. In winter, due to a broken drain in the basement, a fever broke out. "Miss Nightingale procured a house, had it cleaned and furnished; she organized a plan to give employment to soldiers' wives . . . she started a school for the children and got a chaplain to visit them and help them." Nightingale wrote later (according to Tooley), that as improvements in the system were made which the war suggested, that care should be taken that the wives and the children of soldiers not be forgotten. Florence Nightingale "was . . . possessed by the idea of the district nurse as a health missioner . . . [these missioners were to] introduce to village mothers particular knowledge [such as in the area of] sanitation and skillful hands" (Cook, 1913, p. 383). "The movement for district nursing was always dear to Miss Nightingale's heart. She regretted "that once district nursing came, it was too late for her to help" (Cook, 1925, p. 340).

The quotation from Tooley contains all the elements of the concept family: Nightingale recognized family members, husbands, wives, and children; she mentioned needs of both mothers and infants, and in her own words she used the relationship terms wife and child, and implied (as soldier) husband and father. The last quotation hints at a regret on the part of Nightingale that she had not further developed the branch of nursing, which at that time dealt mostly with families. Because all the documents referred to by Tooley and Cook were not available for independent examination, original works of Nightingale were examined. They essentially corroborated the secondary sources.

For example, Nightingale (1863) wrote about the need to improve hospital accommodations for the sick wives and children of the soldiers, and she advised of the need for a separate delivery room. In a letter dated August 6, 1855, she sent a soldier's widow to a friend so that the widow might receive some dark clothing as a sign of her mourning. She discussed the privacy and financial needs of families when they joined the soldier at military camp (Nightingale, 1858). Nightingale graphically depicted the treatment of the women and children in military camps and offered detailed directions to the army for improvement of these conditions.

1890–1910

Journal articles written about the time of Tooley's work were reviewed for references in either title or text for the term family or family unit as well as for relationship terms. In the *Trained Nurse*, Brooks (1890) stated, "Caring for the insane in their homes will relieve their families" and Stewart (1908) made note of a nurse who "ministered to three ill children and two who were not stricken" with diphtheria. Stewart also noted that in one family the parents were very frightened by the children's illness, and it was two hours before they "could decide what was best to do." After seeing the older boy successfully treated, "the parents decided I should treat the baby."

Wald (1904) set forth general principles as to how to "nurse in the home," including advice about how to enter the family, that is, before removing "children lying upon the bed of the sick mother" and "washing their faces," the nurse should first "establish herself" (p. 430). Wald recommended evaluating whether a family can care for "an invalid" without becoming "demoralized." She also discussed the relationship of the family to their neighbors and to service agencies. Several case studies were given in which the nurse assessed the ability of the family to care for the ill member, wherein the nurse taught a family member to give care and/or put the family in touch with community agencies (pp. 603–606).

1910–1930

Beard (1915) noted that the ideal of bringing nursing to every home was "an idea that is little more than thirty years old." She had read a report of a home nursing visit conducted in 1890 in which the "child had double pneumonia" and the nurse gave instructions "to the mother about medication and nourishment" (p. 47). Beard quoted Nightingale (no reference given) as stating that success in nursing is "to keep whole families out of pauperism" by "nursing the breadwinner back to health."

By 1917 Beard had extended her discussion and stated that the public health nurse must have as "her [*sic*] conviction, that upon her observation and foresight depends the health of their whole family." The family "as a unit more than any other individual member of it must be her thought . . . the correction of defects may be the pivot upon which family health turns" (p. 247). Beard described several cases in which the family was approached as a unit by the public health nurse (pp. 249–250).

The 1917 *Standard curriculum for schools of nursing* was prepared by the committee on Education of the National League for Nursing Education (NLNE). In the outline of the subject matter, it stated that students were to receive instruction in "Household Science," which pertained to "housekeeping problems of an industrial family." The overall objective of this course was to prepare "pupils who intend to go into families either as a public health or as a private duty nurse" (p. 62). The most satisfactory teaching method was to "have the pupil study individual families" (p. 62).

Laird (1923) was primarily concerned with the control of communicable disease, when she identified that "any plan of health education which does not include the whole family is not adequate" (p. 40). While a patient was hospitalized, she wondered, "What about the other members of the family? Even though the patient is adequately cared for . . . may not his progress be dependent on the condition and attitude of his in the home?" (p. 40).

In presenting several case studies, Faville (1925) identified the necessity to consider the family in terms of all relationships. "The public health nurse visiting homes has the priceless opportunity for seeing the family as a whole, for securing the solution of many of the social maladjustments at the root of illness" (p. 22).

As a result of major revision, the NLNE 1927 edition of *A curriculum for schools of nursing* tended to exclude many of the references to preparation of nurses for work with families; the thrust of the guide was thus different from the 1917 edition. For example, in the section "Practical Objects for Nursing Education," no mention was made of families. In addition, the section "Household Science" was removed. Perhaps a clue to these changes is the introductory statement that there is no need to separate the preparation of "bedside" nurses from that of "public health nurses."

1930–1950

The NLNE (1937) published a third curriculum guide in which "The Modern Family" was a major unit of study, having 10 to 15 hours allocated. An emphasis in this edition was on the development of "the 'normal' family and the influence [that modern life] is tending to make in the functions and organization of the family" (p. 216).

On the subject "Nursing and Health Services in the Family," the text declared, "The entire program outlined in this curriculum is based on the assumption that the participation in health conservation and prevention of disease is inherent in the whole concept of nursing . . . also that the patient should not be considered as an individual only, but as a member of a group" (p. 510). In addition, courses that were directed toward family health care were not "specific preparation for public health nursing." It was intended to round out the nursing students' "experience, to meet more common situations found in family health" (p. 510). This theme continued in the statement that "the nurse must consider the family as a unit. This may involve making study of the family" (p. 513). Thus the increased discussion of the family and analysis of the family as a unit was well established by 1937.

A textbook from 1931 by Chayer stated, "The visiting nurse must be given the credit for pioneering work in the education of parents . . . Before public schools went into the home, the visiting nurse was there" (p. 206). Chayer also commented that it had "taken 50 years for Florence Nightingale's vision [to come about] of the Health Nurse going into homes in the community" (p. 4).

A textbook that dealt primarily with medical-surgical nursing (Harmer, 1935) stated, "Very often patients although pronounced cured, require further care. When this is the case, the nurse in charge of the social service department will see that patients are properly cared for. As previously stated the patient can never be rightly understood or adequately cared for considered apart from the family . . . in the homes of rich and poor alike, rural or army nursing includes all of this" (p. 367).

Zabriskie (1934) addressed aspects of family care in her textbook. "A thorough study of the cause and effect relationships entails not only a knowledge of the factors operating as determinants in the parent's attitude toward the child . . . but accepting the fact that the child reacts to given situations in the family" (p. 199). She continued, "In families where the parental adjustment to each other is inharmonious, the conflict problem for the child becomes markedly increased."

Bean and Brockett (1937) titled an article, "The family as a unit for nursing service." They noted that when going into a home, the public health nurse should not only give nursing care to individuals, but address the health needs of the entire family and work out a health plan for its members. The authors also identified ways to ascertain if nurses were carrying out the commitment to care for the entire family. They described a one-year survey by the United States Public Health Service (USPHS) conducted at three county health departments. The purpose was, "In view of the emphasis that has been placed on the principle of 'the family as a unit' for nursing service, it seemed appropriate to investigate the degree to which nurses in actual practice broadened their visits to include the entire family" (p. 1924). A review of over 3000 records revealed that in 62 percent of the cases, nurses addressed problems other than those for which they first came into the home. The authors concluded, however, that the visits tended to be confined to services for just a few family members on any one visit. This did not meet their criteria for total family service.

1950–PRESENT

Because of increased numbers of sources found in the nursing literature since 1950 that discuss addressing the family as a unit or a system, only a few articles were reviewed. (In 1975, for example, more than eight nursing articles discussed the family as the unit of service.) Beasley (1954) reported on service to families who had a mentally ill member, stating, "It was this concept of supportive services to the families of the mentally ill that became the basis for an experimental program" (p. 482). The function of public health nurses in this regard was in part to help the family accept the patient's illness and understand the patient's need to be hospitalized, to help the patient be accepted back into the home, and to arrange for several families to meet together to discuss common problems. Beasley noted that the emphasis of service was placed purposefully on the family needs rather than on the patient.

Garside (1958) stated, "The home visit provides for a closer observation of intangibles such as family relationships and intergroup personality reactions" (p. 153). She also indicated that school nurses tended to address the needs of school-age children and thereby unintentionally neglect family health. She stated further that the health of individual family members must be addressed "in order to protect the family as a whole" (p. 155). The need to approach the family unit as the client was found in many other articles (Kvarness, 1959; Reinerston, 1963; Hess, 1966; Mereness, 1968; Smiley, 1973). The issue at this time was not whether the family was the client, but how to address a multi-person group.

STANDARDS OF PRACTICE

As one might expect, the interest in the family was evident in the American Nurses' Association's (ANA) *Standards of community health nursing practice* (ANA, 1973a). The opening statement said, "Nursing practice is a direct . . . service to the individual, the family, and the community during health and illness." Consumers may be "individuals or families," and "active involvement of the individual, family, and community is necessary in attainment of positive health." The word family was used approximately seven times in this standard.

Standards of gerontologic nursing practice (ANA, 1976) did not use the word family at all. Instead, the term "significant others" indicated relationships. For example, standard 3 states, "A plan for nursing care is developed in conjunction with the older adult and/or significant others." The reasons and implications for the exclusion of the term family must be considered further.

Standards of maternal-child health nursing practice (ANA, 1973b) mentioned family more than 25 times. One standard stated, that maternal and child health nursing practice is aimed at promoting and maintaining optimal health of each individual . . . and of the family unit. Included in several places was the idea that the nurse develops services to promote "family solidarity."

Standards of medical-surgical nursing practice (ANA, 1974) mentioned the family approximately five times. The nurse is to "ensure patient and family participation in health promotion." In addition, "goals are formulated by the patient and his family" and the nursing care plan "is communicated to the patient and family."

In *Standards of pediatric oncology nursing practice* (ANA, 1978), the family was mentioned more than 20 times. "Nursing care given to the pediatric oncology patient . . . incorporates the needs of the individual child and family." Standard 1 stated, "The collection of data about . . . the individual child and his family is systematic," and "nursing actions reflect consideration and appreciation of the integrity of the family unit."

Standards of psychiatric mental health nursing practice (ANA, 1982) referred to the family approximately 12 times. It defined family therapy as "any intervention that focuses on the family system as a unit and promotes change toward adaptation in that system." The standard on intervention noted that the nurse "utilizes advanced clinical expertise in . . . family psychotherapy" (p. 13).

NURSING MODELS

King's 1981 edition of "A Theory for Nursing: Systems, Concepts, Process" indexed the family extensively. On the first page she stated that most persons begin life as a part of a family and learn ways to meet basic needs in families, and that the family constitutes one of the groups in which one performs a certain role. King noted that the family demonstrates the features of a social system, that is, structure, status, role, and social interaction. King later noted that the family as a social system as well as health as a goal for nursing, are two major concepts in her framework (1983, p. 178). She discussed "family-nurse interactions" as well as the need to assess "the family's perceptions," thus treating the family as a unit.

In 1979 Newman did not index or discuss the family as such; however, in 1983 she restated the assumptions of her earlier work in terms of families, noting that health could be described as "fluctuating patterns of energy exchange . . . that are part of the developing consciousness of the family" (p. 169).

She discussed the family unit in terms of a whole or single entity and focused on the interactions of all members and how this related to family health. Newman's focus in her discussion of families is thus definitely a family unit in terms of the nurse approaching the family as a unit of care.

Although Orem's 1971 text did not index the term family, she did indicate that the nurse "learns to work in cooperation with patients and their families" (p. 119) and that in terms of achieving goals "one had to be aware of family implications" (p. 71). In the 1980 edition of this work the term family is indexed as appearing on several pages. Orem stated in this later edition that, "In search of valid ways to provide health care to families . . . it has been recognized that it may be essential to work with all members of the unit" (p. 200). Orem (1983) extended the discussion of family as a unit of analysis, stating, "First, accept the family as a system . . . and the family culture as basic conditioning factors for all family members. . . . The system of family support should be examined and adjusted as needed and then incorporated into the family system of living" (pp. 367–368). This last statement indicated that family interactions and the family system as a whole are a unit of analysis.

In 1970 and 1980 Rogers did not reference or discuss the family as such. In 1983, however, she stated, "The proposed paradigm is as applicable to families as it is to individual human beings . . . an irreducible, four dimensional, negentropic family energy field becomes the focus of study" (p. 226). Rogers continued the point that the family could logically be the focus of analysis in her model by applying to the family as a unit the concepts of pattern and organization and energy fields. She stated that families may or may not live in the same household, and may or may not be related by blood or by law (p. 226).

Roy in 1976 addressed the family primarily as it related to the individual. Roy and Roberts in 1981 stated, however, "The client of nursing may be a person, a family, a group, a community, or society" (p. 42).

In 1983, however, Roy explicated the family as the client or unit of analysis: "Nursing may focus on an individual person, the family, and group, a social organization, or a community" (p. 262). Families are an adaptive system with input, output, and internal processes (p. 273), and just as nurses assess the person as an adaptive system, so too do they assess the family when a family is the focus of care (p. 275).

SUMMARY

The conclusion is drawn that the family as a unit of care in nursing is by now well established. The historical and current literature is clear in terms of this conclusion.

The literature review verified the position taken at the outset that the discussion of family proceeds from discussion of family position terms to the discussion of the family as a whole or as the unit of care. The review also identified several trends: (1) public health or district nursing was the first practice area that clearly focused on the family as a unit of care; (2) later, other practice areas reflected this focus; and (3) certain nursing models tended to focus less on family in their initial statements.

ACKNOWLEDGMENTS

The author thanks Dr. Rosemary Ellis and Dr. Evelyn Barbee for their suggestions that were incorporated into this paper, and Dr. Jacqueline Fawcett for suggesting the term "recipient of care." This paper was presented on September 29, 1983, at the Nursing Theory Think Tank, Chicago, Illinois.

REFERENCES

American Nurses' Association. (1973a). *Standards of community health nursing practice.* Kansas City, MO: Author.

American Nurses' Association. (1973b). *Standards of maternal-child health nursing practice.* Kansas City, MO: Author.

American Nurses' Association. (1974). *Standards of medical-surgical nursing practice.* Kansas City, MO: Author.

American Nurses' Association. (1976). *Standards of gerontologic nursing practice.* Kansas City, MO: Author.

American Nurses' Association. (1978). *Standards of pediatric-oncology nursing practice.* Kansas City, MO: Author.

American Nurses' Association. (1982). *Standards of psychiatric mental health nursing practice.* Kansas City, MO: Author.

Bean, H., & Brockett, G. (1937). The family as a unit for nursing service. *Public Health Report, 52,* 1923-1931.

Beard, M. (1915). Home nursing. *Public Health Nursing Quarterly, 7,* 44-51.

Beard, M. (1917, October). The family as the unit of public health work. *Modern Hospital,* (1954), 247-251.

Beasley, F. (1954). Public health nursing services for families of the mentally ill. *Nursing Outlook, 2,* 482-484.

Brooks, J. (1890). Nursing the insane. *Trained Nurse, 4,* 10-12.

Chayer, M. (1931). *School nursing.* New York: Teachers College Press.

Cook, E. (1913). *The life of Florence Nightingale* (Vol. 2). London: Macmillan.

Cook, E. (1925). *The life of Florence Nightingale* (rev. ed.). London: Macmillan.

Faville, K. (1925). The nurse as counselor in troubled homes. *Red Cross Courier, 4,* 14-15.

Fawcett, J. Hallmarks of success in nursing theory development. In P. L. Chin (Ed.) *Advances in nursing theory development.* Rockville, MD: Aspen Systems, pp. 3-18.

Feetham, S. (1984). Family research in nursing. In H. H. Werley & J. J. Fitzpatrick (Eds.) *Annual review of nursing research* (Vol. II). New York: Springer.

Garside, A. (1958). The school nurse as a family counselor. *Journal of School Health, 28,* 153-157.

Gillis, C. (1983). The family as a unit of analysis: Strategies for the nurse researcher. *Advances in Nursing Science, 5,* 50-59.

Harmer, B. (1935). *Textbook of the principles and practice of nursing.* New York: Macmillan.

Hess, G. (1966). Family nursing experience. *Nursing Outlook, 14,* 51-53.

King, I. (1981). *A theory of nursing: Systems, concepts, process.* New York: John Wiley & Sons.

King, I. (1983). King's theory of nursing/analysis and application of King's theory of goal attainment. In I. Clements & F. Roberts (Eds.), *Family health: A theoretical approach to nursing care.* New York: John Wiley & Sons.

Kvarness, M. (1959). The patient is the family. *Nursing Outlook, 7,* 142-146.

Laird, M. (1923). The value of follow-up work in the family. *American Journal of Nursing, 24,* 4043.

Logan, B. (1979). The nurse and the family: Dominant themes and perspectives in the literature. In K. Knafl & H. Grace (Eds.), *Families across the life cycle: Studies for nursing.* Boston: Little, Brown.

Mereness, D. (1968). Family therapy: An evolving role for the psychiatric nurse. *Perspectives in Psychiatric Nursing, 6,* 259.

National League for Nursing Education. (1917). *Standard curriculum for schools of nursing.* Baltimore: Waverly Press.

National League for Nursing Education. (1927). *A curriculum for schools of nursing.* New York: Author.

National League for Nursing Education. (1937). *A curriculum guide for schools of nursing.* New York: Author.

Newman, M. (1979). *Theory development in nursing.* Philadelphia: F. A. Davis.

Newman, M. (1983). Newman's health theory. In I. Clements & F. Roberts (Eds.), *Family health: A theoretical approach to nursing care.* New York: John Wiley & Sons.

Nightingale, F. (1855). Letter to Lady Alicia Blackwood. Written at Scutari, 8/6.

Nightingale, F. (1858). *Notes on matters affecting the health, efficiency, and hospital administration of the British army.* London: Harrison & Sons.

Nightingale, F. (1863). *Notes on hospital.* London: Longman, Green.

Orem, D. (1971). *Nursing: Concepts of practice.* New York: McGraw-Hill.

Orem, D. (1980). *Nursing: Concepts of practice* (2nd ed.). New York: McGraw-Hill.

Orem, D. (1983). The self-care deficit theory of nursing: A general theory/analysis and application of Orem's theory. In I. Clements & F. Roberts (Eds.). *Family health: A theoretical approach to nursing care.* New York: John Wiley & Sons.

Reinerston, B. (1963). The patient is part of a family. *American Journal of Nursing, 63,* 106–107.

Reisner, W. (1980). The historical development of the conceptualization of family within the context of nursing care of well children. Unpublished master's thesis, Frances Payne Bolton School of Nursing. Case Western Reserve University, Cleveland, Ohio.

Roberts, S. (1983). The American family. In I. Clements & F. Roberts (Eds.). *Family health: A theoretical approach to nursing care.* New York: John Wiley & Sons.

Rogers, M. (1970). *An introduction to the theoretical basis of nursing.* Philadelphia: F. A. Davis.

Rogers, M. (1980). Nursing: A science of unitary man. In J. Riehl & C. Roy (Eds.). *Conceptual models for nursing practice,* 2nd ed. New York: Appleton-Century-Crofts, 1980.

Rogers, M. (1983). Science of unitary human beings: A paradigm for nursing. In I. Clements & F. Roberts (Eds.). *Family health: A theoretical approach to nursing care.* New York: John Wiley & Sons.

Roy, C. (1976). *Introduction to nursing: An adaptation model.* Englewood Cliffs, NJ: Prentice-Hall.

Roy, C., & Roberts, S. (1981). *Theory construction in nursing: An adaptation model.* Englewood Cliffs, NJ: Prentice-Hall.

Roy, C. (1983). Analysis and application of the Roy adaptation model. In I. Clements & F. Roberts (Eds.), *Family health: A theoretical approach to nursing care.* New York: John Wiley & Sons.

Smiley, O. (1973). The family-centered approach—A challenge to public health nurses. *Int Nurs Rev, 20,* 49–50.

Stewart, H. (1908). In quarantine with diphtheria. *Trained Nurse, 41,* 92–94.

Tooley, S. (1905). *The life of Florence Nightingale* (2nd ed.). London: Macmillan.

Wald, L. (1904). The treatment of families in which there is sickness. *American Journal of Nursing, 4,* 427–428, 515–519, 602–606.

Walker, L., & Avant, K. (1983). *Strategies for theory construction in nursing.* Norwalk, CT: Appleton-Century-Crofts.

Zabriski, L. (1934). *Nurses' handbook of obstetrics.* Philadelphia: J. B. Lippincott.

CHAPTER 2

The Concept of Family Nursing

Marie-Luise Friedemann

A system-based conceptualization of family nursing is suggested, with family nursing practised on three system levels. The level of individual family members views the family as the context of the individuals. The interpersonal level addresses dyads and larger units and the family system level includes the structural and functional system components interacting with the environment. Intervention on a higher system level includes the lower levels. While family nursing falls within the practice scope of all nurses, intervention aimed at system change requires holistic understanding of the intricate relationships between family system components and the skills of clinical specialists.

INTRODUCTION

The aim of this paper is to propose a new working definition of family nursing that integrates the differing nursing views of the family without creating a conflict. The family is seen as a human social system with distinct characteristics that is composed of individuals whose characteristics are equally distinct.

Family nursing has been taught in nursing schools since the early days of our profession. Public health nurses first recognized the family as an important factor in an individual's growth and development or recovery from illness (Ford 1973). With the

Reprinted from *Journal of Advanced Nursing, Vol. 14,* 1989, pp. 211–216. Used with permission of Blackwell Scientific Publications, Ltd., and the author.

advent of systems theory that was adapted to living systems in the 1930s by von Bertalanffy (1966) and introduced into nursing in the 1960s, the concept of family nursing has been generally understood as nursing care given to the total family system or unit (Miller-Ham & Chamings 1983). Consequently, family nursing practice has accepted as a fact the understanding that the client of a family nurse is the family system rather than the individuals in the family. However, nursing scholars have encountered problems in integrating the concept of family nursing into their conceptual thinking.

Nursing conceptual thinking has been advanced considerably by the recent formulation of a nursing metaparadigm (Fawcett 1983). In the term metaparadigm 'meta' describes that which is beyond the ordinary dimensions, the global and most abstract understanding of phenomena. The term 'paradigm' is synonymous with the word model that is defined as a configuration of integrated concepts. The development of a metaparadigm in nursing is based on a common understanding that the concepts of person, environment, health and nursing are the essential components of the discipline (Fawcett 1984). This understanding has existed throughout nursing history and has led nursing leaders to single out the four concepts to define the phenomena of their interrelationship in the most abstract and general nature (Kuhn 1977). In fact, the most central proposition in nursing and the essence of the metaparadigm is nursing's concern with the health of the person who is continuously interacting with the environment (Donaldson & Crowley 1978). Consequently, Fawcett (1984) suggests a 'structural hierarchy of knowledge' that places the metaparadigm at the top in order to provide general direction. The nursing discipline, while subscribing to the metaparadigm, is free to develop multiple conceptual models and numerous theories that aim at describing nursing phenomena in detail.

Family nursing scholars have successfully formulated family theories for a multitude of nursing situations. In addition, they have made significant progress in applying to families the most widely used nursing conceptual frameworks originally proposed for nursing of individuals (Clements & Roberts 1983, Fawcett 1975, Whall 1986). However, family theorists have encountered serious problems in reconciling the concepts of family and family nursing with the nursing metaparadigm (Murphy 1986).

FAMILY, FAMILY NURSING AND THE NURSING METAPARADIGM

The main problem rests on the question of whether the family should be viewed as part of the concept of person (client who receives the nursing intervention) or the concept of environment (context that influences the individual's health), a combination of the two, or a separate concept (Murphy 1986). Nursing theorists maintain differing views of the family and family nursing. According to Whall (1981) there are four ways in which the concept of family has been defined by nurses: the family as the environment for individuals; the family as a group of interacting dyads, triads and larger groups; the family as a single unit with defining boundaries; and the family as a unit transacting with the environment.

Orem (1985) subscribes to Whall's (1981) first definition of the family. She maintains that nurses direct their care towards individuals, that the concept of self-care is applicable to individuals only, and that the family serves as context or environment for these individuals. Her understanding of family nursing implies that if individuals are nursed with the goal of strengthening their self-care agency, the system in which these individuals function will be equally enhanced. Based on these assumptions, some nursing leaders have begun to question the existence of family nursing or whether actual nursing practice is in fact family oriented (Barnard 1980).

In contrast, King (1983) sees the family as interacting individuals or groups and assumes that family nursing consists of helping these individuals to reach goals through improved interaction or communication. This definition of family nursing differs from Orem's in that it includes interpersonal issues on the nurse's problem and goal list. The nurse is encouraged to define interpersonal conflicts such as those based on role conflicts, parenting issues and developmental changes.

The last two family concepts on Whall's (1981) list, the family as a single unit and the family transacting with the environment are most clearly represented by Martha Roger's theory (Johnston 1986). The family nurse is seen as an energy field, one with the environment, and continuously interacting with the family and the environmental fields.

It is the belief of this author that all four definitions of the concept of family are applicable and necessary. If the whole family system is viewed as the 'person' who receives the care, the focus on each individual in the family is lost. In contrast, the view of the family as the 'environment' of the person who is the client precludes nursing interventions directed at the total family system. The family needs to be understood as part of both, the concepts of person and of environment, or the nursing metaparadigm could be expanded to include two more concepts, family and family nursing.

DEFINITION OF FAMILY NURSING

The concept of family nursing encompasses three levels of the family system: nursing of the system of individuals, the system of dyads, triads and larger groups, and the entire family system. The system of individuals and the interpersonal system of multi-person units can be conceptualized as subsystems of the total family system. The following attempts to clarify the concept of family nursing on all three system levels as well as the links between the system levels. However, before family nursing can be described clearly, one needs to address the issue of the scope of family nursing.

The Scope of Family Nursing

It is generally accepted that the nurse generalist practises family nursing when treating individuals and includes to some extent the interpersonal communication process. Each nurse at graduation is expected to exhibit proficiency in communication techniques, family and group processes. Interpersonal family nursing, however, can be practised only by a nurse who sits together with more than one family member and guides the communication process through appropriate channels. The nurse leads family members to express thoughts, and guides them towards workable goals and necessary strategies. Such interventions are clearly within the scope of community health nurses, nurses in maternal-child health settings, and hospice nurses, and should be practised by all nurses who have access to their patients' family members.

The depth of family interventions, however, varies greatly and seems positively correlated with the five levels of proficiency outlined by Benner (1984). Benner describes the 'novice' nurse (1) as an inexperienced nurse who functions by following rules, and the 'advanced beginner nurse' (2) as a nurse with some experience who is able to detect and predict repetitive patterns in nursing situations. The 'competent' nurse (3), according to Benner, is one who can define the difference between significant and insignificant aspects of nursing care and begins to feel a sense of mastery, and the 'proficient' nurse (4) is a professional who is able to perceive situations holistically and understands the relative importance of the variables involved. The 'expert' nurse (5) is one who has acquired an intuitive comprehension of situations and can unerringly identify the most essential factors.

Benner's (1984) framework is helpful in defining the scope of family nursing. The nurse generalist with a baccalaureate degree, namely the 'novice', the 'advanced beginner' and the 'competent' nurse, directs nursing actions mainly towards individuals in a family and towards individual and family goal achievement through the interpersonal process. Total system changes in this process are not brought on intentionally. Nurses in these stages of professional development do not yet have the ability to predict reactions of complex family systems that result from the change induced by nursing actions. Instead, system change is a byproduct of improved individual health and well-being of family members, and of improved interpersonal communication between family members.

A cut-off between family nursing as practised by a generalist versus a specialist may fall within the category of a 'competent' nurse. High level 'competent', 'proficient' or 'expert' nurses who perceive nursing situations in a holistic way and are willing to explore and gain understanding of the relationships between individual, family and environmental factors can practise interactional family nursing with the intention to change family patterns and the total family system. To accomplish this goal, they predict, at least with some confidence, how changes at the individual and interpersonal system levels and changes in the environment might influence the family system and its structure.

Taking these differences in skills into account, the following are attempts to clarify the concept of family nursing as well as the links between the system levels by focusing on the role of the family nurse.

Individually Focused Family Nursing

The nurse establishes a relationship with each individual in the family and treats each individual as a client. Individuals are seen as subsystems of the total family system.

The family system is the immediate, joint environment of each client subsystem. Nursing goals are focused on the individuals (i.e. improved diet or exercise, effective home care of an ill person). While one individual is seen as the client, the function of the other individual subsystems is one of a supportive network in helping the client to make changes. All family member subsystems can become clients at various times, depending on their needs. For example, in the case of ill family members, these patients are clients when the nurse teaches them to care for themselves and counsels them in coping with their illness. Other family members become clients when they are taught to perform caretaking tasks or to attend to their physical and emotional needs in order to prevent excessive stress and illness. The ultimate goal of individually based family nursing is personal well-being of the individuals in the family.

In order to assure congruence between individual subsystems and the family system as a whole, all family members are involved together with the nurse in mutual goal setting for each family member so that they understand the treatment plan and provide support. The use of environmental systems may also fall within individually focused nursing if through nursing care the family gains access to new resources, for example medical equipment or supportive care, which enhance individual well-being.

This level of intervention assumes a well functioning family system. Information is fed to individual subsystems who will accommodate the change. Change at the subsystem level is likely to effect change at the family interpersonal level and the family system as whole, but such change will not be the focus of nursing interventions as long as the system maintains crisis free functioning. Helpful theories for family nurses practising on the individual level are stress and coping theories and psychosocial and physical developmental theories.

Interpersonal Family Nursing

Family nursing on the interpersonal level involves the use of communication techniques and addresses family processes such as decision-making, limit setting, and defining family roles. The interpersonal system is considered a subsystem of the total family system and becomes the client for nursing intervention. The interpersonal system consists of two or more individual systems depending on the number of family members interacting with each other at a given time. The need for intervention on the interpersonal level comes about when there is conflict between individuals, a difference in opinion about a nursing issue, or a misunderstanding between family members.

In order to clarify nursing goals and to respect all family members' opinions, the nurse plays the role of a moderator by intervening with the family interaction system. The ultimate nursing goal in addition to individual subsystem changes is mutual understanding and support among family members. This state of interactional harmony provides for the environment in which the individuals can learn and grow.

Thus, family interactional nursing aims at changing the interpersonal system through direct interventions. Nurses must understand the linkages between individuals and primary groups. Theories helpful in conceptualizing interpersonal nursing are parenting theories, theories addressing attachment and bonding, social support, marital relationship, verbal and non-verbal communication, roles, caregiving, and for the advanced practitioner theories in family therapy.

By changing interpersonal relationships nurses anticipate certain individual changes. Predictions of individual reactions related to interpersonal changes are rooted in complex family systems dynamics. For example, in the case of a mother of a delinquent adolescent the nurse will suggest ways to improve the mother's communication with the boy hoping that he will experience support and understanding from his mother and as a result gain an improved self-concept, experience encouragement to work towards constructive goals and decrease his dependence on peers. In order to link the communication changes with the desired personal outcomes of the boy, the nurse needs to understand among other factors the processes which triggered dysfunction in the relationship, the mother's needs and problems, the boy's and the mother's stages of development and related needs, and the influences of other family members on the relationship.

There is risk involved in nursing interventions which are not solidly founded in knowledge and understanding of the family and its interpersonal processes. In the above example, a nurse's decision to suggest to the mother that she enforce limits and become strict with the boy has to be coupled with the knowledge that the mother has the ability to follow the nurse's advice in a consistent manner and knows how to convey to her son that the change in parenting is based on love rather than on revenge. Only then can the nurse predict a change in the son's behaviour without risking harmful consequences.

This example illustrates that family nursing at the interpersonal level is often more than a nurse generalist can handle. The complexity of the subsystem interface surpasses the limited scope in which nurses without advanced education are able to practise family nursing.

Family System Nursing

Nursing of the whole family or transactional nursing of family and environment are creative processes, according to Rogers (Johnston 1986), but such ideas are still hazy and lack consensus (Whall 1981). Family system nursing is practised at the level at which the client becomes the total system. Nursing goals are aimed at changes in the system processes or structure. Nursing actions may also involve the environment within which the system interacts with the purpose of subsequent deliberate change within the family system. Since it is the individuals in the family who act and behave and it is the interpersonal systems that exhibit repeated patterns of behaviour sequences or strategies, nursing actions at the system level alone are not possible. Family system nursing arrives at system changes through interventions which are directed at the individuals and the family interactional system. Contrary to interpersonal family nursing which anticipates system change as a byproduct of interpersonal change, family system nursing plans interpersonal and personal changes as parts of a master system plan. Family development theories, family functioning and therapy theories, including family systems and ecological theories, are helpful in family systems nursing. Theories related to the environment include the community mental health ideology, education and learning theories, sociological theories, administration and work environment theories, peer group and social support theories, and others.

While nursing interventions on the previous two levels are relatively easy to envision, family system nursing is a difficult concept. Family system nursing includes all actions aimed directly at positive system change. Some family therapy techniques are acquired with extensive training and supervision, but family nursing is not a psychiatric nursing concept. Instead, it is practised by experts of all nursing disciplines. Nurses who carry a holistic understanding of families are able to practise interactional nursing interventions on the system level by first assessing a need for system change. For example, in the case of a family giving care to a terminally ill member, there may be a need for reorganization of the system's internal resources and acceptance of external assistance in order to accomplish the difficult task. The design of strategies includes teaching the nursing tasks to family members, setting up a schedule for caring that accommodates the individuals' willingness to help as well as their need to pursue their own interests, counselling the family to accept help from professionals, friends and neighbours and ask for it if they need it. While interventions such as teaching procedures pertain to individually focused family nursing and strategies like joint negotiation of responsibilities are interpersonal nursing actions, the anticipated goal of all interventions is system change.

Change is evaluated continuously at all system levels. Feedback from individuals, interpersonal units and the environment is monitored. Corrections in the master plan are necessary if unhappiness or tension is expressed by family members or the family rejects or is dissatisfied with external resources.

Family system nursing includes the immediate environment. Rogers (1980) describes nursing as creative acts of interchange with the environment. Family system interventions go beyond simple referrals of family members to a support group or a medical clinic. With a system change in mind a nurse specialist negotiates with the family an approach tailored to the family's needs. For the family to follow the approach, the plan needs to be consistent with the general strategies the family uses in daily coping.

For example, the nursing assessment of a family with an alcoholic member includes (1) family system processes—power structure, individual roles and behaviour patterns, emotional bonds; (2) interactional processes—individual reaction to the drinking behaviour, enabling behaviours, compensating behaviours, and family members' perceptions of an ideal interactional system; and (3) individual factors—the individual's motivation to change the drinking behaviour, developmental stages, physical health, individual needs and desires. In addition, the assessment includes the interpersonal and the family system as they interact with the environment. These data are collected through direct questioning of family members and observations of interpersonal dynamics, support systems of the extended family and friends, spacial arrangements, physical surroundings, and use of family time. The analysis and synthesis of the data will lead to a definition of goals.

Effective nurses are aware of their values and avoid formulating goals which are based on their own norms rather than the family's needs and values. Initially, nursing goals often cannot be mutually negotiated due to problem denial or problem misperception. As soon as family members are ready to accept them, however, goals need to be verified with them. The timing of goal sharing is carefully evaluated. Prior to enacting goal directed interventions, the nurse may have to spend time on individually focused actions for the purpose of improving an individual's self-concept and motivation for positive change. Depending on the family's needs, goal directed actions involving the environment in the above sample may include inpatient treatment of the substance abuser, support groups for family members, and collaboration with the children's teacher. Often families have serious economic or health problems which are foremost on their minds. A sensitive family nurse specialist will help the family to receive from the environment what it needs to survive, reinforce its positive interaction patterns with environmental systems and learn new interaction patterns in order to sustain better system functioning. All these actions are part of a master plan that leads ultimately to a system which is in better harmony with its members and its surroundings.

IS FAMILY NURSING UNIQUE?

Most family interventions are not unique to nursing but instead are shared with other disciplines. This is understandable since the basic family understanding is also shared. There is no question that experts as defined by Benner (1984) exist in other disciplines as well and that they also give holistic care. For example, the family therapist Salvador Minuchin demonstrates and makes visible on video-tape expert intuition which leads to an almost instant diagnosis of actual family problems, irrespective of the problem presented by the family.

There are two premises, however, that are basic to nursing practice. The first is the basic focus of nursing on health rather than pathology. Families are extremely sensitive to becoming a target of blame. While family therapy was derived from the assumption that individual pathology is directly related to system pathology, nursing need not subscribe to the same thinking. Even an explanation of shared blame for emotional or physical symptoms is counterproductive in gaining families' cooperation. All family nursing needs to be rooted in an attitude of acceptance and genuine concern for each family member. Family nursing must consist of actions that reinforce the family's strengths and changes can be brought about by increasing the use of existing positive family strategies as well as adopting new strategies the family recognizes as beneficial.

The second premise involves the access nurses have to families. Historically, nurses have gained entry into homes which have refused access to any other professionals, sometimes even physicians. Many families respond to social workers with anger and feelings of being intruded upon and to other mental health professionals with mistrust; they see nurses as helpers who truly understand their situation.

Nurses do have an additional advantage over other professionals in that their education includes exposure to the most significant events in human life, namely birth, tragedy and death, human development at all stages of life, the states of health and illness, and the most basic emotions of joy, anxiety and sorrow. This exposure to physical and emotional human events gives nurses a greater scope of human understanding and makes it easier for them to become experts. Such family experts may use some of the same interventions as other disciplines, but always with a focus on health. For example, the family therapy technique of refraining can be useful in nursing in that it provides positive interpretations of individual and family dynamics and eliminates guilt. While family system nursing is practised with clearly dysfunctional families, dysfunction is believed to diminish if positive system changes elicit subsystem feedback which encourages further positive changes.

While the above supports the legitimacy of the concept of family nursing, more work is needed in incorporating the concept in nursing conceptual models. The most comprehensive work in synthesizing family therapy theory and practice from nursing models with a focus on individuals has been recently published by Whall (1986). In contrast, this article has attempted to describe family nursing by using an inductive thinking process based on clinical experience. In order for family nursing interventions to become unique to the nursing profession, the concept of family nursing has to be made congruent with a nursing conceptual model that is applicable to all possible nursing situations. The construction of a framework for families is beyond the scope of this article, but it is hoped that the suggested definition will become a basis for professional discussion.

CONCLUSIONS

Family nursing can and should be practised by all nurses. Nurse generalists are equipped to nurse relatively well functioning families at the individual level and the interpersonal level. Family system nursing and advanced interpersonal nursing of families with dysfunctions are reserved for advanced clinical specialists of all nursing specialties who have knowledge and skills in family theory and practice.

Family nursing is practised on three levels, the individual level with the family seen as the context of the individual; the interpersonal level with the family consisting of dyads, triads and larger units; the system level on which the family is a system with its own structural and functional components interacting with environmental systems and its own subsystems. A family nurse who practices on a higher level also includes the lower level(s).

The goal for practice on the individual level is physical health and personal well-being of family members. Interpersonal change and system change are by-products. The family nurse at the interpersonal level has as the main goal mutual understanding and support of the family members. Personal change is anticipated and the interaction between personal and interpersonal factors is understood and included in the nursing care plan. System change is anticipated by advanced practitioners so that harmful situations are avoided.

The goal for the nurse who practises at the system level consists of change in the family system as a whole and increased harmony between system and subsystems as well as between system and environment. Changes at all system levels are carefully predicted, monitored and corrected if the need arises. Nursing practice at the system level is focused on family health and strengths, is holistic and implies knowledge of complex interactions of a multitude of family factors at all system levels.

REFERENCES

Barnard, K.E. (1980) Knowledge for practice: directions for the future. *Nursing Research, 29*, 208–212.

Benner, P. (1984) *From novice to expert: Excellence and power in clinical nursing practice.* Menlo Park, CA: Addison Wesley.

Donaldson, S.K., & Crowley, D.M. (1978) The discipline of nursing. *Nursing Outlook, 26*, 113–120.

Fawcett, J. (1983) Hallmarks of success in nursing theory development. In *Advances in nursing theory development* (Chinn, P.L., ed.), Rockville, MD: Aspen.

Fawcett, J. (1984) *Analysis and evaluation of conceptual models of nursing.* Philadelphia: F.A. Davis.

Ford, L. (1973) The development of family nursing. In *Family health care: General perspectives* (Hymovich, D., & Barnard, M., eds), New York: McGraw-Hill, pp. 3–17.

Johnston, R.L. (1986) Approaching family intervention through Rogers' conceptual model. In *Family therapy theory for nursing: Four approaches* (Whall, A.L., ed.), Norwalk, CT: Appleton-Century-Crofts, pp. 11–32.

King, I.M. (1983) King's theory of nursing. In *Family health: A theoretical approach to nursing care* (Clements, I.W., & Roberts, F.B., eds), New York: John Wiley, pp. 177–188.

Kuhn, T.S. (1977) Second thoughts on paradigms. In *The structure of scientific theories,* 2nd ed. (Suppe F., ed.), Chicago: University of Illinois Press.

Miller-Ham, L., & Chamings, P.A. (1983) Family nursing: historical perspectives. In *Family health: A theoretical approach to nursing care* (Clements, I.W., & Roberts, F.B., eds.), New York: John Wiley, pp. 33–43.

Murphy, S. (1986) Family study and nursing research. *Image, 18,* 170–174.

Orem, D.E. (1985) *Nursing: Concepts of practice,* 3rd ed. New York: McGraw-Hill.

Rogers, M.E. (1980) Nursing: a science of unitary man. In *Conceptual models for nursing practice* (Riehl, J.P., & Roy, C., eds.), New York: Appleton-Century-Crofts.

Von Bertalanffy, L. (1966). General system theory and psychiatry. In *American handbook of psychiatry,* Vol. 1 (Arietti S. ed.), New York: Basic Books, pp. 1095–1117.

Whall, A.L. (1981) Nursing theory and the assessment of families. *Journal of Psychiatric Nursing and Mental Health Services, 19,* 30–36.

Whall, A.L. (1986) *Family therapy theory for nursing: Four approaches,* Norwalk, CT: Appleton-Century-Crofts.

CHAPTER **3**

Trends in Nursing
of Families

Lorraine M. Wright, Maureen Leahey

The authors describe their observations of three trends in the nursing of families: namely, increased diversity in nursing practice; increased research; and increased family content in academic settings. These trends have major implications for nursing practice, research and education. The authors speculate on the implications and their effect on the families for whom nurses care.

FAMILY CENTRED NURSING

Family centred care has always been a part of nursing but is now receiving unprecedented attention. The purpose of this paper is to discuss three major trends occurring in the nursing care of families: increased diversity in clinical practice; increased family research; and increased family content in academic settings. Implications for the future of the nursing of families will also be addressed.

TREND: INCREASED DIVERSITY IN
CLINICAL PRACTICE

Nurses are theorizing about and involving families more in health care. Partial evidence for this statement is found in the nursing literature (Leahey & Wright 1987a,

Reprinted from *Journal of Advanced Nursing, Vol. 15,* 1990, pp. 148–154. Used with permission of Blackwell Scientific Publications, Ltd., and the author.

1987b, Wright & Leahey 1987), conference programmes and interviews with clinical staff. Such terms as 'family centred care' (Cunningham 1978), 'family nursing' (Friedman 1986, Leahey & Wright 1987a, 1987b, Wright & Leahey 1987, Gilliss *et al.* 1989), 'family focused care' (Janosik & Miller 1979) and 'family interviewing' (Wright & Leahey 1984) are frequently cited in nursing journals and textbooks.

As nurses theorize about and involve families more in health care, they are altering and/or modifying their usual patterns of clinical practice. The outcome of this change in behaviour is the trend of increased diversity in clinical practice with families. One way to determine how and if patterns of practice are changing is to analyse *how* nurses are involving families in health care. From our observer perspective and from our own clinical practice, two major types of nursing practice involving families now exist. The present trend in nursing is to either focus on the individual in the context of the family or to focus on the family with the individual as context. However, there is an emerging trend of family systems care, i.e. where the family is the unit of care. The senior author has made a distinction between these two clinical nursing practices and named them: *family nursing* and *family systems nursing.*

Family Nursing

Family nursing can be conceptualized in two ways. It is the focus on the individual in the context of the family, i.e. where the individual is the figure and the family is the ground (Figure 1). An alternative conceptualization is the focus on the family with the individual as context, i.e. the family is the figure and the individual is the ground (Figure 2). Family nursing practised in either of these ways is normally based on developmental theory, social-learning theory and family studies.

Example of Family Nursing: Individual as Focus

An example of this approach occurs when a nurse interviews a diabetic patient in the context of the family. The nurse focuses on the individual's experience with a particular illness in his family. Some questions that the nurse might ask the individual and the family include the following:

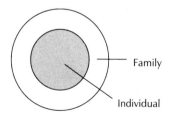

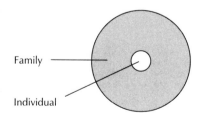

FIGURE 1. Family nursing: individual as focus.   **FIGURE 2.** Family nursing: family as focus.

To the patient: What is your understanding of the insulin? The diet? How do you explain your diabetes to others? How is your life different now that you have been diagnosed as diabetic? What is your experience coping with diabetes in your family?

To the mother: What is your understanding of John's diabetes? His diet?

To the father: What is your understanding of John's diagnosis? The amount of exercise that he can tolerate?

Example of Family Nursing: Family as Focus

An example of this type of family nursing occurs when a critical care nurse interviews family members to discuss their experiences as caregivers coping with their family member's coronary. Some possible questions that the nurse might ask family members include the following:

To the wife: What is your experience in coping with your husband's heart attack? How has it been for you to have your husband in hospital?

To the adult daughter: What is it like for you to assist your father with his physical care?

Family Systems Nursing

In contrast to family nursing which focuses on *either* the individual or the family, family systems nursing can be conceptualized as focusing on the whole family as the unit of care (Figure 3). Concentration is on *both* the individual *and* the family simultaneously. The focus is always on the interaction and the reciprocity. It is not 'either/or' but rather 'both/and'. Family systems nursing is the integration of nursing, systems, cybernetics and family therapy theories (Figure 4).

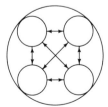

FIGURE 3. Family systems nursing: family as unit of care.

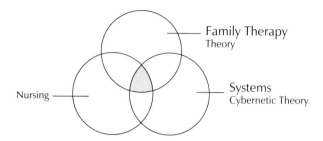

FIGURE 4. Family systems nursing.

Example of Family Systems Nursing: The Family as the Unit of Care

This type of nursing practice occurs when nurses focus on interaction among family members. To gather information about the interaction between all family members, the nurse will ask questions that focus on relationships. It may be relationships or connections between family members' behaviours, beliefs, or affect. For example:

To the patient's older sister: What happens between your parents when your younger brother forgets to take insulin? What does your brother do when your parents remind him about his insulin? What does he do when they don't remind him? How does this affect you? Other family members?

To the patient: Who worries the most in your family about you and your diabetes? Do you think they worry the right amount, or should they worry more or less?

Implications of Increased Diversity in Clinical Practice

The first general implication of the trend towards increased diversity in clinical practice with families is that more nurses will involve families in health care. It is our prediction that this will occur irrespective of which type of family practice nurses choose. As nurses begin to discuss the distinctions between family nursing and family systems nursing, there will be a ripple effect. Nurses who previously dismissed nursing care of families as nothing new and suggested that 'we have been doing this all along' (e.g. Lillian Wald at the Henry Street Settlement, births in the home, etc.) will now need to examine the diversities that presently exist in family practice. In so doing, they will begin to analyse their own practice with families to either defend, expand or abandon it.

It is also our prediction that nurses will exert more leadership to invite families to interviews. These will likely not be seen as threatening either to the family or to other health professionals' sense of territory. Rather, the family will welcome the opportunity to come to a meeting not 'because something is wrong with us' but rather 'because the health care agency is interested in us'. Furthermore, nurses will begin documenting their clinical work with families. Charts, kardexes, computer print-outs, etc., will all have space for family data. As nurses gain confidence and skill in family work, they will document more of their nursing practice with families which in turn will lead to increased ideas for family intervention.

A more specific implication of increased diversity in practice is that nurses involved in family systems nursing will conceptualize and assess interaction at all systems levels. Just as it has been commonplace for nurses to accept multiple systems levels within an individual (molecule, organ, organ system, interaction between organ systems, etc.), it will become common for family systems nurses to conceptualize the interaction between an illness and the individual patient. They will understand the reciprocal influence of the patient in maintaining, aggravating or ameliorating the illness. Family systems nurses will concentrate on the interconnections between illness, the individual and the family. They will reflect on studies (Minuchin *et al.* 1975, Selvini-Palazzoli *et al.* 1978) which illustrate these interconnections and will conduct research to explore, explain, and support their work. Interaction at all systems levels, as well as across systems levels, will be assessed by family systems nurses, i.e. from the micro level of fluid and electrolytes to the macro level of the family, the community and society (Figure 5).

Having assessed a health problem from an interactional perspective, family systems nurses will intervene at the system level with the greatest leverage for change. For example, if the presenting problem is electrolyte imbalance, then the primary unit of treatment would be the individual patient with attention to the cellular level. If the presenting concern is a husband's understanding of the diabetic regime, then the primary unit of treatment would be the family for health teaching about diet, exercise and insulin. If the diabetic patient is a school-aged child, then the primary unit of treatment might also include, in addition to the family, the community (i.e. school) because this is where the child spends a large majority of time.

Another implication of the trend towards increased diversity in clinical practice is that family systems nurses will request more one-way mirrors in their facilities in order to work collaboratively with other disciplines and to receive feedback on their clinical work from their nursing colleagues and other health care professionals who specialize in systems practice.

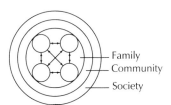

Family
Community
Society

FIGURE 5. Systems embedded within systems.

One implication having negative consequences for family practice would be potential competition between nurses involved in family nursing and those involved in family systems nursing. There is presently a phenomenon in nursing of becoming so committed to focusing on the family as the unit of care that focusing on the individual in the context of the family or focusing on the family is viewed as an inferior or a secondary level of practice. In our view, this constitutes a serious epistemological error. The practice of family nursing as compared to family systems nursing is no less inferior, no less important, only different. More often, the type of family practice will be determined by the context of nursing care and the competency level of the nurse. For example, in emergency rooms, intensive care units, and some adult care units, family nursing is the appropriate practice of choice.

TREND: INCREASED FAMILY RESEARCH

Despite families being so important in health care, they have often been neglected in research. However, nursing has awakened to the need to understand the connection between family dynamics and health and illness. Within nursing, there is an enthusiastic increase in the clinical and theoretical interest in the family. In addition, there is a beginning trend to increase the amount of family nursing research (Murphy 1986). This has not been an easy task when both nursing and North American society have been primarily focused on the individual. Since the 19th century, North Americans have developed a culture of individualism whereby the welfare of individuals supersedes commitment to social groups. Yet the family is the most intimate social environment, being both a major source of stress and social support.

Research on the family and mental health is much further advanced than that on the family and physical health (Campbell 1987). This is an area where nurse researchers could and are beginning to make a significant contribution.

Studies of the family's impact on physical health have predominantly been from a social epidemiological view. Family interactions have only been examined in studies of diabetes (Campbell 1987). Poor diabetic control is associated with chronic family conflict and poor organization, but studies disagree as to whether these families have low or high cohesion. In a more recent study by a nurse family researcher, Duhamel (1987) examined family interaction and hypertension. One of the significant hypotheses generated from this study was that hypertensive patients suppress anger and hostility and the suppression of these feelings leads to unresolved marital conflicts that reciprocally reinforce the suppression of anger and hostility.

Other recent studies on family and physical health have identified marital status and support by the spouse as the most potent family factors affecting overall mortality and cardiovascular disease. Family support, especially by the spouse, has a protective effect that is not specific to any disease process (Campbell 1987).

Family interventions, such as involving a spouse in the care of a coronary patient, can have a major impact and have been demonstrated to lower overall mortality. In hypertension the effect of family involvement is primarily increased compliance with antihypertensives and diet (Campbell 1987).

An interactional phenomenon that is needing study is how family members' reactions influence the course of an illness. Nurses and other health care professionals know that individuals' responses to a life-threatening illness vary (for example, denial or anger). However, some family clinicians now propose that patients respond more to their family's responses to the illness than to the condition itself (Wright *et al.* 1989, Wright & Watson 1988). The research of Reiss *et al.* (1986) suggests that affected families who are too emotionally close may precipitate death in the sick family member. Death represents an 'arrangement' between the family and the patient—the patient dies so that 'the family may live'. This is often an extreme but perhaps the only 'reasonable' patient response to the family's feelings of grief and burden.

Implications

Three implications of this trend of increased family research are:

1. Family assessment techniques will be further developed. In the family research literature, less than 5% of the articles on family and health are empirical studies (Campbell 1987). Therefore, nursing can make a tremendous contribution to this neglected area. Attention should be given to self-report methods as well as direct observation methods, and the results of these two approaches should be compared.
2. Research on the reciprocal relationship between family functioning and the course and treatment of an illness will gain prominence. This will be partly due to the difficulty of demonstrating that family factors precede the development of an illness but mostly due to nursing being more aware of this important connection.
3. The efficacy of family treatment will become paramount as health care providers become more concerned with what type of health care services are most appropriate for specific situations. For example, family nursing interventions, such as education and providing family support, should be compared with other types of nursing interventions. As well, more complex interventions, such as 'prescribing a ritual' or 'externalizing the symptom' should be examined for their effectiveness for treatment of family conflicts related to health problems.

This increase in nursing research will profoundly expand knowledge of the impact and long-term consequences that serious illnesses have on family members and on the family unit. As well, the far-reaching influence that family interaction has on the development, perpetuation, aggravation or amelioration of physical illness will be better understood and in turn more effective and comprehensive family care will be given.

TREND: INCREASED FAMILY CONTENT IN ACADEMIC SETTINGS

Family content has been substantially integrated into nursing curriculums over the past 10 years. Until now, however, very little information has been available to provide evidence about the quantity and quality of family content in university nursing curriculums. Even less has been known about nursing students' clinical practice with families or the methods of supervision of family interviewing skills. However, two recent studies, one by Hanson & Bozett (1987) conducted in the United States and another by Wright & Bell (1988) conducted in Canada suggest similar preliminary findings and substantiate this trend.

Family Content in Nursing Curriculums

Although family content varies dramatically from school to school, it has become an integral part of most undergraduate programmes. Many nursing programmes teach about families within the parent/child, community health or mental health part of the curriculum. Also, family content is frequently embedded in other courses. There is a wide variance of family content in graduate programmes, with many providing only cursory attention while others are providing specialization in family nursing.

One very interesting finding in the preliminary results of these two studies is that nursing adopts a variety of family assessment models. These models tend to be eclectic, wide ranging and often list specific concepts from family development and family therapy. A few nursing authors have taken on the challenge of integrating significant concepts from nursing, family developmental theories, communication theories, systems theory, cybernetics and family therapy (Friedman 1986, Gilliss et al. 1989, Leahey & Wright 1987a, Wright & Leahey 1984, 1987).

Clinical Practicums Involving Families

Clinical practicums, as reported in the Wright & Bell (1988) study, presently focus on family nursing with emphasis on either the individual or the family. Very infrequently is the focus on family systems nursing, where the family is viewed as the unit of care. Family nursing practicums address various family dimensions such as roles or problem-solving abilities, whereas family systems nursing practicums focus on relationships and interaction. Baccalaureate level nurses tend to experience family nursing practicums, whereas masters and doctorally prepared nurses tend to experience specialized practicums in either family nursing or family systems nursing.

Methods of Supervision

From the two surveys conducted (Hanson & Bozett 1987, Wright & Bell 1988), it is apparent that students receive clinical experience working with families in a variety of settings (e.g. home, clinic and hospital). However, the amount and type of supervision varies dramatically. The Wright and Bell study reports the predominant method of supervising the student's family interviewing skills is clinical case discussion and/or verbal and written process recordings. In the authors' experience, these methods have been the least effective for aiding the development of executive skills, i.e. the therapeutic interventions that the nurse actually carries out in an interview (Wright & Leahey 1984). The new trend emerging is audiotape and videotape supervision and in a few instances, live supervision. Audiotape supervision is extremely valuable in that it corrects the distortion of traditional verbal and/or written content. However, it omits extremely valuable data concerning non-verbal behaviour.

Although direct observation has been a common method used for the development of nurses' psychomotor skills, live supervision of interactional skills has not been pursued as vigorously. The underuse of live supervision, even though the most effective method for the development of executive family interviewing skills, is due in part to a dearth of one-way mirrors in many facilities.

At the undergraduate level, nursing students more often receive supervision of their family nursing skills through case discussion rather than audiotape or videotape supervision. Rarely do undergraduate nursing students have their work with families supervised directly. The result is that the most inexperienced nursing students receive the least powerful and effective methods of supervision. Graduate students receive more audiotape and videotape supervision and, in a few instances, live supervision.

Faculty Practice

Whether faculty members practise family nursing or family systems nursing, it should be at an advanced level. The knowledge and skill level of the advanced practitioner should approximate each other (Calkin 1984). At the present time it appears that a gap exists between the knowledge and skill level of faculty working with families. However, clinical practice by faculty members would decrease this gap (Stainton *et al.* 1989). As there are few nurse educators/clinicians who specialize in family nursing or family systems nursing, most nurses have to go outside of nursing to receive supervision in family assessment and intervention skills. The implication for students, who are not supervised by a competent faculty member in a nursing context, is that they will likely not internalize the significance of the family within the discipline of nursing (Wright & Leahey 1988).

However, there does appear to be a trend that increasing numbers of nurse educators are seeking advanced family work by studying in programmes outside of nursing such as family studies, family social sciences, and family sociology. In addition, there is a growing movement within nursing to establish departments of family nursing at the graduate level within universities. Whether these programmes be in nursing or in other disciplines, emphasis tends to be on family theory and research and only secondarily or not at all on clinical practice. However, it is encouraging to speculate that within a few years there should be a substantial increase of faculty members with advanced family theory and research knowledge and skills. The next step will be to strengthen faculty resources *within nursing* to become advanced family clinicians. In so doing, the gap will be reduced between knowledge and clinical skills in faculty practice with families.

Implications

Preliminary findings in the Hanson & Bozett (1987) and Wright & Bell (1988) surveys are that nursing courses seldom identify family content as such in the course titles. However, the trend of more nurse educators being proficient in family nursing and/or family systems nursing will result in more nursing courses titled to accurately reflect their family content and increased integration of concepts from the social sciences, family development, biology, etc.

Another implication of evolving faculty competence in the practice of family nursing and/or family systems nursing is that more focus will be given to interventions as well as assessment. Despite the proliferation of family assessment models within nursing curricula, little emphasis has been given to family intervention and the processes by which change takes place. Sound interventions are based on sound assessment and clear identification of problems/concerns/risks, but most nursing curriculums and texts stop at this level. Very few nursing texts consider what types of intervention are appropriate for what types of families with what types of health problems (Leahey & Wright 1987a, 1987b, Wright & Leahey 1984, 1987). As more nurse educators become advanced family clinicians, the nursing literature will reflect this significant development with more emphasis on family interventions.

Finally, as the trend continues for more clinically competent nurse educators to work with families, the implication will be that more direct supervision, either videotape or live, will be provided for both undergraduate and graduate nursing students.

CONCLUSIONS

Family-focused care has always been a part of nursing but now needs to further entrench itself in academic and clinical settings. Whether nurses elect to involve the family as the context for care or as the unit of systems care, their nursing practice must be real, observable and teachable. Whether nurses choose to integrate family nursing or family systems nursing into academic or clinical settings, they must *demonstrate* their work to students, families and colleagues. In faculty and family meetings, student and clinical interviews, academic and clinical family conferences, nurses need to discuss the work that they are and have been doing for years with families. As the trends discussed in this paper become more commonplace, major contributions to nursing knowledge will accumulate, further research ideas will be generated and clinical practice with families will be more efficacious.

REFERENCES

Calkin, J.C. (1984). A model for advanced nursing practice. *The Journal of Nursing Administration,* *14*(1), 24–30.

Campbell, T.L. (1987). *Family's impact on health: A critical review and annotated bibliography.* National Institute of Mental Health (Series DN No. 6, DHHS Pub. No. ADM 87-1461), US Government Printing Office, Washington, DC.

Cunningham, R. (1978). Family-centered care. *Canadian Nurse 2*, 34–37.

Duhamel, F. (1987). Essential hypertension, family functioning and family therapy. Unpublished doctoral dissertation, University of Calgary, Calgary.

Friedman, M. (1986). *Family nursing: Theory and assessment,* 2nd ed. Norwalk, CT: Appleton-Century-Crofts.

Gillis, C.L., Highley, B.L., Roberts B.M., & Martinson I.M. (1989). *Toward a science of family nursing.* Menlo Park, CA: Addison-Wesley.

Hanson, S.M.H., & Bozett, F.W. (1987). *Family nursing curriculum survey.* Unpublished manuscript, Oregon Health Sciences University, Portland; and University of Oklahoma, Oklahoma City.

Janosik, E., & Miller, J. (1979). Theories of family development. In *Family health care: General perspectives* (Hymovich, D., & Barnard, M., eds), Vol. 1, 2nd ed. New York: McGraw-Hill, p. 346.

Leahey, M., & Wright, L.M. (1987a). *Families and life-threatening illness.* Springhouse, PA: Springhouse Corporation.

Leahey, M. & Wright, L.M. (1987b). *Families and psychosocial problems.* Springhouse, PA: Springhouse Corporation.

Minuchin, S., Baker, L., Rosman, B., Liebman, R., Milman, L., & Todd, T. (1975). A conceptual model of psychosomatic illness in children. *Archives of General Psychiatry, 32* (8), 1031–1038.

Murphy, S. (1986). Family study and nursing research. *Image: Journal of Nursing Scholarship, 18*(4), 170–174.

Reiss, D., Gonzalez, S., & Kramer, N. (1986). Family process, chronic illness, and death: On the weakness of strong bonds. *Archives of General Psychiatry, 43,* 795–804.

Selvini Palazzoli, M., Boscolo, L., Cecchin, G. & Prata, G. (1978). *Paradox and counterparadox: A new model in the therapy of the family in schizophrenic transaction.* New York: Jason Aronson.

Stainton, M.C., Rankin, J.A., & Calkin, J.D. (1989). The development of a practising nursing faculty. *Journal of Advanced Nursing, 14,* 20–26.

Wright, L.M., & Bell, J.M. (1988). Survey of family nursing education in Canadian universities. Unpublished manuscript, The University of Calgary, Calgary.

Wright, L.M., & Leahey, M. (1984). *Nurses and families: A guide to family assessment and intervention.* Philadelphia: F.A. Davis.

Wright, L. M., & Leahey, M. (1987). *Families and chronic illness.* Springhouse, PA.: Springhouse Corporation.

Wright, L.M., & Leahey, M. (1988). Nursing and family therapy training. In *Handbook of family therapy training and supervision* (Liddle, H.A., Breunlin, D.C., & Schwartz, R.C., eds), New York: Guilford Press, pp. 278–289.

Wright, L.M., & Watson, W.L. (1988). Systemic family therapy and family development. In *Family transitions: continuity and change over the life cycle* (Falicov, C.J., ed), New York: Guilford Press.

Wright, L.M., Bell, J.M., & Rock, B.L. (1989). Smoking behavior and spouses: A case report. *Family Systems Medicine, 7*(2), 158–171.

CHAPTER 4

Family Nursing Research, Theory and Practice

Catherine L. Gilliss

The absence of critical dialogue regarding what constitutes family nursing prevents the further development of the specialty area of family nursing. In this essay, the author issues nine challenges faced by those who would contribute to the development of family nursing.

Interest in the family continues to grow within nursing, as evidenced by attendance at "family nursing" meetings and publication of papers about the family. Yet the diverse community of interested nurses lacks common nomenclature, common understanding about the focus of family nursing, and agreement about preparation for the role of family nurse. Although the lack of definition of the field of family nursing promotes recruitment to the movement, it interferes with critical dialogue that would refine the field. The time has come to bring definition to our field, to make clear statements about what family nursing is and is not and then to engage in intellectually sophisticated and clinically pragmatic dialogue about priorities and resources.

In this paper, nine specific challenges are issued regarding family nursing research, theory and practice. The overarching challenge is to begin a critical dialogue about the field. We need to take positions on important issues and debate the usefulness of these positions. Such discussion will sharpen our vision of the content and future directions of family nursing.

From *IMAGE: Journal of Nursing Scholarship, Vol. 23* (No. 1), Spring 1991, pp. 19–22. Reprinted by permission of the publisher.

NINE CHALLENGES

To begin, we must examine an issue fundamental to the field of family nursing: namely, we must clarify the nature of family nursing.

Family Nursing Defined

We have traditionally viewed nursing as family-based or family-centered (Whall, 1986b) and seldom attempted to clarify how family nursing differs from this traditional family-centered nursing. A nonsystematic review of several standard nursing texts offers insight into the problem. The idea described in these texts is that the patient should be treated in the context of the family group. As nursing is a humanistic, caring profession, there can be little argument that good, contemporary nursing practice is contextual. In fact, it is in the family-as-context perspective that nursing care has been traditionally offered.

By contrast, family nursing, or in the language of Wright and Leahey (1987), family systems nursing, is nursing intervention deliberately and consistently targeted at the level of the family unit. The failure to differentiate clearly between family-as-context and family-as-client has caused considerable confusion to the further development of the field of family nursing. In many current texts the units of assessment, intervention and evaluation are frequently interchanged. What begins as a discussion of family-as-client quickly dissolves into assessment, intervention or evaluation of individual members of the family or family-as-context. The distinction between family-as-context and family-as-client is important, and our nomenclature should address this distinction. Although the family-as-context perspective is significant to family nursing, it does not constitute family nursing. Family nursing should consistently address the family group throughout assessment, planning, intervention and evaluation.

Is Family Nursing a Specialty or Generalist Practice?

For some time we have politely discussed whether family nursing is a generalist or specialist practice in nursing. The significance of this issue is now more apparent. By denying that any significant difference existed between family-as-context and family-as-client, we in family nursing have annexed a large community of nurses and by that have gained additional voices and visibility. But however well the family-as-context approach is represented in nursing, it does *not* constitute specialty practice in family nursing. The family-as-context is a generalist practice view that may be used in another area of nursing specialty, for instance, in pediatrics or community health. Specialty practice in family nursing is targeted at the family unit and involves specialty preparation in family nursing. In the words of the American Nurses Association (ANA, 1980):

Generalists in nursing provide most of the care for most of the people served by nursing . . . The care provided by these nurses should be available to people wherever they may be at a given time and whatever may be their situation in terms of health, disease, illness, or injury at the time. The nurse generalist has a comprehensive approach to health care and can meet the diversified health concerns of individuals, families, and communities. (p. 19)

In contrast, according to the ANA (1980) nurse specialists are experts in providing care focused on specific clusters of phenomena drawn from the range of general practice. Specialized practice represents a refinement of interests, either by focusing on a part of the whole of nursing practice or by focusing on relations among the parts. Further, the phenomena of specialty concerns may relate either to a specialized field or to the relationship among specialized fields.

A nurse who views the family-in-context may be a generalist in family nursing and a specialist in another field of practice. Conversely, those nurses who practice family nursing are specialists in family care and generalists in other areas of practice. (See Figure 1.)

Preparation of a Specialist in Family Nursing

The Social Policy Statement of the ANA also suggested how new specialties arise and listed the criteria for specialty nursing practice. Clearly, graduate-level preparation is required for specialist practice in family nursing.

Preparation for specialty practice involves the study of theories about the area of specialization and faculty-supervised clinical practice. Therefore, any program preparing specialists in family nursing should be expected to provide, at a minimum, academic coursework on theories of family behavior, intervention with families and supervision of clinical work with families. Many other topics could or should be covered, for example, health care economics, culture and families, and family self-care.

Anyone who is clinically grounded has already asked: "But where will the family nurse specialist practice? What work can this nurse do within the existing health care system?" And this leads to the next problem. Based on the current structure of the health

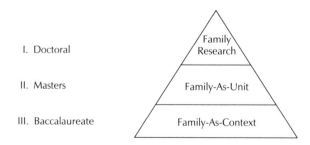

FIGURE 1. Levels of preparation for Family Nursing.

care system and the system for reimbursement of practice activities, there are very few places for experts in family nursing. The existing opportunities are those where the presenting problems are constituted as family problems, for instance, in psychiatric nursing.

Specialists in family nursing also must be specialists in another traditional area of nursing practice. Recently, a large West Coast school closed a program for "Family Clinical Specialists." The program met the school requirements for the masters degree and attracted well-qualified nurses who knew the importance of studying family nursing. Yet, the new graduates sought positions by describing themselves as clinical specialists in a traditional area of practice (e.g., maternal child health or cardiology) who had a special interest in families. No graduate-level practice supervision had occurred in any of the areas in which they claimed expertise, but, because no positions for family nurses were available, the graduates fitted themselves to the demands of the marketplace.

The Phenomena of Interest and Related Concepts

The phenomena of concern in nursing are human responses to actual or potential health problems (ANA, 1980). According to Meleis (1985), the phenomena may first be articulated as questions. For instance, why do some families experience stress during recovery from a life-threatening illness? How can families manage the care of a chronically mentally ill child at home? How do couples participate in the regulation and control of diabetes in their child? Is vigilance an adaptive coping style in families? Meleis indicated phenomena are not "things," per se, but are organized around perception. To develop the phenomenon, Meleis suggested noting its timing and physical placement, dimensions and boundaries, relationships to other phenomena, variations and related circumstances. She suggested besides describing the phenomenon, we need to ask whether the phenomenon falls within the domain of nursing.

As phenomena are organized and labeled, concepts emerge. As the building blocks of theory, concepts are more precise and generally have some empirical referent (i.e., a concrete demonstration of how that concept occurs in reality). Our progress in concept delineation in family nursing is quite limited.

Several barriers hinder our progress. At the level of concept development we confuse the unit of analysis. The confusion occurs for two reasons. First, we have precious little language to describe what we do for families and so we rely on familiar language with well-worn images that do not capture the nuances of the family phenomena. Naming, creating the new vocabulary for new images is very hard creative work. All scholars are not equally suited for this work. Second, our mental and visual images of nursing practice are formed in our interaction with individuals, and with family members, not family groups. Thus, when we begin to operationalize our ideas, when we think of what we would *do,* we begin to think of activities that relate more directly to family members than to families.

To continue our work in concept development about the family in health and illness, we must rigorously attend to the unit of analysis, maintaining a consistent focus on the family and clarity about what is empirically based in the individual and what in the family. One of the best examples of family phenomena delineation to date is a paper by Robinson and Thorne (1984) in which they discuss "family interference," a strategy of the family system to communicate with the hospital nursing staff. More work such as this will advance our field.

Another obstacle to progress is the absence of a scholarly forum to address our particular interests in a readily accessible, visible way. Although it has been argued that by remaining in the general nursing literature we would have an effect on the practice of others, in fact this approach has diluted our own discussion. Through ongoing reviews of the general literature, several authors (Gilliss, 1989; Wright & Leahy, 1990) have noted an increase in family and family-related topics. This may mean the general level of awareness and interest in families has increased. But for those whose interest is in the family, the literature is diverse and difficult to survey. Papers are sometimes not adequately reviewed by peers outside family nursing, and little printed discourse occurs that pertains to families or the development of the field. The challenge to begin a journal focused on family nursing is embedded in this observation.

Evaluation of the Utility of Theories Arising from the Social Sciences Against Those Developed in Nursing

Progress in paradigm development is inextricably connected to our progress in explication of phenomena. Paradigmatic diversity abounds; however, the usefulness of those paradigms needs closer examination. Many theories addressing family nursing in health and illness are borrowed from other fields. Frequently, the nursing theories addressing the family have simply replaced "individual" client with "family" client, failing to capture and address the unique complexity presented by the family unit. A major advance toward the science of family nursing will be accomplished when we are more attentive to the development of paradigms and theories that adequately address the nurse and the family together.

There are at least two positions regarding the issue of how to develop or use theory in family nursing. Fawcett and Whall (1990) have taken the position that either existing or new nursing theories should serve as the basis for our theory-testing work in nursing. Further, they believe it inappropriate to use or test sociological theories of family behavior in nursing science. Fawcett's own work employed Rogers' model to examine spouses' body image before and after pregnancy (Fawcett, 1977; Fawcett, Bliss-Holtz, Haas, Leventhal & Rubin, 1986; Fawcett & York, 1986).

The contrasting view proposes that social science theories are useful within nursing, and, though some adaptations may be required, these theories merit our review and use. Mercer (1989) supported this approach when she stated that, although some classical theories may not apply and will require alternative hypotheses, "family theorists have gone too far not to take advantage of the trial and error of other scientists" (p. 31).

Examples of the two approaches exist in our literature. Clements and Roberts (1983) collated, for undergraduate nursing students, theories from the social sciences and nursing and demonstrated their application in nursing. Within this text, nurse theorists Roy, Rogers, Orem, King, Newman, Neuman, Roberts and Black attempted to extend and apply their work to the family. Often, this extension involved substitution of family for client. Whall (1986a) has similarly shown the use of social science and nursing theories to the area of family therapy. Although she makes clear that nursing has responsibility for the development of theory to guide practice, she supports the use of conceptual models from outside nursing, observing that their users are required to make some conceptual leaps. The work of Wright and Leahey exemplifies how this can be accomplished (Leahey & Wright, 1987a, 1987b; Wright & Leahey, 1984, 1987). Drawing heavily from the work of Karl Tomm, they adapted family systems theories to nursing practice as family systems nursing. Their work applies family systems nursing to situations of life-threatening illness, chronic illness and to psychosocial problems.

Meleis (1985) explicated an approach to theory development that involves what she referred to as primitive and derived concepts. Primitive concepts are introduced in the theory as new and defined within the theory. Derived concepts come from outside the theory and take on a new meaning within the new theory. The wisdom of Mercer, guided by the strategies of Meleis, offers direction to continue development of concepts relevant to the phenomena of interest. Use of existing theories permits introduction of primitive or derived concepts into these existing theories. The applications will be unique within our discipline and in time it is likely the developments will be so distinct from their origins as to be "a theory of family nursing." After all, what we view as a distinct theory of nursing in the Roy (1974) model was developed as an adaptation of general systems theory, based on Helson (1964), who was a physiologic psychologist.

Accumulate Knowledge About Families and Nursing Practice with These Families

Few compendia exist that address the accumulated knowledge about families and health. Campbell's monograph for the National Institute of Mental Health (1986a, 1986b) makes a highly significant contribution to this problem. Campbell, a family physician, abstracted research reports addressing some aspect of family health and contributed a thoughtful and rigorous research critique of the reports and an analysis of the state of our knowledge about the impact of the family on health.

In the family nursing literature several summative documents exist (Feetham, 1984; Gilliss, Highley, Roberts & Martinson, 1989). These reviews accumulated research in nursing and catalogued the work according to focus, design and methods.

We need to specify what we know about families in health and illness and how to care for them. We must attempt to study populations seldom studied in family nursing (e.g., vulnerable families). To that end, state-of-the-art papers that address a substantive area within the field of family nursing are needed. Woods, Yates and Primono (1989) recently published such a paper on supporting families during chronic illness. Such works are needed so the gains and the gaps in our accumulated knowledge are clearly specified.

Setting Priorities for Research in Family Nursing

Based on an analysis of the accumulated knowledge, we should set priorities for research in family nursing and communicate these to funding agencies, notably the National Center for Nursing Research. This challenge is particularly important to our efforts in family nursing. Research resources are scarce, competition is fierce. Current reimbursement strategies for nursing practice suggest no one realizes we have a contribution to make. Although we have expended great energy theorizing about how important the family is to problems of illness and maximization of health, thus far there exists precious little evidence for our claims. Critical to the further development of the field is a successful demonstration of our work. Two areas demand our attention.

We must demonstrate the practice of family nursing and its outcomes. This can be accomplished through case studies similar to the examples shared throughout the ongoing regional meetings on family nursing sponsored by the Oregon Health Sciences University (Krentz, 1987, 1988a, 1988b). Such case studies should highlight the phenomena of interest, begin to label concepts and explain nursing care of the family. Similarly, clinical trials of family care can be undertaken. A recently concluded trial of nursing care with families following cardiac surgery (Gilliss, Gortner, Shinn & Sparacino, 1989) demonstrated that nursing care improved recovery outcomes for patients. Despite the stated intention to improve outcomes for the family, there was no clear evidence the investigators accomplished this goal. Some fault lies with inadequate family measures. However, very little data in family nursing exists to suggest nursing interventions affect families. Rather, we have been successful in showing that when we intervene with families we improve outcomes for individuals. Improving individual health may be reason enough to intervene with families as clients, but we need more well-conceptualized family nursing intervention studies in which the outcome for the family is adequately measured before we abandon our claims of influencing the family.

A priority of parallel importance is the further development of methods of data collection about the family. Presently our methods are so primitive we cannot be sure whether our practiced interventions are effective. Data collection strategies often target the individual, make no adjustment for this in the analytic technique selected and claim to produce a family outcome. Frequently we find ourselves wishing to tap into some aspect of family life for which there is no known measure, for instance, reciprocity between family members in a caregiving situation. Without adequate approaches to capturing data about the family, certain critical questions cannot be answered. It is time to elaborate a research agenda for family nursing.

Evaluation of Family Nursing Practice

It is important to practice family nursing as described earlier and then critically evaluate it for pragmatics and outcomes. This challenge invites the reader to address the framework for family nursing proposed at the outset. Can a nurse focus on the family while dealing with individuals? What facilitates or detracts from this focus? To accomplish family nursing, what skills are required beyond changing the thinking patterns of the practicing nurse? How receptive are family members to the care offered the family? What influences this receptivity? What institutional characteristics enhance the delivery of family nursing services? Most important, what are the significant outcomes of family nursing?

Evaluation of Data for Policy Implications

We must evaluate our clinical work and research data for its policy implications. Meister (1989) has articulately set forth a strategy for policy analysis of clinical data in which review of case load data is a first step in the development of a family policy. This makes policy analysis the job of every nurse.

When examining the practice of family nursing, consider the financial aspects of care delivery and the indirect costs or savings of the outcomes achieved. For example, in analyzing the cost of family caregiving, consider not only actual costs and costs of replacement services but also costs of lost opportunities (e.g., missed days from work or failure to complete one's education). We face another unit of analysis problem as we analyze and report our findings to government policy makers, as outcomes of interest to policy makers are generally outcomes of the individual (e.g. immunization rates, sick days, income levels, insurance coverage). Although we may need to convert our outcomes to demographics of the individual, let us continue to search for relevant markers of the quality of health of the family group.

CONCLUSION

We need to sharpen our developing field of family nursing by entering thoughtful, analytical debate with one another about the nature and scope of our work. We must begin by clarifying the nature of and preparation for specialty practice in family nursing. Next, we must move beyond the declaration of our practice intentions to demonstrate family nursing practice and its *real* outcomes. Our theoretical explanations of family nursing need refinement; observing practice outcomes offers considerable promise for theory development.

REFERENCES

American Nurses Association. (1980). *Nursing: A social policy statement.* Kansas City, MO: The Association.

Campbell, T. (1986a). The family's impact on health: A critical and annotated bibliography. Washington, DC: U.S. Government Printing Office. (DHHS #ADM861461).

Campbell, T. (1986b). The family's impact on health: A critical review. *Family Systems Medicine, 4*(2&3), 135–328.

Clements, I., & Roberts, F. (Eds.) (1983). *Family health: A theoretical approach to nursing care.* New York: Wiley.

Fawcett, J. (1977). The relationship of identification and patterns of change in spouses' body image during and after pregnancy. *International Journal of Nursing Studies, 14,* 199–213.

Fawcett, J., Bliss-Holtz, V.J., Haas, M.B., Leventhal, M., & Rubin, M. (1986). Spouses' body image changes during and after pregnancy: A replication and extension. *Nursing Research, 35,* 220–223.

Fawcett, J., & Whall, A. (1990). Family theory development in nursing. In J. Bell, W. Watson, & L. Wright (Eds.), *The cutting edge of family nursing.* (pp. 17–23). Calgary, Canada: University of Calgary.

Fawcett, J., & York, R. (1986). Spouse's physical and psychological symptoms during pregnancy and the postpartum. *Nursing Research, 35,* 144–148.

Feetham, S. (1984). Family research: Issues and directions for nursing. In H. Werley, & J. Fitzpatrick (Eds.), *Annual Review of Nursing, 2,* 3–25. New York: Springer-Verlag.

Gilliss, C., Gortner, S., Shinn, J., & Sparacino, P. (1989). Final Report: *Improving Recovery from Cardiac Surgery* (2-RO1-NR1031).

Gilliss, C. (1989). Family research in nursing. In C. Gilliss, B. Highley, B. Roberts, & I. Martinson (Eds.), *Toward a science of family nursing.* (pp. 37–63). Menlo Park, CA: Addison-Wesley.

Helson, H. (1964). *Adaptation level theory.* New York: Harper & Row.

Krentz, L. (Ed.) (1987). *Nursing of families in transition.* Portland: Oregon Health Sciences University.

Krentz, L. (Ed.) (1988a). *Nursing and the promotion/protection of family health.* Portland: Oregon Health Sciences University.

Krentz, L. (Ed.) (1988b). *Nursing of families with acute or chronic illness.* Portland: Oregon Health Sciences University.

Leahey, M., & Wright, L. (1987a). *Families and life-threatening illness.* Springhouse, PA: Springhouse.

Leahey, M., & Wright, L.. (1987b). *Families and psychosocial problems.* Springhouse, PA: Springhouse.

Meister, S. (1989). Health care financing, policy and family nursing practice: New opportunities. In C. Gilliss, B. Highley, B. Roberts, & I. Martinson (Eds.). *Toward a science of family nursing.* (pp. 146–155). Menlo Park, CA: Addison-Wesley.

Meleis, A. (1985). *Theoretical nursing.* Philadelphia, PA: Lippincott.

Mercer, R. (1989). Theoretical perspectives on the family. In C. Gilliss, B. Highley, B. Roberts, & I. Martinson (Eds.), *Toward a science of family nursing* (pp. 9–36). Menlo Park, CA: Addison-Wesley.

Robinson, C., & Thorne, S. (1984). Strengthening family "interface." *Journal of Advanced Nursing, 9,* 597–602.

Roy, C. (1974). The Roy adaptation model. In J. Riehl & C. Roy (Eds.), *Conceptual models for nursing.* (pp. 135–144). New York: Apple-Century-Crofts.

Whall, A. (1986a). *Family therapy theory for nursing.* Norwalk, CT: Appleton-Century-Crofts.

Whall, A. (1986b). The family as the unit of care: A historical review. *Public Health Nursing, 3.* 240–249.

Woods, N., Yates, B., & Primono, J. (1989). Supporting families during chronic illness. *Image: Journal of Nursing Scholarship, 21,* 46–50.

Wright, L., & Leahey, M. (1984). *Nurses and families.* Philadelphia: F.A. Davis.

Wright, L., & Leahey, M. (1987). *Families and chronic illness.* Springhouse, PA: Springhouse.

Wright, L., & Leahey, M. (1990). Trends in nursing of families. In J. Bell, W. Watson, & L. Wright (Eds.), *The cutting edge of family nursing.* (pp. 5–16). Calgary, Canada: University of Calgary.

CHAPTER **5**

Closing the Gap Between Grand Theory and Mental Health Practice with Families. Part 1: The Framework of Systemic Organization for Nursing of Families and Family Members

Marie-Luise Friedemann

This paper proposes a nursing framework for individuals and families that was inductively derived from existing knowledge and the author's personal experience. The framework is based on the premise that all things are organized as systems. Individuals, family systems, and the environment are interrelated and the congruence of patterns and rhythms between systems and subsystems signifies health. Nursing involves assisting individuals and families to reduce anxiety by weighing against each other the two major dimensions of system control and congruence or spirituality with the aim of maintaining a dynamic equilibrium.

The family focus in nursing practice has existed ever since Florence Nightingale wrote instructions for district nurses and home missioners in 1876 (Miller-Ham & Chamings, 1983). Recently, all nursing disciplines have adopted an increasingly holistic perspective that includes the family system and the community (Murphy, 1986). Even though nursing conceptual frameworks are focusing primarily on individual clients and the nurse-client relationship, significant progress has been made in broadening the accepted nursing metaparadigm to include family system concepts (Clements & Roberts, 1983; Fawcett, 1975, 1977); and in applying these concepts in family practice (Whall, 1981, 1986).

Nevertheless, there is still a gap between grand theory and practice models, between nursing of physical illness and psychosocial problems, and between practice that

From *Archives of Psychiatric Nursing, Vol. III* (No. 1), February 1989, pp. 10–19. Copyright © 1989 by W. B. Saunders Company. Reprinted by permission of the author and W. B. Saunders Company.

encompasses various focal systems such as the personal, the interpersonal and the social systems (King, 1981). The following two articles propose (a) a conceptual framework that integrates the concepts of family and family health and guides the thinking of all nurses involved with families, and (b) a practice model based on this broad conceptual framework. The suggested practice model is especially useful for family mental health nurse specialists and nurse family therapists.

The framework of systemic organization, originated at Wayne State University, presents a view of the world relative to nursing and suggests a way to perceive the nature of individuals and families as well as their basic processes of functioning within the environment. During a recent presentation at Wayne State, the nurse theorist Rose-marie Parse (1988) said that it is naive to believe that nursing conceptual frameworks are created from knowledge unique to nursing and that, once formulated, they do not change. Instead, all viable conceptual frameworks are constantly evolving through both inductive and deductive thinking processes, critical examination of the relationships between constructs, and assimilation of new knowledge over time. Consequently, nursing conceptual frameworks are a synthesis of the creator's personality and life experience, context, and relevant existing knowledge leading to a unique perception of the relationships between the acting components of the process of nursing. The evolution of the framework of systemic organization has been no different. Bits and pieces of the thinking and writing of scientists and practitioners in nursing such as Martha Rogers (1980) and Margaret Neuman (1979, 1983), and family specialists from related disciplines, among others David Kantor and William Lehr (1975), Salvador Minuchin (1974), Jay Haley (1976), W. Robert Beavers (1976, 1981), and Larry Constantine (1986), have been reformulated and become part of this author's universe of discourse.

The framework of systemic organization has been taught to several classes of undergraduate nursing students. In the clinical setting, undergraduate students have helped families and managers of residential facilities to better manage the chronically mentally ill and prevent further need for hospitalization. Upon follow-up after discharge, family members have made many favorable comments: for example, about improved patient compliance with the medication regime or increased willingness of patients to assume responsibilities. The framework was also used by graduate students in a family therapy course. Of 10 dysfunctional families all showed significant improvement in parenting and interpersonal relations. The therapy of four families was recorded in a case study format and improvement in family functioning was documented (Friedemann, Jozefowicz, Schrader, Collins, & Strandberg, 1988). The students involved have evaluated the framework as helpful in guiding the analysis of complex mental health problems and directing them toward logical goals for the family. Such evidence has inspired this author to share the promising theoretic base.

ENVIRONMENT

Propositions

1. All existing things are organized as open systems of energy and matter in movement.

2. The basic order of the universe encompasses the organization of all systems on Earth.
3. The order of the universe is ruled by conditions largely unknown to humans. It is timeless and limitless, and its power is awesome.
4. The organization of systems on Earth follows a secondary order; the laws of the earthly conditions of time, space, energy, and matter.

The environment is the inescapable context in which humans are living. The environment consists of all things outside a person's physical boundary. All matter and energy are organized in systems: microsystems, such as atoms and cells, material systems as in rocks or metals, living systems of plants and animals, social systems such as schools or the work place, and macrosystems including political systems, economic systems, ecosystems, and nature as a whole, the total organization of this planet's resources ruled by nature and by man, and, finally, the universal systems. All systems are defined by rhythms and patterns. Rhythm involves the time of revolutions of matter and the flow of energy around a system's center of gravitation, whereas pattern describes the system's use of space.

The view of the universe as systems purports that all that exists is complex and organized. General systems theory is applicable here since it deals with organized complexity (Weinberg, 1975). The system view is global in that it looks at phenomena in their totality and explains process in its full complexity. It does not reduce the whole to simpler parts but instead explains the parts by the function they perform as part of the total system (Constantine, 1986).

Since all systems are open systems that exchange matter and energy with each other, they are interrelated and interdependent and form a terrestrial system. The terrestrial system is specific to Earth since it depends on the specific earthly conditions of time, space, energy, and matter. The terrestrial system is subordinated to a universal system that is timeless, limitless, and ruled by conditions largely unknown to humans. Its functions are predetermined and its power is awesome.

HUMANS

Propositions

1. Humans define their identity and the nature of their environment by the relationships they have with the human, material, and other living systems in their environment.
2. Human reality is limited to human perception.
3. Human knowledge is limited to the earthly conditions of time, space, energy, and matter.
4. The human ability to recognize the dependency on natural forces and to foresee death has the potential to evoke a human system disturbance that disrupts the organizational congruence with subsystems and primary and secondary environmental systems.

5. Humans have the need and the capacity for transcendence in their attempt to reestablish organizational congruence with their environment and the universe.
6. Humans who realize their vulnerability and dependency on natural forces have the need to create and maintain a sense of power in a manmade environment or civilization.
7. Civilization is becoming increasingly complex through the transmission of culture to new generations and the incorporation of new knowledge in the human way of life.

Since forces that move electrons around the nucleus of an atom also move planets around their suns, human system organization is universal organization and as a result humans are intrinsically one with their environment and the universe. Humans have direct relationships with primary environmental systems in that they continuously exchange energy and matter with them. Humans have indirect relationships with all other systems that are part of the terrestrial subsystem and the universe.

The terrestrial subsystem of the universe is determined by the earthly conditions of time, space, energy, and matter. As part of the terrestrial subsystem and equal to all other systems on Earth, the human system of body and mind, created and constantly evolving, is dependent on the earthly conditions. Therefore, the human system is responding to a perception of reality relative to its senses and nervous system and its movement is determined by anatomic structure, shape, and gravity. Human knowledge of the environment is restricted to the secondary organization of terrestrial energy and matter evidenced as bodies, shapes, colors, sounds, and odors.

From birth on, humans are forming their personal identity in relation to a reality perceived through their senses. Objects are not defined by their universal meaning but by the meaning relative to the objects' relationship with the human system. For example, a cup is a cup because humans drink from it and its atomic structure or its relationship to all matter that forms the Earth's crust is irrelevant to human thinking. Similarly, fellow humans are defined by their relationship to the individuals with whom they interact, or to their reference groups. For example, fellow humans who become part of a defined interpersonal relationship are parents, friends, spouses, or playmates, and people whose relationship is determined by services they offer are carpenters, teachers, or doctors. Consequently, human understanding of the functions of the total universal system is limited. Human knowledge does not encompass universal truth since knowledge of one small part of the system, the terrestrial subsystem, cannot explain the whole.

While humans, equal to other living systems, are generally absorbed by their own limited reality of things to touch, taste, see, hear, and smell, they distinguish themselves by their ability to realize their physical limitations and their dependency on conditions such as the availability of food, drink, and shelter, temperature and weather, rhythms and patterns of day and night, the seasons, or human growth and development. In addition, humans foresee their end. They experience a glimpse of the universal truth in becoming aware of the process of transformation of all matter and the law of decay of all living things on Earth. The resulting sense of helplessness and vulnerability may effect tension that has the potential to destroy the given organization of the human system and subsystems. Human systems under tension may experience a disturbance in their spatial and temporal patterns, their rhythms, and their structure and process. Since systems are interdependent, tension will affect all human subsystems ranging from those of microscopic dimension to the organic organization of the human body. Ultimately, ongoing tension may result not only in incongruence between the human body subsystems but also between the human system, other human systems, and primary and secondary environmental systems. Humans have two defenses against tension and system incongruence: spirituality and control.

Spirituality is a need and practice unique to humans. While all material objects, plants, and animals in nature have an organization that is undisturbed and inherently congruent with other earthly subsystems, humans continuously need to reestablish system congruence that is being destroyed by tension each time vulnerability becomes evident.

Humans living in primitive conditions are relatively unprotected against the forces of nature and spirituality is their major defense against helplessness and system tension. Even though the need for protection may be less pronounced in humans of modern civilizations, system incongruence leads all humans to search for meaning in life through spirituality or submission to the awesome and incomprehensive universal order. Humans have the capacity for transcendence and a mode of perception that goes beyond logical reasoning and leads to a sense of unity with the universe and a sensation of inner peace.

Control is the second measure humans use in defending themselves against their vulnerability and their dependency on such terrestrial and extraterrestrial conditions. In controlling external forces, humans have established elaborate systems such as economic systems for the supply of food, clothing, and shelter, political systems to enforce and control leadership, and subordination and social systems to assure cooperation and division of labor. As a result, modern humans have achieved considerable control over their dependency through a superimposed civil system or civilization, and a sense of power that allows them to deny the awesome power of the universe. Within their civil system humans perceive themselves as the center of world action and reduce their need for spirituality.

Civilizations or civil systems are the purposeful organization of culture, and culture can be defined as the totality of the human way of life that includes control of natural forces through the knowledge of terrestrial laws as well as the institutionalization of spiritual practices. Culture is passed on from generation to generation. Consequently, the ongoing development of civil systems depends on two processes: transmission of culture and increase of knowledge. New knowledge, as it becomes incorporated into a generation's way of life, becomes culture with each new generation. Consequently, over time the civil structure adopts characteristics of its own and becomes increasingly incongruent with the subsystem of nature and the universe. This makes it more difficult for humans to achieve spirituality or congruence with universal order.

As various civil systems around the globe have become increasingly independent of nature, they are also turning more interdependent and complex. An individual person's contribution to the total civil system has become insignificant and no longer provides personal gratification. Many individuals have lost their sense of control even over small segments of their environment such as their workplace. Ironically, with the increased ability to control natural forces, the civil systems have become so complex and intertwined that their reactions to changes are hard to predict even by experts. This has made individuals painfully aware of their powerlessness and dependency not only on the natural and universal forces, but on their own civil system now ruled by forces beyond human control. Consequently, the civil system created to relieve tension has become a new source of tension and human system disturbance.

This leads to the realization that modern humans are in ever increasing need of a system, namely the family, that allows them to experience some control over a small portion of their environment and to practice spirituality.

FAMILIES

Propositions

1. The family functions in conjunction with the human civil structure in transmitting culture, the most basic human patterns and values.
2. The family shares with the civil structure the responsibility to provide physical necessities and safety, to procreate, to teach social skills to its members, to provide for personal growth and development, to allow emotional bonding of members, and to promote a purpose for life and meaning through spirituality.
3. The family satisfies its members' needs for control over their environment and guides them in finding through system congruence comfort with each other and a meaning for life.
4. All family processes include collectively accepted and coordinated behaviors that aim at regulating the earthly condition or access conditions of space, time, energy, and matter in order to gain the target conditions of stability, growth, affect, and meaning for all family members.
5. The family strives to keep the four process dimensions in a dynamic equilibrium: system maintenance, system change, togetherness, and individuation.

While families early in history were the only civil system available to humans this is no longer true. As the body of knowledge and its organization has become too complex for any one person to understand, knowledge now belongs to the larger civil system incorporated in community systems and governments. Likewise, the human socialization process once unique to the family occurs to a great extent in schools and in social and recreational organizations. Even basic tasks such as reproduction, physical care for family members, or the management of finances are often carried on outside family boundaries by persons other than family members.

It follows that the family functions, the provision of physical necessities, and safety, procreation, and the socialization of the young today are complementary to those of the larger civil structure. However, the family is no less important in that it is often the only system capable of meeting directly the individuals' needs for control and spirituality, or congruence with other systems. Individuals in a functioning family experience a sense of control based on the order and predictability of family processes and they sense a glimpse of the universal order by tuning into each other's systemic organization through emotional bonding. In addition, free-flowing energy connects the family system and each individual with the environment, nature, and the universe.

The family needs to be understood first as a unit with its own organization that interacts with its environment. Second, the family is a system with interpersonal subsystems of dyads, triads, or larger units defined by emotional bonds. Third, the family is a system of individuals, personal subsystems who have their own distinct relationships with the primary environmental systems, the family system, and other family members. The purpose of the family is the transmission of family culture, namely the most basic human patterns and values that represent the backbone of culture at large.

Family-specific culture is the sum of all family processes. A representation of the pathways of family processes is pictured in Figure 1. Family processes are aimed at regulating the earthly conditions, or accessing conditions of time, space, energy (Kantor & Lehr, 1975), and matter (Constantine, 1986) in order to achieve control and congruence

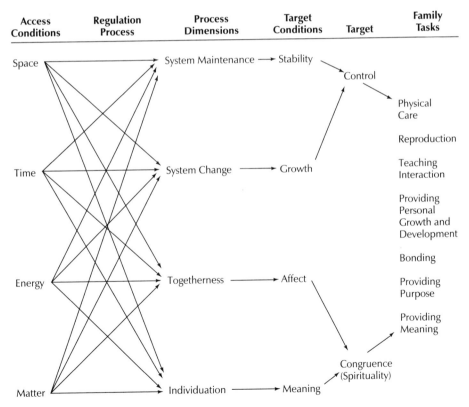

FIGURE 1. Family processes; transmission of family culture.

for each individual within the system. As is true for culture transmission at large, family culture transmission consists of two processes: transmission of patterns and values and the acquisition of new knowledge. Therefore, the target of control is achieved by meeting two target conditions: (a) stability that refers to stable patterns transmitted over generations and (b) growth made possible through the incorporation of new knowledge into the system. The target of congruence, the goal of spirituality, is aimed at each individual. It is equally divided into two target conditions: (a) affect or emotional bonding based on interactional patterns and values learned from previous generations, and (b) meaning individuals acquire through critical thinking and opening of the mind that leads to new knowledge and new realizations (Kantor & Lehr, 1975).

The regulation process consists of strategies or collective family behaviors. For example, in the attempt to regulate space with the purpose of achieving the target condition of affect and, consequently, congruence, a family may institute a weekly gathering at the grandmother's house. Another family may attempt growth necessitated by a family member who has a crippling illness. Regulating matter, the family may buy books for information or acquire equipment such as a wheelchair; regulating energy, family members may ask for help from a visiting nurse agency.

The family processes are organized along process dimensions relative to each target condition. The system maintenance dimension includes family processes that organize and structure the system. A family may set up rules to share space, assign roles to family members, coordinate activities, make decisions, or schedule family time. The organizational structure is consciously controlled and preserved as family values and learned patterns are passed on to new generations. Family maintenance processes lead toward the target condition of stability that provides individuals with a sense of control and the family system with an identity.

The process dimension of system change includes processes that lead to the incorporation of new knowledge and assumption of new family behaviors. The family allows a free flow of energy and material out of the system to the environment and adjusts its time and spatial arrangements in response to environmental feedback. Thus, the family system reaches the control target by accommodating changes from within, such as new developmental needs of family members, and from the environment. Over time, the system focusing on the target condition of growth develops into a unit with new characteristics.

The process dimension of togetherness includes all processes that lead to family system-personal system congruence. It consists of a series of learned behaviors based on a set of firm values that permit energy to flow freely between family members and regulate space and time in such a way as to bring members together. The target condition is affect or emotional bonding between members that leads to a sense of commitment to the family unit and individual satisfaction with the family system.

Individuation is the second process dimension relative to the congruence target, this time environmental systems-personal systems congruence or spirituality. Individuation processes in a family encourage the acquisition of new knowledge and values leading to actions that allow individuals to establish their own relationships with external systems. Individuals use their talents and strive for spiritual growth or the target condition of meaning by connecting with systems outside the family unit and with the universe.

All four process dimensions are interrelated. There is a negative correlation between the two dimensions pertaining to each target: control and congruence. Thus, system maintenance and system change are negatively correlated. For example, a family that promotes strict control over its internal environment and limits exchange with external systems will automatically restrict its potential to assimilate new knowledge and respond to changes of the environment. Likewise orientation toward congruence between family members (togetherness) is negatively correlated with the individual's ability to establish congruence with the environment (individuation). For example, a family with extremely high unity requires commitment and sacrifice from the individuals and restricts independent thinking and acting, thereby restraining them from unfolding their full potential. Conversely, of the process dimensions relative to both, control and congruence/spirituality targets, one focuses inward toward the family system, while the other is directed outward toward the environment. Both inward-oriented dimensions (system maintenance and togetherness) and both outward-oriented dimensions (system change and individuation) are necessarily positively correlated, but each maintains enough distinction to exert individual influence on family functioning. The family is thus a unit that transmits culture and keeps in a dynamic equilibrium the four target processes that assist individuals to achieve well-being.

HEALTH

Propositions

1. Health is system congruence evidenced on all levels of an individual's system, the subsystems, and the primary environmental systems.
2. Physical disease is a condition that refers to the organizational disturbance at the organic system level.
3. Physical disease and a high level of health can occur concurrently.
4. The crucial determinant of lack of health is anxiety that results from system incongruence while well-being is the result of high level health.

Health is the maintenance of the human relationship with the universe. Health is the congruence of the universal rhythm and pattern of movement of matter and energy with the pattern and organization inherent in each person. In a person with an ideal state of health the universal rhythm and pattern are one with those of body and mind. The uninhibited movement of energy and matter within and without the person exhibits perpetual rhythms and patterns that are calming and soothing and thus promote a supreme sense of well-being. Such a state is rarely achieved except for limited periods of spiritual tranquility and through meditation.

Disturbances of the internal dynamic organization or the blockage of energy flow between the internal systems and the environment are experienced daily by all humans due to tension and the resulting feeling and sensation of anxiety. Anxiety is basic to all other emotions and is the antithesis of well-being. Both anxiety and well-being are evidenced as a sensation of the dynamic organization of body and mind and as a feeling at the interface of the human system with its environment. The relationship between the two is linear and negatively correlated.

As all parts of a system and all external systems are interrelated, anxiety experienced by the individual at one system level, if uninhibited, will spread and affect all patterns of the individual's subsystems and the primary environmental systems. Simple linear causality is not applicable in systems theory (Constantine, 1986). Instead, causality is circular in that anxiety arising at one system interface is fed back to the personal system where it is interpreted. If it is perceived as a threat to the personal system, anxiety may become the cause of new disturbance and new anxiety to be reinterpreted and reinforced.

In addition to this horizontal circular spread, the effect of anxiety moves vertically to all contact systems and subsystems down to the microscopic system level. For example, anxiety experienced by an individual at the interface between the personal system and the workplace may affect the individual's organic health or emotional connectedness with other family members. These new disturbances may then evoke new anxiety and effect further disturbance in the congruence between the individual and other persons or between the system and its organic subsystems. The search for a cause of anxiety is often in vain. Since patterns of system function that evoke anxiety are transmitted as part of culture, the actual roots of the anxiety may be dated back generations. Prolonged incongruence between system levels may lead to the loss of health and to physical disease or emotional illness.

Physical disease is defined as a malfunction of one or more human organic systems or microsystems. As such physical disease is not equivalent to lack of health or the disturbance of congruence between human systems and their environment, and/or between system levels within the human body. Instead, physical disease may occur in the absence of anxiety. For example, since the process of infectious agents gaining access to a host involves a process that is intrinsic to universal order, physical disease is congruent with universal order and may represent health. Such is the case of a person with a terminal illness who is weakened through age and has accepted mortality through submission of the self to the universe. In most cases physical disease happens concurrently with lack of health in that disease is either evoked by system incongruence and anxiety, or the anxiety occurs when the person interprets the disease as a threat to the personal system, or both. Nevertheless, the concepts of health and disease are separate. Disease takes a major focus where it affects a person's well-being. The treatment of disease includes not only those measures that lead to improved congruency and less impairment of organ and microsystems but also those factors that sustain the improved flow of energy within the body and lead to congruency among the personal, family, and environmental systems.

Consequently, the concept of disease is included in the concept of health. In addition to an assessment of organic system disease, the estimation of health needs to include a measure of the person's level of control in various areas of life and the individual's congruence with the family interpersonal system, the family unit, the larger environment, and the universe. Since system congruence signifies spirituality, the concept of health also encompasses spirituality.

FAMILY HEALTH
Propositions

1. Family health encompasses three criteria: the presence of all four family process dimensions, congruence between the family system and its primary environmental systems, and congruence between all subsystems.
2. The family style is the product of weighing and emphasizing the process dimensions of (a) system maintenance, (b) system change, (c) togetherness, and (d) individuation.
3. Family functioning consists of the processes that families use in pursuing the targets of control and congruence/spirituality.
4. No single family functioning process or family style can be judged as effective or ineffective. Effectiveness of family functioning is equal to the criteria of family health.

Family health is a dynamically balanced state in which all four family process dimensions are present: (a) system maintenance, (b) system change, (c) togetherness, (d) individuation. Consequently, family health is achieved by weighing and emphasizing family structural and organizational processes that lead to family stability against those that lead to growth through exchange with the environment. Family health is also a process of weighing family togetherness and commitment to the family unit against the striving of individuals to develop their own potential. The four target dimensions are emphasized, combined, and balanced in such a way that none of the family members have to compromise their personal growth and sense of well-being for the sake of the family system in their interaction with other family members and with primary environmental systems. Consequently, family health is present if (a) all four target processes are present, (b) the family system is congruent with its primary environmental systems, and (c) there is congruence between all subsystems and between the interpersonal and the personal subsystems; that is, all family members are satisfied with the family system.

Families have many options in achieving a dynamic equilibrium between these seemingly oppositional processes and none can be valued as better than the other. Therefore, the family style, defined as the sum of all family processes involved in weighing and emphasizing the four family dimensions, and family health are separate concepts. Family functioning consists of the processes that families use in pursuing the targets of control and congruence. Neither singular processes of family functioning nor their collective, the family style, can be judged as effective or ineffective by themselves. Only by using all the criteria of family health, including the family's exchange with the environment, can a family's effectiveness be evaluated. Therefore, the effectiveness of family functioning is defined as family health.

NURSING

Propositions

1. Nursing occurs on the various system levels from microsystems to the larger environmental systems in the community.
2. All nursing focused on individuals includes the influence of family and environmental systems on the individual's well-being.
3. All nursing interventions at the level of family systems or the community also heed to individuals and their subsystems.
4. The art in nursing consists of the nurse's creative ability to shift position from the role of a participant and actor in the system to that of a bystander, and to shift from one system level to another.

Nursing is the act of assisting humans in their attempt to reestablish control over their systems and congruence between their own system, their subsystems, and their primary environmental systems. In the sense that the well-being of humans is dependent on the individual's congruence with the family system and the larger environment, community nursing and family nursing are one with individual nursing. Nursing occurs at the interface of system levels. Each system level can become the main focus of nursing interventions; however, the focus is shifted to other system levels as the need arises.

Nursing is a science because its interventions depend on the understanding of system operation and processes. Energy can flow between system levels only if each level operates smoothly. Nursing is an art in that individuals are assisted in seeking congruence with their own subsystems, other humans, nature, and the universe through the nurse's use of self.

Nursing of the individual is the process in which nurses temporarily unite their own personal system with that of clients by letting energy flow between the systems so that patterns and rhythms adjust to each other. In this manner the client becomes receptive to change and interventions can be effective. Interventions include those targeted to act at the microscopic level, such as medications, and at the organic level, such as wound care or relaxation techniques. At the personal level nursing care addresses well-being, anxiety, and other emotions; at the interpersonal level the focus is on relationships with family members and other people; and at the family level nursing is concerned with the person's role and contribution to the family system as well as the family's ability to meet the person's needs for individuality. Nursing at suprasystems levels assesses and assists in changing the client's relationship with environmental systems in terms of using them more fully or reducing conflict. Environmental system interventions also include spiritual care and assisting clients in accepting the unavoidable by the nurse reaching out and sensing together with the client the order of the universe and a moment of peace.

On occasion, nurses will find that the local system incongruency is located at the family system level and has a secondary influence on individual persons in the family. This is true in situations where family demands exceed coping resources, where family cooperation falters and individuals become hurt in interpersonal struggle. Alert nurses will recognize the need for family nursing. Nurses who practice family nursing allow themselves to become a part of the family system. As all system parts maintain their own properties while they contribute to the characteristics of the whole, nurses may fully apply their own self within such systems without losing their own identity. They can sense the energy flow within the system, the rhythms and patterns. The mere presence of nurses in an ailing system will effect change. Consequently, nurses joining family systems have powerful effects on the system unit and, as a result, on each individual.

In summary, nursing is the act of the nurse's frequent shifting from the position of a participant in a client, family, or community system to that of an objective bystander and evaluator. It also involves shifting from lower to higher system levels in balancing and meeting the clients' needs for control and congruence. The act of nursing depends on the art of the nurse's use of self and the extensive knowledge of the science relative to all systems involved in the nursing process.

This leads to the conclusion that all nursing needs to include mental health and spiritual nursing. Physical care alone ends at the organic level and ignores those qualities that distinguish one person from another. A personal system is defined by the ways input and feedback are perceived, processed, and responded to. Each personal system reacts with feelings and behaviors and interprets input by ascribing meaning to it in unique ways. Each of these unique systems in turn interacts with other systems in special ways, again ascribing meaning to each relationship. Nurses need to be aware of the beauty inherent in each individual, in the processes of life, and in the interaction between themselves and others. It is such beauty that reflects the systems of nature and the order of the universe.

REFERENCES

Beavers, W.R. (1976). A theoretical basis for family evaluation. In J.M. Lewis, W.R. Beavers, J.T. Gosset, & V.A. Phillips (Eds.), *No single thread.* New York: Brunner/Mazel.

Beavers, W.R. (1981). A system model of family for family therapists. *Journal of Marital and Family Therapy, 7,* 299–308.

Bradburn, N.M. (1969). *The structure of psychological wellbeing.* Chicago: Aldine.

Clements, I.W., & Roberts, F.B. (1983). *Family health: A theoretical approach to nursing care.* New York: Wiley.

Constantine, L.L. (1986). *Family paradigms: The practice of theory in family therapy.* New York: Guilford.

Fawcett, J. (1975). The family as a living open system: An emerging conceptual framework for nursing. *International Nursing Review, 22,* 113–116.

Fawcett, J. (1977). The relationship between identification and patterns of change in spouses' body images during and after pregnancy. *International Nursing Studies, 14,* 199–213.

Friedemann, M.L., Jozefowicz, F., Schrader, J.L., Collins, A.M., & Strandberg, P. (1988). *Advanced family nursing with the Control-Congruence Model.* Unpublished manuscript. Wayne State University, College of Nursing, Detroit.

Haley, J. (1976). *Problem solving therapy.* San Francisco: Jossey-Bass.

Kantor, D., & Lehr, W. (1975). *Inside the family.* San Francisco: Jossey-Bass.

King, I.M. (1981). *A theory for nursing: Systems, concepts and process.* New York: Wiley.

Miller-Ham, L., & Chamings, P.A. (1983). Family nursing: Historical perspectives. In I.W. Clements & F.B. Roberts (Eds.), *Family health: A theoretical approach to nursing care.* New York: Wiley.

Minuchin, S. (1974). *Families and family therapy.* Cambridge, MA: Harvard University.

Murphy, S. (1986). Family study and nursing research. *Image, 18*(4), 170–174.

Neuman, M.A. (1979). *Theory development in nursing.* Philadelphia: Davis.

Neuman, M.A. (1983). Newman's health theory. In I.W. Clements & F.B. Roberts (Eds.), *Family health: A theoretical approach to nursing care* (pp. 161–176). New York: Wiley.

Parse, R.R. (1988, July). *Man-living-health theory of nursing.* Paper presented at the Summer Conference of the College of Nursing, Wayne State University, Detroit.

Rogers, M.E. (1980). Nursing: A science of unitary man. In J.P. Riehl & C. Roy (Eds.), *Conceptual models for nursing practice* (2nd ed.). New York: Appleton-Century-Crofts.

Weinberg, G.M. (1975). *Introduction to general systems thinking.* New York: Wiley-Interscience.

Whall, A.L. (1981). Nursing theory and the assessment of families. *Journal of Psychiatric Nursing and Mental Health Services, 19,* 30–36.

Whall, A.L. (1986). *Family therapy theory for nursing.* Newark, CT: Appleton-Century-Crofts.

CHAPTER 6

Needs of Spouses of Surgical Patients: A Conceptualization Within the Roy Adaptation Model

Mary Cipriano Silva

Within the framework of the Roy Adaptation Model, three research questions were raised: What individual needs are most important to spouses of patients undergoing major general surgery? What category of needs (factor label) best accounts for spouses' responses to the study questionnaire? Do factors identified from the individual needs reflect the four modes of Roy's model? The study sample was composed of 75 spouses 21 years of age or older whose husbands or wives had undergone cholecystectomy, herniorrhaphy, hysterectomy, or prostatectomy for a benign condition. Spouses were asked to respond to a 46-item Needs of Spouses of General Surgical Patients questionnaire. Individual need items considered most important to spouses were related to reassurance about quality of patient care, availability of hospital staff, and understandability of information provided about the patients' hospitalization and surgery. When the individual need items were submitted to factor analysis, all four modes of the Roy Adaptation Model were reflected, but in a somewhat different patterning than that suggested by the model. Factors were labeled Psychosocial Needs, Physiological Needs, Staff Support/Confidence in Care Needs, and Information Needs. The category of needs that best accounted for spouses' responses were Psychosocial Needs.

Evidence is accumulating that major surgery is often more stressful for individual family members than for patients (DeMonbrun, 1974; Gilliss, 1984; Silva, 1979). Reasons include the wait for surgery (Gilliss, 1984), lack of control over hospital events (Gilliss, 1984), fears about malignancy and the risks of surgery (Silva, Geary, Manning & Zeccolo, 1984; Watson & Hickey, 1984), inadequate information about the length of time patients remain in the operating room (Silva et al., 1984; Watson & Hickey, 1984), lack of information about changes in the patient's condition (Campbell, 1975), and altered lifestyles brought about by the patient's surgery (Gilliss, 1984; Silva et al., 1984). In these instances, the patient's surgery produced needs in individual family members, such as a need for increased control or a need for information. These needs, if unmet, can result in feelings of helplessness, anger, anxiety, and isolation that hinder individual family member's adaptation (Silva, 1977; Watson & Hickey, 1984).

Adaptation is the central concept of the Roy Adaptation Model. Within this model, the person is viewed as an adaptive system composed of *input, control processes, effectors, output,* and *feedback* (Andrews & Roy, 1986, pp. 17–25; Roy, 1984, pp. 28–36). Roy believes that a person's ability to adapt is a function of (1) stimuli, (2) processing of the significance of the stimuli, and (3) responding to the stimuli. Needs (requirements within persons that stimulate responses to preserve integrity) and the ability to adapt are interrelated in that needs are viewed as focal stimuli; that is, stimuli immediately confronting individuals (*input*). In response to internal and external environmental changes that affect satiety, need deficits or excesses occur that trigger-off regulator and/or cognator coping mechanisms (*control processes*). As a result of these mechanisms, responses occur that manifest themselves through the physiological, self-concept, interdependence, and role-function modes (*effectors*) (Roy, 1976, p. 15; 1980, p. 184; 1983, pp. 274–275; 1984, pp. 30–35).

According to Roy (1984, pp. 88–322) and Andrews and Roy (1986, pp. 41–44), the physiological mode primarily encompasses nutrition, activity, rest, oxygenation, elimination, and protection. The basic need underlying this mode is physiological integrity. The self-concept mode encompasses the physical self (body sensations and body image) and the personal self (self-consistency, self-ideal, and the moral-ethical-spiritual self). The basic need underlying this mode is psychic integrity. The interdependence mode encompasses interactions related to the giving and receiving of respect, value, and love. The basic need underlying this mode is affectional adequacy—a feeling of interpersonal security engendered through significant others and support systems. The role-function mode encompasses role development, role performance, and role mastery. The basic need underlying this mode is social integrity. Together, the self-concept, interdependence, and role-function modes are viewed as psychosocial modes, in contrast to the physiological mode. All four modes are interrelated, and adaptation may occur both within and across the modes.

According to Roy (1984, pp. 28–36), the interrelatedness of input, control processes, and effectors determines whether or not a person exhibits adaptive or ineffective responses (*output*). These responses are then fed back into the system (*feedback*). The goal of adaptation nursing is to enhance the individual's adaptive responses and diminish ineffective responses.

Although the Roy Adaptation Model has been used as a basis for research, no studies were found that used the model to structure needs of family members of surgical patients. Investigators, however, have used other frameworks such as loss theory (Breu & Dracup, 1978; Dracup & Breu, 1978; Hampe, 1975) or crisis theory (Bethel, 1981; Molter, 1979a) to identify needs of family members whose relatives underwent surgery or were critically or terminally ill.

Hampe (1975), for example, identified the needs of 27 spouses of terminally ill patients, among them, the need to be with the dying patient, to be informed of the dying patient's condition, to be informed that death was imminent, and to express emotions; a need for support and comfort from family members; and a need for support, acceptance, and comfort from health professionals. Building on Hampe's work, Breu and Dracup (1978) and Dracup and Breu (1978) interviewed 26 spouses of critically ill coronary care unit patients and modified Hampe's list as follows: the need to diminish initial anxiety, to be with the patient, to be informed about the patient's condition, to be of assistance to the patient, and to express feelings and receive support.

Molter (1979a) studied the needs of 40 relatives of critically ill intensive care unit patients. She found the following needs to be "very important" to 35 or more of the respondents: to feel hopeful, to feel that health team members cared about the patient, to be telephoned at home about changes in the patient's condition, to know the prognosis, and to receive daily information about the patient's status. Based on Molter's (1979a) study, a few investigators (Daley, 1984; Rodgers, 1983; Stillwell, 1984) studied needs of individual family members within intensive care units. Overall, their findings were consistent with those of Molter. Hickey (1985) has summarized the preceding research literature on needs of families of critically ill patients.

Based on the studies of both Hampe (1975) and Molter (1979a), Bethel (1981) identified the perceived needs of 19 spouses of patients undergoing elective abdominal surgery. The most important needs to emerge were to be informed of the outcome of the surgery, to be telephoned at home if the patient's condition changed, to know that the patient would receive prompt attention if discomfort was experienced, and to have questions answered honestly in understandable language. A limitation of this study, however, was the small sample size.

From trends found in review of the literature, as well as the tenets of the Roy Adaptation Model, the following research questions were raised: What individual needs are most important to spouses of patients undergoing major general surgery? What category of needs (factor label) best accounts for spouses' responses to the study instrument? Do factors identified from the individual needs reflect the four modes of the Roy Adaptation Model?

Overall, this study differentiated itself from or built upon earlier studies in four ways: (1) It was conceptualized within, and tested theoretical constructs of, a *nursing* model as opposed to testing of theoretical constructs of a model from a related discipline; (2) the subjects were spouses of noncritically ill major general surgical patients rather than relatives of critically ill medical or surgical patients; (3) the sample size was considerably larger than the sample size in the reported studies; and (4) the data were analyzed using a multivariate procedure (factor analysis).

Three assumptions guided this study. First, major general surgery of a husband or wife would generate stress for a spouse. Second, this stress would generate important needs for spouses. Third, spouses would report these needs honestly as they perceived them.

METHOD

Subjects

The subjects were spouses of patients in a 656-bed voluntary, nonprofit community hospital in the eastern United States. The population consisted of spouses who were associated with the hospital over the eight-month period of data collection and who were at least 21 years of age or older, able to read and understand English, not part of the nursing or medical profession or an employee of the study hospital, married to a person undergoing major general surgery for cholecystectomy, herniorrhaphy, hysterectomy, or prostatectomy and expecting a benign outcome to the patient's surgery. The unity of analysis was the individual spouse.

The sample consisted of the first 75 spouses who met these criteria and who consented to participate in and complete the study. (One spouse withdrew before completing the study.) Each spouse who participated was asked to sign an informed consent statement that included, among other information, study purpose, nature of participation, risks, benefits, voluntariness, time involvement, confidentiality of data, and assurance of anonymity.

The sample was composed of 29 women and 46 men who had a mean educational level of 14.63 years (range, 7 to 21 years) and a mean age of 50.11 years (range, 23 to 76 years). All but 6 spouses were Caucasian.

Instrument

Spouses' needs were measured with the Needs of Spouses of General Surgical Patients instrument, a questionnaire adapted from the Needs of Relatives of Critically Ill Patients, a structured interview developed by Molter (1979b). The adaptation consisted of: (1) rewording several items for use with spouses of general surgical patients instead of relatives of critically ill patients, (2) deleting several items that were inappropriate because they focused on the intensive care unit, and (3) adding several items of relevance based on the review of the literature and the Roy Adaptation Model.

In its final form, the Needs of Spouses of General Surgical Patients instrument consisted of 46 individual need items about hospitalization and surgery. The odd-numbered items constituted one equivalent half of the instrument, and the even-numbered items constituted the other equivalent half. When responding to the instrument, spouses were asked to concentrate on how important the need was to them before, during, and after the patient's surgery and not on whether or not the need had been met.

Spouses responded to each of the 46 items by checking one of five categories of need importance that ranged from 1 (need not important) to 5 (need always important). For each item, mean scores, frequency counts, and percents were obtained.

To assess whether or not spouses gave socially desirable responses to items, the range and distribution of scores were assessed. Mean scores for the 46 items ranged from 1.67 to 4.59. Mean scores for the 23 odd-numbered items ranged from 1.75 to 4.59, and mean scores for the 23 even-numbered items ranged from 1.67 to 4.57. The distribution of scores for the 46 items, as well as the distribution of scores for the 23 odd-numbered and the 23 even-numbered items, all closely approximated normal curves. Consequently, it appeared that spouses did not report socially desirable responses. In addition, spouses' responses showed discrimination among item options, with spouses selecting among all five options for 40 of the items and among four of the five options for the remaining six items.

Content validity of the Needs of Spouses of General Surgical Patients instrument was established by incorporating appropriate need items from Molter's (1979b) instrument, as well as other relevant need items identified in the literature and in the Roy Adaptation Model. The instrument was then given to a panel of three nurses with expertise both in the Roy Adaptation Model and in the care of surgical patients and their families. The panel was asked to review the instrument for item relevancy and clarity, adequate sampling of items, comparability of items in each equivalent half, and applicability of items to the four modes (physiological, self-concept, interdependence, role function) of the Roy Adaptation Model. After several revisions of the instrument resulting in a minimum of two-thirds agreement on all mode labels, as well as two pilot studies that included pretesting of the instrument, the instrument was deemed to have good content validity.

Reliability of the 46-item Needs of Spouses of General Surgical Patients instrument was established by using both a split-half method and Cronbach's alpha. Using an odd-numbered versus an even-numbered split, the coefficient of reliability obtained after applying the Spearman-Brown formula was .98. Using Cronbach's alpha, coefficient alpha was .90 for the 23 odd-numbered items and .91 for the 23 even-numbered items. Coefficient alpha for the 46-item instrument was .95.

Because of the high reliabilities and consistency of reliabilities, results of this study are reported primarily using only data from the 23 even-numbered items. (These items were chosen by random selection.) The decision was made to eliminate the reporting of redundant results (as for every odd-numbered item, there was a comparable even-numbered one) and to facilitate factoring of items that were not linearly dependent—a requirement for factor analysis.

Procedure

Two research assistants obtained daily surgery schedules to identify those patients scheduled for the designated surgeries. They then contacted spouses in the patients' rooms, told them the purpose of the study, and screened them for inclusion into the study based on the study criteria. Spouses who met the criteria were taken individually by a research assistant to private conference rooms within the hospital where their informed consents were obtained. They then were asked to complete the Needs of Spouses of General Surgical Patients instrument. Spouses were told that the research assistant would remain in the room and would be willing to answer questions about the instrument's directions but not about individual items until after the study was completed. Following completion, the research assistant study was completed. Following completion, the research assistant answered any questions and then collected the instruments. Because of the overall inaccessibility of spouses, data collection took eight months and occurred between the patient's first postoperative day and day of discharge from the hospital.

RESULTS

Most Important Individual Need Items

To identify individual need items that were most important to spouses of surgical patients, mean scores, frequencies, and percentages for the 23 even-numbered need items were obtained using the frequencies procedure with appropriate statistics of the Statistical Package for the Social Sciences (SPSS) (see table).

Of the even-numbered items, the highest individual item mean scores, out of a possible mean score of 5.0, were 4.57 (I needed to feel that hospital personnel were taking good care of my relative) and 4.53 (I needed to know I would be called at home if my relative's condition changed). These two need items, in comparable form, were also the most important need items to emerge on the odd-numbered half of the Needs of Spouses of General Surgical Patients instrument.

In addition to mean scores, frequency counts and percentages were also obtained for each of the 23 even-numbered need items. As shown in the table, need items reported by spouses as "always important or almost always important" to them were the need to feel that hospital personnel were taking good care of their relative (68 out of 75, 91%), and the need to be told about their relative's surgery and hospitalization in words they could understand (65 out of 74, 88%). These two need items, in comparable form, were also among the four odd-numbered need items most frequently selected by spouses on the Needs of Spouses of General Surgical Patients instrument.

Factoring of Individual Need Items and Their Relationship to Modes of the Roy Adaptation Model

To determine what category of needs best accounted for spouses' responses and also to determine whether or not the 23 even-numbered individual need items, when reduced, reflected the modes of the Roy Adaptation Model, factor analysis was performed with SPSS, using principal axes factoring, with squared multiple correlations used as communality estimates. For inclusion each factor had to have an eigenvalue reaching 1.0 or greater, and the factor had to account for 5% or more of the explained variance (Kachigan, 1986, p. 387; Polit & Hungler, 1983, p. 550). Using the Kaiser normalization technique, four factors were extracted that met these criteria. These factors were rotated orthogonally using the Varimax® solution.

TABLE 1
Assigned Factors, Mean Scores, Numbers, and Percentages of Spouses of Surgical Patients Who Identified the Need Items as Important ($N = 75$)

Item Number	Item	Assigned Factor(s)	Mean Score for Item[a]	No. and % of Spouses Identifying Item as "Always Important or Almost Always Important"
2*	I needed to feel I could talk freely with staff taking care of my relative.	3,4	3.99	53 (71%)
4	I needed to have a place to be alone in the hospital.	1	1.84	8 (11%)
6	I needed to feel aware of how to locate hospital services.	1	3.31	34 (45%)
8*	I needed to have my questions answered about my relative's surgery and care.	4	4.32	60 (80%)
10*	I needed to know about my relative's progress throughout the hospitalization.		4.43	61 (81%)
12*	I needed to know how to contact hospital staff if I wanted help.	3	3.64	44 (59%)
14	I needed to feel able to help with some of my relative's care.	1	2.81	22 (29%)
16*	I needed to know I would be called at home if my relative's condition changed.		4.53	64 (86%)[b]
18	I needed family nearby for support during my relative's hospitalization.		2.59	19 (25%)
20	I needed to follow my regular eating habits during my relative's illness.	2	2.20	10 (13%)
22	I needed to attend to my own physical problems during my relative's illness	2	2.52	20 (27%)
24	I needed to feel the doctors, nurses, and other staff accepted me.		2.73	27 (36%)
26	I needed to have the name of someone to call at the hospital when I was busy elsewhere.	1	2.67	24 (32%)
28*	I needed to know in what places I could wait during my relative's operation.		3.59	47 (63%)
30	I needed to talk with someone about my feelings in regard to my relative's surgery.	1	2.53	19 (26%)[b]

(continued)

TABLE 1 (continued)

Item Number	Item	Assigned Factor(s)	Mean Score for Item[a]	No. and % of Spouses Identifying Item as "Always Important or Almost Always Important"
32*	I needed to be told about my relative's surgery and hospitalization in words I could understand.	4	4.42	65 (88%)[b]
34	I needed information about what I could do for my relative when I was with him/her.		3.39	38 (51%)[b]
36	I needed to see my relative more frequently than visiting hours allowed.	1	2.53	17 (23%)[b]
38*	I needed to feel that hospital personnel were taking good care of my relative.	3	4.57	68 (91%)
40	I needed friends to be with me during my relative's illness.	1	2.13	7 (9%)
42	I needed to get some rest for myself while my relative was sick.	1,2	2.31	16 (21%)
44	I needed to pay attention to my routine bowel and bladder patterns during my relative's illness.	2	2.37	14 (19%)
46	I needed to adjust to different room temperatures in the hospital.		1.67	4 (5%)

*Individual need items most important to spouses.
[a] 1.00-1.50, need not important; 1.51-2.50, need seldom important; 2.51-3.50, need sometimes important; 3.51-4.50, need almost always important; 4.51-5.00, need always important.
[b] $N = 74$, 1 spouse did not respond to this item.

To determine which items were associated most strongly with each factor and, therefore, were retained in the analysis, the following criteria were used: Each item had to attain a factor loading of .50 or greater, and each factor had to contain three items with factor loadings of .50 or greater to be retained. In naming the factors, items with the highest loadings were given more consideration than items with lower loadings, and no item was ignored in the naming of a factor because it did not seem to fit conceptually with the other items loading on a factor (Waltz & Bausell, 1981, p. 304).

Cronbach's alpha coefficients were computed on the retained items for each factor. These coefficients reflected high internal consistency for Factors 1 and 2 (.86 and .85, respectively) and moderately high internal consistency for Factors 3 and 4 (.70 and .74, respectively). In addition, as previously noted, there was good internal consistency for each split-half, as well as the total Needs for Spouses of General Surgical Patients instrument.

Factor 1 was characterized primarily by a variety of psychosocial needs that were personal to spouses. As a result, Factor 1 was labeled *Psychosocial Needs*. Although the percent of explained variance (63.6%) was the greatest for Factor 1, it was a difficult factor to name because of the diversity of needs it represented. Factor 2 clearly was characterized by basic physiological needs. As such, Factor 2, which accounted for 19.8% of the explained variance, was labeled *Physiological Needs*. Factor 3, which accounted for 9.2% of the explained variance, was characterized by needs related to the availability of hospital staff and the quality of the care they provided. As such, Factor 3 was labeled *Staff Support/Confidence in Care Needs*. Factor 4 was characterized primarily by information-attaining needs. As a result, Factor 4, which accounted for 7.3% of the explained variance, was labeled *Information Needs*. Factor numbers for items retained appear in the table.

In assessing these factors as they relate to the four modes of the Roy Adaptation Model, the following interpretations were made. Factor 1 primarily represented the interrelationship of some aspects of the self-concept, interdependence, and role-function modes of the Roy Adaptation Model. This interrelatedness of the modes has been addressed by Andrews and Roy (1986, p. 43). Factor 2 clearly reflected the physiological mode of the Roy Adaptation Model. Both Factor 2 and the Roy Adaptation Model encompass basic physiological needs of, for example, nutrition and elimination. Factor 3 appeared to reflect that aspect of the interdependence mode that focuses on interpersonal security related to support systems (Andrews & Roy, 1986, p. 152). In this instance the support was from hospital staff as opposed to other types of support reflected in Factor 1. Factor 4 reflected the theoretical basis of the self-concept mode of the Roy Adaptation Model that focuses on the relationship between principles of learning and the development of the self-concept (Roy, 1984, pp. 260–261). It did not, however, reflect the two major constructs of the self-concept mode: the physical self (body sensations and body image) or the personal self (self-consistency, self-ideal/ self-expectancy, and moral-ethical-spiritual self). The most likely reason for this is that most of the items on the instrument relevant to the self-concept mode focused on information. The items relevant to the self-concept mode that did not focus on information showed up in Factor 1. The role-function mode of the Roy Adaptation Model did not emerge as a separate factor, but was incorporated in Factor 1. Some possible reasons for this finding include the fact that there were fewer items related to role function within the Needs of Spouses of General Surgical Patients instrument than items related to the other three modes, and that the need items perceived to be role related may have represented a broader (or different) concept than role function.

DISCUSSION

Within the boundaries of the Needs of Spouses of General Surgical Patients questionnaire, the conclusions of this study are as follow:

1. Individual need items most important to spouses of patients undergoing major general surgery are related to reassurance about quality of patient

care, availability of the hospital staff, and understandable information about the patients' hospitalization and surgery.
2. The category of needs that best accounts for spouses' responses is Psychosocial Needs (Factor 1).
3. Factors identified from individual need items within the Needs of Spouses of Surgical Patients instrument reflect all four modes of the Roy Adaptation Model, but in a somewhat different patterning than that suggested by the model.

That is, within the model, all four modes are conceptualized to be interrelated (Andrews & Roy, 1986, pp. 43–44). These study data suggest that certain needs related to the self-concept, interdependence, and role-function modes are indeed interrelated as reflected in Factor 1; however, other needs theoretically related to these modes appear to be independent factors (i.e., Factors 3 and 4). In addition, Factor 2 appears to be relatively independent of Factors 1, 3, and 4.

The preceding conclusions must be viewed in light of the limited generalizability of the results due to nonrandom sampling, the homogeneity of the sample regarding ethnicity, and the inadequate sample size to meet ideal conditions for factor analysis (Kachigan, 1986, p. 384), although adequate to meet practical considerations (J. Hickey, statistician, personal communication, December 2, 1985).

When this study is viewed within the context of similar studies, it is found to most closely resemble the Bethel (1981) study. In that study, subjects were spouses of patients undergoing elective abdominal surgery as opposed to subjects who were relatives of critically or terminally ill patients as reported in other need studies (e.g., Breu & Dracup, 1978; Hampe, 1975; Hickey, 1985; Molter, 1979a; Rodgers, 1983). The most important individual needs to emerge in the Bethel (1981) study were for information about the surgery and the patients' condition, quality care for the patient, and clear communication. These needs are consistent with the findings of the present study, and with findings in those studies focusing on critically and terminally ill patients. With critically or terminally ill patients, however, other needs of family members such as the need for hope and the need to be with the patient also surfaced as important.

Despite these consistencies, the following question must be raised: If the individual needs reported in the preceding studies were factor analyzed, would the most important individual need items also be representative of the factors that accounted for most of the variance? The present study suggests that this may not be the case. Although five of the most important individual need items were retained in the factor analysis, they were all associated with either Factors 3 or 4—factors that accounted for the least amount of the explained variance. Conversely, individual need items that made up Factors 1 and 2 and accounted for most of the explained variance were not the most important individual need items that surfaced. Therefore, individual needs, when reduced to factors, may represent a different construct than when viewed alone.

When the study results are examined within the framework of the Roy Adaptation Model, individual needs are viewed as focal stimuli (Roy, 1983, p. 275). In this study, then, the 23 individual need items constituted focal stimuli. Of those study spouses who perceived one or more of these needs to be sometimes, seldom, or not important, it is conjectured that the occurrence of the patient's surgery most likely did not generate need deficits or excesses for these relatively important or unimportant needs. Of those study spouses who perceived one or more of the 23 need items to be almost always or always important, it is conjectured that the occurrence of the patient's surgery most likely did generate need deficits or excesses for these important needs.

According to Roy's (1984, pp. 28–36) model, a person's responses to these deficits or excesses manifest themselves through the physiological, self-concept, role-function, and interdependence modes. In this study, results of the factor analysis show that, with regard to needs of 75 spouses of surgical patients, spouses' responses to assumed need deficits or excesses manifested themselves through Psychosocial Needs, Physiological Needs, Staff Support/Confidence in Care Needs, and Information Needs. The factor analysis supports Andrews' and Roy's (1986, pp. 41–44) assertion that there is a construct (Factor 1) that interrelates parts, but not all of, the self-concept, role-function, and interdependence modes. The physiological mode, however, appears to be relatively independent of the psychosocial modes.

Using the Roy Adaptation Model, one can surmise that if the needs of spouses related to their husbands' or wives' hospitalization and surgery are unmet, then spouses may exhibit ineffective behaviors such as anxiety. Since the goal of nursing within the Roy Adaptation Model is to enhance adaptive responses and diminish ineffective ones, several implications for nursing exist that are based on the model and the study results.

First, nurses must interact with spouses to identify their needs during hospitalization and surgery. Because investigators (Silva et al., 1984) have found limited contact between nurses and spouses throughout patients' hospitalization and surgery, efforts must be directed toward establishing mechanisms through which nurses (and other health team members) can interact with spouses and family members to identify needs of importance to them.

Second, nurses must create environments in hospitals that facilitate meeting needs of importance to spouses. According to these study results, such an atmosphere is one that reassures spouses that the patient will be well cared for and provides opportunities for spouses to talk with staff and others about the hospitalization and surgical experience. Special attention must be given to keeping spouses informed of the patient's condition and talking to them in language that they understand.

Finally, because major surgery often affects the family unit, unmet needs affecting the spouse may adversely affect the patient. This premise is congruent with tenets of the Roy Adaptation Model (1983) in which the family as an adaptive system is emphasized and, as such, events occurring to one family member often affect the adaptation of other members. Therefore, not only must needs of importance to individuals within families be studied, but also needs of importance to the family as a unit must be studied.

Based on the preceding discussion, recommendations for theory, research, and practice include:

1. Refinement of the Needs of Spouses of General Surgical Patients instrument to reflect more clearly the self-concept and role function modes of the Roy Adaptation Model.

2. Refinement of the modes of the Roy Adaptation Model to reflect more clearly the interrelated (and independent) areas of the modes.
3. Identification of personal and institutional barriers that interfere with hospital staff's ability to meet needs of importance to spouses of general surgical patients.
4. Assessment of need patterns of both patients and family members to determine how met and unmet needs related to hospitalization and surgery simultaneously affect both groups' adaptive responses.

In addition, because of the overall consistency of individual needs across the reviewed studies, it is recommended that the needs of importance to relatives be used to plan nursing care and that the relationship between these needs and nursing models, such as the Roy Adaptation Model, be emphasized. Only through the continued emphasis on the interrelationships of theory, research, and practice will nursing science be best served.

ACKNOWLEDGMENTS

This research was supported in part by a George Mason University grant from the Center for Research and Advanced Studies and through funding by the George Mason University School of Nursing and College of Professional Studies. It was part of a larger study entitled: "Spouses' Responses to Major General Surgery: A Replication and Extension." The extension part of the study is reported here. The author thanks J. Sorrell and P. Zeccolo for library and computer assistance, M. L. Geary and C. Manning for data collection, and J. Hickey for statistical consultation.

REFERENCES

Andrews, H. A., & Roy, C. (1986). *Essentials of the Roy adaptation model.* Norwalk, CT: Appleton-Century-Crofts.

Bethel, P. L. (1981). *An exploratory study of perceived needs of spouses of surgical candidates in the hospital setting.* Unpublished master's thesis, Columbus: The Ohio State University.

Breu, C., & Dracup, K. (1978). Helping the spouses of critically ill patients. *American Journal of Nursing, 78,* 50–53.

Campbell, G. W. (1975) . . . haunted by the spectre of what might have been . . . (Letter to the editor). *American Journal of Nursing, 75,* 393, 395.

Daley, L. (1984). The perceived immediate needs of families with relatives in the intensive care setting. *Heart & Lung, 13,* 231–237.

DeMonbrun, M. R. (1974). Effects of preoperative teaching upon patients with differing modes of response to threatening stimuli (Doctoral dissertation, The Catholic University of America, 1974). *Dissertation Abstracts International, 35,* 914B.

Dracup, K. A., & Breu, C. S. (1978). Using nursing research findings to meet the needs of grieving spouses. *Nursing Research, 27,* 212–216.

Gilliss, C. L. (1984). Reducing family stress during and after coronary artery bypass surgery. *Nursing Clinics of North America, 19,* 103–112.

Hampe, S. O. (1975). Needs of the grieving spouse in a hospital setting. *Nursing Research, 24,* 113–120.

Hickey, M. (1985). What are the needs of families of critically ill patients? *Focus on Critical Care, 12*(1), 41–43.

Kachigan, S. K. (1986). *Statistical analysis: An interdisciplinary introduction to univariate and multivariate methods.* New York: Radius.

Molter, N. C. (1979a). Needs of relatives of critically ill patients: A descriptive study. *Heart & Lung, 8,* 332–339.

Molter, N. C. (1979b). Needs of relatives of critically ill patients. In M. J. Ward & C. A. Lindeman (Eds.), *Instruments for measuring nursing practice and other health care variables* (Vol. 2, pp. 741–747). (DHEW Publication No. HRA 78–54). Hyattsville, MD: U.S. Department of Health, Education, and Welfare.

Polit, D. F., & Hungler, B. P. (1983). *Nursing research: Principles and methods* (2nd ed.). Philadelphia: Lippincott.

Rodgers, C. D. (1983). Needs of relatives of cardiac surgery patients during the critical care phase. *Focus on Critical Care, 10*(5), 50–55.

Roy, C. (1976). *Introduction to nursing: An adaptation model.* Englewood Cliffs, NJ: Prentice-Hall.

Roy, C. (1980). The Roy adaptation model. In J. P. Riehl, & C. Roy, *Conceptual models for nursing practice* (2nd ed., pp. 179–188). New York: Appleton-Century-Crofts.

Roy, C. (1983). Roy adaptation model. In I. W. Clements & F. B. Roberts (Eds.), *Family health: A theoretical approach to nursing care* (pp. 255–278). New York: Wiley.

Roy, C. (1984). *Introduction to nursing: An adaptation model* (2nd ed.). Englewood Cliffs, NJ: Prentice-Hall.

Silva, M. C. (1977). Spouses need nurses too. *The Canadian Nurse, 73*(12), 38–41.

Silva, M. C. (1979). Effects of orientation information on spouses' anxieties and attitudes toward hospitalization and surgery. *Research in Nursing and Health, 2,* 127–136.

Silva, M. C., Geary, M. L., Manning, C. B., & Zeccolo, P. G. (1984). Caring for those who wait, *Today's OR Nurse, 6*(6), 26–30.

Stillwell, S. B. (1984). Importance of visiting needs as perceived by family members of patients in the intensive care unit. *Heart & Lung, 13,* 238–242.

Waltz, C. F., & Bausell, R. B. (1981). *Nursing research: Design, statistics and computer analysis.* Philadelphia: Davis.

Watson, S., & Hickey, P. (1984). Cancer surgery: Help for the family in waiting. *American Journal of Nursing, 84,* 604–607.

Response to "Needs of Spouses of Surgical Patients: A Conceptualization Within the Roy Adaptation Model"

Sister Callista Roy

Nurse scholars conducting research on models for practice address issues of both the content and process of clinical investigation in the discipline. As a respondent for the paper "Needs of Spouses of Surgical Patients: A Conceptualization Within the Roy Adaptation Model," by Silva, I have the opportunity to address the contribution of this work within the context of such issues. The paper will be discussed in relation to knowledge of development within the Roy Adaptation Model, both the phenomena addressed and the methodology used. A specific framework for scholarly inquiry for nursing practice is the basis for this response.

The author of the research holds the basic premise that nursing science will be best served only through the continued emphasis on interrelationships among theory, research, and practice and her work clearly demonstrates this premise. The nursing model points to relevant phenomena for study and the perspective for examining those phenomena. A model for nursing practice provides a specific description of persons in interaction with their environment. Conducting theory building and research about these interactions leads to knowledge that is the *basic science of nursing.* Further, the model's delineation of the concepts of health and of nursing provides the basis for developing knowledge that is the *clinical science of nursing* (Roy, 1983a, pp. 456–459; Roy, 1985). With any nursing model, and specifically with the Roy Adaptation Model, the concepts of person, environment, health, and nursing are derived from the theorist's

From "Response to 'Needs of Spouses of Surgical Patients: A Conceptualization Within the Roy Adaptation Model,'" by Sister Callista Roy, in *Scholarly Inquiry for Nursing Practice: An International Journal, Vol. 1* (No. 1), 1987, pp. 45–50. Copyright © 1987 by Springer Publishing Company. Used by permission of Springer Publishing Co., Inc., New York 10012.

experience in nursing practice. Throughout the processes of theorizing and research, the basic concepts are clarified and tested in practice and further used to guide advances in nursing practice.

The content of Silva's research includes two concepts of the Roy Adaptation Model, needs and the adaptive modes. The model describes the goal of nursing as promoting adaptation in the changing environment. Environment is defined as both internal and external stimuli. The clinical science based on the model, then, will explore and classify relevant stimuli for various populations. Silva has chosen to focus on the needs of spouses of surgical patients using an instrument that reflects the four adaptive modes. The finding that the most important needs are related to reassurance about quality of patient care, availability of the hospital staff, and understandable information about the patients' hospitalization and surgery is useful for nurses working with families of patients having general surgery. Within the limitations of the research noted by the author, clinical science now has some specific knowledge of a phenomenon identified by the model, that is, relevant stimuli for a given population.

From the perspective of the basic science of adaptation nursing, however, we must recognize a concern in the use of the concept of need. The theorist's treatment of the concept differs from early to later work. The conceptualization and data collection of the study being reviewed were completed prior to the 1984 edition. In the 1976 text (Roy, p. 24) it was stated that when a change in the environment causes a deficit or excess in the need, then the appropriate adaptive mode is activated. The coping mechanisms were considered the functional or working units of the adaptive modes. The later discussion of the person as an adaptive system (Roy, 1984, pp. 30–36) expands on the descriptions of the coping mechanisms as the processors of the changing environment. The four adaptive modes, then, provide the particular form or manifestation of coping mechanism activity. The notion of needs has been omitted from the 1984 discussion of the person as adaptive system, and the omission was purposeful.

Clarification of the assumptions of the model have focused on a scientific base of systems theory and Helson's Adaptation Level Theory (Andrews & Roy, 1986; Roy, 1983). As theorist I am convinced that exploring the input of adaptive systems in the light of the focal stimulus and adaptation level is essential for nursing knowledge development. A clarity of focus on these scientific assumptions, as well as on the philosophical ones, is necessary in the full and authentic development of this model. Such a focus can allow one to avoid unproductive controversies about needs, drives, and other motivational constructs (Helson, 1964, p. 376). This is not to say that the concept of need is not useful to the clinical science of nursing, nor that a relevant theory about needs may not be derived as a part of the basic science of adaptation nursing. Still, needs is not a central concept in this model, and the place of a needs theory within the model is yet to be developed. Silva has labeled her work correctly in viewing needs as focal stimuli. In fact, her research questions might be framed in terms of the model without using the concept of need; for example, what stimuli are likely to be focal to spouses of patients undergoing major general surgery?

The second concept in the content of Silva's research is that of the Roy model adaptive modes. Silva accurately notes the development of the modes within the model as the effectors or manifestations of cognator and regulator activity. What knowledge about the adaptive modes does this report of Silva's work contribute to the basic science and clinical science of adaptation nursing? Answering this question will also raise issues related to factor analysis as a methodology for research related to nursing models.

The use of factor analysis in investigations of human behavior has a long and controversial history. Major questions relate to both the philosophy of science rationale reflected in this method and to the operational decisions based on this rationale and on varying mathematical solutions. Coan (1964) notes that the basic arguments regarding the reality and interpretability of factors are related to preferences for different modes of verbal formulation and for different types of theoretical constructs, as well as a lack of clarity about the function and generality of constructs. Using factor analysis to establish taxonomic systems or to develop causal explanation is another issue that has been confronted by other disciplines. As the American Academy of Nursing addressed the future of nursing science at its 1985 meeting, a plurality of methods was endorsed. The membership particularly noted that the interface of methodologies is crucial, with rigor used for each method. Furthermore, they called upon scholars in the discipline to pursue the excellent use of different approaches so that we can evaluate how appropriate each is for studying the phenomena of nursing. Silva's work begins pursuing factor analysis as a methodology for research based on the Roy Adaptation Model.

Some of the features of factor analysis make it an appealing method for developing both the basic and clinical science of nursing, in spite of its limitations as a linear/spatial model. The method assumes structural theories that view a phenomenon as an aggregate of elemental components, such as atomic elements or genes in the chromosomes, interrelated in a lawful way. The phenomena of nursing have been identified as "patterns of human environment interactions that enhance health" (American Academy of Nursing, 1986). It would seem, then, that factor analysis might be useful in investigating the patterns of human-environment interactions. Mulaik (1972) notes Thurstone's caution, however, that factor analysis is not a method for discovering full-blown structural theories about a domain. The analogy is given of the child's experiences of dismantling an alarm clock. With the gears, springs, and screws scattered around, the child has learned at least two things—how to take a clock apart and what is inside of it. But this knowledge fails to answer the mystery about understanding the theory of how clocks in general work. Accordingly, in psychology the more substantial contributions of factor analysis have been made when researchers postulated the existence of certain factors and used the technique to reveal the factors as clearly as possible.

In Silva's factor analytic research, the four adaptive modes postulated by Roy were used both in instrument construction and interpretation of findings. The author set out to determine what category of needs best accounted for spouses' responses and whether or not the need items when reduced reflect the four modes. Her analysis revealed a factor with an explained variance of 63.6%, but which was difficult to name because of the diversity of needs it represented. She chooses to call this first factor Psychosocial Needs and notes that it represents the interrelationship of some aspects of the self-concept, interdependenc, and role function modes.

In reviewing the instrument items and their factor loadings, a new perspective on the interrelatedness of two of the modes may be emerging. Items 4, 30, 40, and 42 can be viewed as responses related to maintaining integrity of self. The remaining items of Factor 1, that is, 6, 14, 26, and 36 all relate to role in that the items focus on doing something from the position of spouse of the surgical patient. The finding that these two sets of items form one factor may reflect a particular dynamic of the adaptive modes of the spouses, namely, as one focuses on the ill spouse, self-concept needs and role needs merge together. This might be expressed by saying that the spouse adapts to the situation by "being for" the other. It would take considerably more research to confirm this insight as part of the basic science of adaptation nursing. Still the method of factor analysis has served to bring this possibility to light. Factor 2 seems to be a clear aggregate of physiological needs, while Factor 3 reflects a particular case of interdependence needs relative to the appropriate support system.

Silva notes that Factor 4 (Information Needs) reflects some principles discussed by Roy in the theory and development of self-concept, but does not reflect the two major constructs of the mode, physical self and personal self. Two points may be made about this use of the self-concept mode. First, the essence of the Roy Model assumes that persons have ways of expressing adaptation that relate to the integrity of who they are. The theories that can describe the components and development of self are multiple and may change over time and in different situations. Secondly, even if self-concept theories based on the assumptions of the model are fully and unchangeably articulated, it cannot be assumed that all components of self will be represented in any particular pattern of behavior sampled, such as in Factor 4. Rather it is postulated that all components would be represented in a given person. The needs expressed in Factor 4, rather, might be interpreted as related to input for the cognator. This observation leads to the more general comment that further work will have to consider how the instrument response items handle the relationship of behaviors to stimuli.

A second feature of factor analysis that is appealing for nursing knowledge development is the summarizing of interrelationships in a concise manner to aid conceptualization. This feature is useful for both theory building and research, as implied above, and for clinical practice. Factor 1 can serve as the example here as well. The nurse would find it difficult and superfluous to keep in mind in all contacts with surgical patients all items within the factor. Having in mind a factor label, however, is most useful in both planning care and in each interaction with patients and their families. I would question, though, whether there has been an advance in clinical science by labeling this factor Psychosocial Needs. Rather it seems that a label that refers to the interrelatedness of self-concept and of role function would be both richer and more accurate in connotation.

Silva's paper, then, has contributed some specific knowledge for the clinical science of adaptation nursing, that is, the identification of focal stimuli for spouses of surgical patients. But perhaps, more importantly, the author contributes to both the content and methods for the basic science of adaptation nursing by providing insights into the interrelatedness of the adaptive modes, by sharpening the focus on distinguishing the essential concepts of the model from the developing theories stemming from the model, and by beginning to explore the usefulness of factor analysis in explicating and testing the Roy Adaptation Model for Nursing Practice. Finally, in this discussion of the research reported by Silva we have demonstrated scholarly inquiry for nursing practice based on both clinical and basic science of nursing.

REFERENCES

American Academy of Nursing. (1986). *Setting the agenda for the year 2000: Knowledge development in nursing, 1985.* Kansas City, MO: American Nurses' Association.

Andrews, H., & Roy, C. (1986). *Essentials of the Roy adaptation model.* Norwalk, CT: Appleton-Century-Crofts.

Coan, R. W. (1964). Facts, factors, and artifacts: The quest for psychological meaning. *Psychological Review, 71,* 123–140.

Helson, H. (1964). *Adaptation-level theory.* New York: Harper & Row.

Mulaik, S. (1972). *The foundations of factor analysis.* New York: McGraw Hill.

Roy, C. (1976). *Introduction to nursing: An adaptation model.* Englewood Cliffs, NJ: Prentice Hall.

Roy, C. (1983a). Theory development for nursing: Proposal for direction. In N. Chaska (Ed.), *The nursing profession: A time to speak* (pp. 452–457). New York: McGraw Hill.

Roy, C. (1983b). Roy adaptation model. In I. W. Clements & F. B. Roberts (Eds.), *Family health—A theoretical approach to nursing care* (pp. 255–278). New York: Wiley.

Roy, C. (1984). *Introduction to nursing: An adaptation model* (2nd ed.). Englewood Cliffs, NJ: Prentice Hall.

Roy, C. (1985). Practice in action: Clinical research. In K. E. Barnard & G. R. Smith (Eds.), *Faculty practice in action: Second annual symposium on nursing faculty practice* (pp. 192–201). Kansas City, MO: American Academy of Nursing.

CHAPTER 7

An Interpretation of Family Within Orem's General Theory of Nursing

Susan G. Taylor

This article offers an interpretation of family from the perspective of Orem's theory of nursing. The family is conceptualized within this theory from three perspectives: (a) as a factor that conditions an individual's requirements for care and ability to provide care for self; (b) as a dependent-care unit; and (c) as a unit of service. The meaning of these perspectives to the nurse is examined. The different assessment questions are identified. The family is seen as having functions related to the members' development of self-care agency and the establishment of appropriate dependent care systems in such a way as to promote the health of the entire family.

Individuals are the object of nursing. Although humans are described as individuals, separate and unique, they live and survive by a series of interdependent relationships. Nursing has long recognized the need for involving families in a patient's care. Furthermore, it is conceivable that there is a need for intervention at the family level in order to promote health. Within nursing theory, however, the interpretation of family has not been made specific. The purpose of this article is to show how a theory of nursing which has individuals as its proper object also has utility for nurses working with families.

When extant nursing theories describe the subject domain in terms of characteristics of the individual, it is left to the theory user to determine the extension or application of these theories to families. Schultz (1987) cogently presents the core problem in using nursing theories when multiperson units of service are viewed as clients:

Reprinted from *Nursing Science Quarterly, Vol. 2* (No. 3), 1989, pp. 131–137. Copyright © 1989 by Williams & Wilkins. Used with permission of Chestnut House Publications.

... if families, groups, organizations, and communities as interactional units with a plurality of persons as components are conceptually appropriate extensions of the concepts of client and person in nursing, then all other domain concepts, including all steps of the nursing process, need to be specified to reflect these extended definitions. (p. 79)

Every human service has a special concern for some aspect of human functioning that defines and differentiates that service from others. Orem's self-care deficit nursing theory (S-CDNT) has as its objective focus the self-care needs and abilities of individuals. Within Orem's theory, the condition that validates a need for nursing is described as the "absence of the ability to maintain continuously that amount and quality of self-care which is therapeutic in sustaining life and health" (Orem, 1985, p. 55). For children, it is the inability of the parent or guardian to provide that level of care. The proper object of nursing, from the perspective of S-CDNT, is the human being in need of assistance with self-care, that need being the result of the person's "inability to provide continuously for self the amount and quality of required self-care because of the situation of personal health" (Orem, 1985, p. 19). Orem also included within the proper object "dependent-care situations where the limitations of the dependent care givers are associated with the health state and the care requirements of the dependent person" (Orem, 1985, p. 30) whose self-care agency is not adequate for knowing or meeting their own therapeutic self-care demand.

Nursing is defined as a contemporary helping service directed toward the patient's self-care system with its two component theoretical elements: self-care agency and therapeutic self-care demand. Orem (1985) has stated that only individuals have human needs that can be met through nursing. She does, however, describe units of service different from the individual which involve a plurality of persons. These are referred to as multiperson units. Further, she has stated that "when the multiperson unit is the patient, the individual member as well as the unit as a whole ultimately benefits from nursing" (Orem, 1985, p. 136). While initially this seems contradictory, it should be noted that multiperson units of service are collections of individuals in some functional relationship one to the other. Although these functional relationships may be enhanced as a result of nursing, it is the individuals within the unit who have the human needs that can be met through nursing.

The focus on the individual as an active agent, the importance placed upon contextual factors such as family and culture, and the identification of the family as a unit of service make S-CDNT useful as an organizing framework for family nursing. Family is conceptualized within this theory from three perspectives: (a) as a factor that conditions an individual's requirements for care and ability to provide care for self, as a basic conditioning factor; (b) as a dependent care unit; and (c) as a unit of service. The term unit or unit of service is used to denote a functional entity composed of one or more persons, with the unit of service being that entity for which the nurse has care responsibility. The term system, as in independent care system, refers to the action system that has been or is being produced. The concept of family as a unit of service includes dependent care situations, with the elements of dependent care agency and dependent care systems and their inclusion within the conceptualization of family structure and function. Other factors included in the concept of family as a unit of service are the self-care systems of all family members, material resources, and time and energy requirements.

THEORY ELABORATION

The proper object of a discipline is that knowledge which distinguishes one discipline from another. The extension or elaboration of a theory of nursing begins with the recognition of the proper object of nursing as specified by that theory of nursing. The extension of any theory of nursing must be explicitly and logically related to the specified proper object and must take into consideration the nature of the units to which the theory is being extended. That is, if the development is to be within the domain of nursing, it must be defined in terms of the relationship of the new theoretical constructs to the proper object. If this is not done, it is not possible to demonstrate logically that the new theory is within the domain of nursing.

Elaboration of the concept of family from the perspective of S-CDNT has begun. Reutter (1984) extended Orem's theory by incorporating self-care requirements into family functions. Her approach uses the elements of self-care and begins to address the differences in the nature of the units, that is, the individual and the family. Reutter does not develop the relationship between the theoretical element of dependent care and the family. Furthermore, she fails to recognize that knowledge is changed when two concepts or theoretical elements are merged, such as family functions and self-care requirements. The result should be something more than the incorporation of the nursing concept into the concept of family systems. Whall (1982) in a discussion of the relationship between family systems theory and nursing models, identified the need to reformulate theories from other disciplines and suggested that

> the congruence between Orem's model and a family systems theory might be approached from her nursing perspective, that is, nursing systems are formed when nurses use their abilities to provide for groups by performing systems of action. (p. 82)

Whall then described the "Orem therapist" by incorporating Orem's theoretical elements into Haley's family system theory. Thus, Whall reformulates Orem's theory rather than Haley's. The unique object of nursing becomes a part of the goal of the family therapist. The relationship of Orem's theory to family is not explored and a unique concept of family nurse or family nursing is not developed.

Tadych (1985) suggested that self-care is a subset of family function and that the purpose of nursing the family as a unit includes "modifying family structure, regulating family function and removing barriers to family normative developmental processes" (p. 53). The relationship of these purposes to self-care is not made explicit.

Chin (1985) described "family universal self-care requirements." Chin's work presents some conceptual problems inasmuch as Orem's theory has specified that only individuals have self-care requirements. The use of the term in reference to family as a unit is not appropriate since the family is not an individual. Furthermore, the universality of the self-care requirements identified by Chin is not validated. The requirements listed are modifications of family functions and may not be essential for the healthy functioning of the family as a unit or for meeting the therapeutic self-care demands of individual family members; therefore, they are not truly requirements. Furthermore, the requirements were not described from the perspective of self-care and dependent care and the relationship to the theory is, therefore, not made explicit.

THEORETICAL ELEMENTS OF OREM'S THEORY OF NURSING

The nursing system is the action system designed and produced by nurses. Its purpose is to ensure that the client's therapeutic self-care demands are met, that his or her self-care agency is protected or developed, or that the exercise of self-care agency is regulated. The self-care system is the set of actions that the person takes to meet his or her own self-care requisites. Included in the concept of this system of action are the constructs of therapeutic self-care demand and self-care agency. Therapeutic self-care demand is the totality of actions the person needs to take to maintain health; the components are referred to as action demands. Self-care agency is the capacity of the person to act with regard to those demands. When the action demand for self-care exceeds the person's capacity to act because of health-related factors, a self-care deficit exists and a need for nursing can be established. Dependent care is that care which members of social groups provide for persons who, for reasons of age, developmental state, or health state, are unable to provide for themselves.

When the nurse anticipates developing a nursing system that includes the family, the first step is to determine the unit of service. The question to be answered is: Will the nurse be responsible for providing nursing to an individual who is a member of a family, to a dependent person who has a care giver, or to the family as a unit? Figure 1 illustrates the three approaches to family described above.

FAMILY AS BASIC CONDITIONING FACTOR

When an individual is the unit of service for the nurse, the family has meaning to the nurse as a factor which conditions the therapeutic self-care demand and the self-care agency of the patient. The family system within which the individual is functioning is a major factor in setting the parameters of the requirements for care and the development of effective systems of care for the individual who is the patient. Self-care is learned within the family. The nature of self-care requisites is conditioned by the family. For example, the size of the family, family expectations of the individual members, and the resoures available for use by the individual family members all have a conditioning effect on the self-care requirements of an individual. The person raised in a large family may have very different requisites for solitude and social interaction than does the person raised in a small family and may need to develop different action strategies to

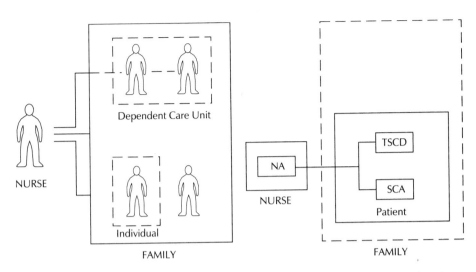

FIGURE 1. Units of service.   **FIGURE 2.** The individual as unit of service.

meet their demand for solitude. The family may be a resource available to be used for and by the patient in managing his/her care requirements. Conversely, in some situations the family may be seen as having a negative effect on the health and self-management of the patient. As expressed by Orem (1985):

> Patients, members of their families, or others who are acting for patients may or may not be interested in the need or psychologically able to accept the need for collaboration with nurses or the need for being active participants in their own self-care or the care of their dependents. (p. 230)

When an individual (i) is the unit of service for the nurse, the nursing system (NS) is a function (F) of the relationship between the individual's self-care agency (SCA), his or her current or projected therapeutic self-care demand (TSCD), and nursing agency (NA). This is illustrated in Figure 2 and can be expressed as

$$NS_i = F(TSCD \cap SCA)_i \cap NA$$

The nursing process focuses on determining the therapeutic self-care demand, establishing the presence and characteristics of a self-care deficit, and designing a nursing system for the purpose of meeting the therapeutic self-care demand and protecting, developing, or regulating the exercise of self-care agency. The primary assessment question related to family system elements is: How do family system factors condition the patient's self-care requisites, methods of meeting self-care requisites, and self-care agency? A second question would be: To what extent can, will, or should the family members be involved in the care of the patient? The nursing diagnosis, when the individual is the unit of service, is related to the nature of the self-care deficits of the patient. Prescriptions may include actions to be taken by family members to accomplish the goals of meeting the therapeutic self-care demands of the patient and to the regulation of self-care agency.

FAMILY AS SETTING FOR
THE DEPENDENT CARE SYSTEM

Dependent care can be considered a specialized family operation that requires management. The family is seen as the setting that conditions the dependent care system and within which dependent care systems are produced. The dependent care unit may be composed of two or more persons, one of whom is dependent on the other(s) for assistance with self-care. The unit may be a dependent-responsible person dyad or a larger unit. It may be the family or a subunit of the family. The dependent care unit may be a stable unit, that is, the same two or three persons are involved over time, or it may fluctuate on a regular or irregular basis.

Dependent care systems are those care systems composed of actions performed by responsible persons, usually adults, to meet the components of their dependents' therapeutic self-care demands. The specific functions of the dependent care giver are directly related to the therapeutic self-care demand and self-care deficits of the dependent. The kind of care needed varies according to the nature of the dependent care unit and the reasons for the dependency, which may be related to age, developmental state, or health state. Dependent care agency refers to the ability of the responsible person or family members to care for other persons or family members with regard to regulation of their health states. Dependent care agency is analogous to self-care agency in that it is a three dimensional construct. The major distinction is that the actions are directed toward meeting the care requirements of another person, not one's own self-care. Rather than self-care operations or power components of self-care, the dimensions would be labeled as dependent care operations or power components of dependent care. The need for reconceptualizing these dimensions can be illustrated by considering the differences in thought processes and actions when one has to decide or offer counsel on seeking health care for a child as compared to making decisions for one's own care. One of the power components of self-care agency is motivation for self-care. In describing dependent care agency, there would be a need to be motivated to care for others as well as to care for self. It is quite possible that one could be an effective self-care agent and and ineffective dependent care agent or vice versa.

Dependent care agency, broadly considered, can also be thought of as analogous to nursing agency and described in terms of individuals' capabilities for knowing, judging, and deciding about dependents' therapeutic self-care demands and self-care agency and the abilities to use the methods of helping to meet the therapeutic self-care demands, develop the self-care agency, or regulate the exercise of the self-care agency of dependents. For example, limitations in dependent care agency may relate to the inability of the dependent care giver to transpose existing knowledge and skill necessary for a set of actions for self in performing those for another person or a particular person.

Dependent care may range from providing custodial care to actively participating in a complex care system. When a dependent care system is needed because of health deviations, specific factors which condition dependent care agency include the severity of illness, the complexity of the technology in use or to be used, the intensity of the dependent's suffering, the meaning of the dependent care relationship, and the tolerance for involvement in personal care measures for others on the part of the care giver.

Neville (1987) described dependent care systems involving two adult family members. She concluded that the quantity and quality of dependent care assistance required by an individual is a function of the complexity of the individual's self-care demand and the nature of the self-care limitations. Other types of dependent care systems could include parent and minor child and the adult child and elderly parent. The nature of the relationship that exists between the dependent person and the care giver is a major conditioning factor in the establishment of the dependent care system and may form the basis for a classification system for dependent care systems, for example, parent-child or spouse-spouse.

When the care giver is unable or unwilling to provide the necessary care, a need for nursing may exist. When the unit of service is the dependent care unit, whether that unit is composed of the whole family or a part of the family, the assessment would include the family as basic conditioning factor to both the dependent and the responsible person or care giver. It is necessary to distinguish the family as a factor that conditions the dependent care system from the family as unit of service because the primary objective of care in dependent care systems is the therapeutic self-care demand of the dependent one, not of all family members.

Whether the unit of service for the nurse is a dependent-responsible person dyad or a larger dependent care unit, assessment includes the determination of the therapeutic self-care demand of the dependent, determination of the nature of the self-care agency of the dependent, and the determination of the care capabilities of the care giver(s). The nursing diagnosis is the statement of the dependent care deficit expressed in terms of the care givers' limitations for action as they relate to helping the dependent. Included in this diagnosis is the statement of the nature of the self-care deficit of the dependent. For example, the dependent patient may be limited in her ability to perform the complex actions required to care for a tracheostomy. The spouse as caregiver might be diagnosed as limited in his ability to assist his wife in caring for the tracheostomy because of fear of injuring a loved one and lack of experience with providing personal care to another person or to a particular person.

In most instances, meeting the dependent care giver's therapeutic self-care demand is not an objective of the nursing system; however, the care system that is prescribed must take into account the care giver's need to care for self at the same time he or she is providing dependent care. The nurse would assess the care giver's therapeutic self-care demand and self-care agency as factors that condition the care giver's ability to provide the care as well as conditioning the dependent's requirements for care. From the perspective of the nurse, the stability of the dependent care unit is a major factor in the prescribing of the care system for the dependent. If there is a different dependent care giver each time the nurse interacts with the patient, as in a home visit, the care system needs to be reevaluated and adjustments made to account for the variations in dependent care agency.

When the dependent care unit (DCU) is the unit of service, the nursing system (NS) which is designed is a function (f) of the relationships of the elements of therapeutic self-care demand (TSCD) and self-care agency (SCA) of the dependent (D), the dependent care agency (DCA) of the dependent care giver (DCG), and the nursing agency (NA). This is illustrated in Figure 3 and can be shown as

$$NS_{DCU} = f(TSCD \cap SCA)_D \cap DCA_{DCG} \cap NA$$

The nurse works with both the dependent care giver and the dependent to varying degrees. The purpose for nursing is to meet the therapeutic self-care demands of the dependent through the development of and regulation of the exercise of the dependent care agency. When appropriate, the nurse is also seeking to develop the self-care agency of the dependent. The nurse may be engaged in direct care to the dependent or may assist the care giver in providing the care to the dependent.

NURSING THE FAMILY UNIT

When the family is the client, that is, when the nurse has accepted the responsibility for nursing for not only individual family members or dependent care units but also the family as a unit, there is another variation in the application of the theory. This difference is related to the belief that the family is a unit, a whole, that is more than the sum of the parts. The family has certain functions related to self-care and dependent care that exceed or are different from meeting each individual's self-care requirement. The basis for this is the recognition that the family has a nonmaterial unity which leads to structure and functions that are substantially different from those of the individual.

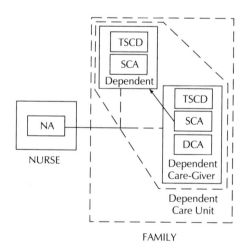

FAMILY

FIGURE 3. Dependent care unit as unit of service.

From the perspective of nursing within self-care deficit nursing theory, the family functions of primary concern to nursing are:

1. The socialization of family members as self-care and dependent care agents.
2. The recognition of therapeutic self-care demand of individual family members and the development of strategies to meet these demands including:
   (a) awareness of changes occurring in the person and environment.
   (b) knowledge of conditioning effects of these changes on the health state.
   (c) knowledge of ways of meeting therapeutic self-care demands and skills and motivation to meet these.
   (d) awareness of the conditioning effect of the interrelationship of family members on the therapeutic self-care demands and abilities of each individual family member.
3. Access to, control, and management of resources needed to meet therapeutic self-care demands and health care needs of family members.
4. The integration of the aspects of self-care and dependent care into an overall satisfactory plan of living and development for the family.

The nursing data base would include the calculated therapeutic self-care demand for each individual family member, the quality and nature of the self-care agency and dependent care agency of each family member, and the current system of meeting the therapeutic self-care demands of the family members, within the context of the family system (Fig. 4). Of special concern is the interrelationship between the self-care requisites and self-care abilities of the individual family members and the resulting interdependence in providing for the care of each other. The assessment question of primary interest when the family is the unit of service is: Is the family system functioning in a manner such that the four functions related to self-care are being adequately met or does family functioning interfere with the meeting of the health-related therapeutic self-care demands of some or all of the family members? What are the interrelationships of the self-care and dependent care systems within the family?

Knowledge about family systems is essential antecedent knowledge for nursing. The description of a nursing model for family assessment by Whall (1981) is helpful in structuring the assessment of the family. Whall identified four assessment dimensions: individual subsystems; family interaction patterns; unique characteristics of the whole; and environmental field considerations. Although her analysis is structured within the framework of Martha Rogers' theory, the relationship of the elements is appropriate to Orem's theory. The individual subsystems to be assessed are the self-care systems of each of the individual family members. The interaction patterns would include the dependent care systems which have been established to meet the therapeutic self-care demands of the dependent family members. In addition to the dependent care systems, there may also be other collaborative or compensatory arrangements between family members which have been established or have evolved to assure that the therapeutic self-care demands of each other are met. These interaction patterns along with the way the family is carrying out the functions related to self-care would constitute the unique

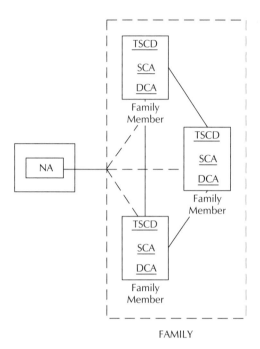

FIGURE 4. Family as unit of service.

characteristics of the whole. Environmental field considerations would be analogous to the assessment of the basic factors which condition both the requirements for self-care and self-care agency and would include such factors as sociocultural orientation, health state, health care system elements, and family system elements.

The condition that establishes the basis for nursing the family as a unit would arise when the functioning of the family unit is being affected by actions taken or not taken to carry out functions related to self-care or dependent care. Nursing diagnostic conclusions related to the family focus on the four identified functions and the effects of meeting the therapeutic self-care demands of individual family members on other members and on family structure and function. Nursing for families is a function of the current or projected therapeutic self-care demands of individual family members, their self-care agency and dependent care agency, and the effects of meeting the therapeutic self-care demands of individual members on other members and on family structure and function. When the family is the client, nursing diagnostic statements will include reference to the individuals' self-care deficits and dependent relationships as well as reference to the functions of the family (Fig. 4). In the design of the nursing system, concern shifts from the self-care requisites and abilities of each individual member to the interrelationship of the family and the impact of this interrelationship on the self-care demands and self-care agency of each of the family members.

The following situation is presented as an example. The Burke family is composed of a mother, father, and two siblings, one of whom is chronically ill. During a home visit, the nurse assessed the individual members and the family system elements and noted that the mother was spending all her energy meeting the therapeutic self-care demand of the ill child and well sibling, but not attending to her own care. Mr. Burke, the father, was meeting his own demands but was not able to assist in care of other family members. Mrs. Burke was experiencing deficits in maintaining adequate intake of food, balance between rest and activity, and solitude and social interaction. As a result, she was not meeting affectional needs with her husband. He was not participating in meeting the dependent care needs of the children or in assisting his wife to meet her self-care and other personal needs. Affectional functions of the family are disrupted because of the dependent care and self-care situations. This family situation, then, constitutes a legitimate nursing situation in which interventions are directed toward the mother's self-care deficits and the ill child's self-care demands. Appropriate interventions might range from increasing the father's dependent care agency directed toward the wife and children to removing the ill child from the home setting to decrease demands on the family. If, after these self and dependent care demands are resolved, the affectional functions of the family remain disrupted, the situation would likely require the assistance of a family counselor rather than nursing.

CONCLUSION

Family can be interpreted within Orem's self-care deficit nursing theory in three major ways. The family may be a factor that conditions the therapeutic self-care demand and self-care agency of the family member who is the identified patient; it may be the setting within which dependent care is provided, or it may be the unit of service for which nursing is provided. When the family is viewed as a basic conditioning factor, the nurse is concerned with the identification of the effect of the family on the patient's need for self-care and the extent to which the family can assist the family member who is the patient in meeting his self-care demands and needs for assistance. When the family is viewed as the setting within which dependent care is given, the nurse is concerned with the conditioning effects of the family on both the dependent and the dependent care givers. When the family is the unit of service, the nurse is concerned with the interactive existent or projected effects of the meeting of the therapeutic self-care demands of the individual family members on the overall family functioning.

The family is seen as having functions related to the members' development of self-care agency and the establishment of appropriate dependent care systems in such a way as to promote the health of the entire family. Assessment occurs at the level of each individual's self-care system, the interaction of the various family members' self-care systems, and the effect of these interactions on the broader dimensions of family functioning.

One of the values derived from the use of S-CDNT is the recognition of the need to identify the unit of service for which nursing is being provided. When making this determination it is necessary to identify with whom the nurse will be interacting. It is interesting to note that while the nurse may view the family as the unit of service, she/he may have little or no contact with some of the family members. The nurse is still able to contribute to the self-care systems and dependent care systems of all family members.

ACKNOWLEDGMENTS

The author wishes to acknowledge Dorothea E. Orem for her critical review of the manuscript and instrumental role in the development of the ideas. Acknowledgment is also given to K. McLaughlin, E. Geden, and J. Noack for their critical reviews and comments.

REFERENCES

Chin, S. (1985). Can self-care theory be applied to families? In J. Riehl-Sisca (Ed.), *The science and art of self-care* (pp. 56–62). Norwalk, CT: Appleton-Century-Crofts.

Neville, S. (1987). *A descriptive study of three dependent-care systems.* Unpublished master's thesis. University of Missouri-Columbia, School of Nursing, Columbia, MO.

Orem, D. E. (1985). *Nursing: Concepts of practice.* (3rd ed.). New York: McGraw-Hill.

Reutter, L. (1984). Family health assessment: An integrated approach. *Journal of Advanced Nursing, 9,* 391–399.

Schultz, P. R. (1987). When client means more than one: Extending the foundational concept of person. *Advances in Nursing Science, 10*(1), 71–88.

Tadych, R. (1985). Nursing in multiperson units: The family. In J. Riehl-Sisca (Ed.), *The science and art of self-care* (pp. 49–55). Norwalk, CT: Appleton-Century-Crofts.

Whall, A. (1981). Nursing theory and the assessment of families. *Journal of Psychiatric Nursing, 19,* 30–38.

Whall, A. (1982). Family systems theory: Relationship to nursing conceptual models. In J. Fitzpatrick, A. Whall, R. Johnston, J. Floyd (Eds.), *Nursing models and their psychiatric mental health applications,* Bowie, MD: Brady.

CHAPTER 8

Family Transformation: Parse's Theory in Practice

Mary Jo Butler

This article illustrates how the principles and practice dimensions of the theory of man-living-health were used to change the health situation of a family facing the loss of the family patriarch who had experienced major neurosurgery. Theoretical structures from the theory of man-living-health are elucidated through describing nursing care with the family. The article demonstrates the value of theory-based nursing practice by describing how care based on the theory of man-living-health transformed a family situation as the family members struggled to live their value priorities.

One essential task for evaluating nursing theory is to determine whether the theory can be translated from the abstract to an appropriate level for guiding practice (Fawcett, 1984; Fitzpatrick & Whall, 1983; Parse, 1981; Stevens, 1979). By using theory to guide practice, the nurse participates in evaluating the function of theory. If a nursing theory has functional value, it will provide propositions that explain research and practice methodologies.

Parse's (1981, 1987) nursing theory, man-living-health, offers three principles and three theoretical structures for shaping nursing practice. Dimensions and processes of Parse's practice methodology translate the theory from the abstract to guide nurses' participation in the changing health process. In Parse's model, the person, more than and different from the sum of parts, is viewed as an open being free to choose meaning

Reprinted from *Nursing Science Quarterly, Vol. 1* (No. 2), 1988, pp. 68–74. Copyright © 1988 by Williams & Wilkins. Used with permission of Chestnut House Publications.

in situation. Human beings are recognized by patterns cocreated in relationship with the environment. The health process is an unfolding, the living experience of choosing value priorities. Health is a continuously changing process that is cocreated.

The nurse practicing from Parse's (1981, 1987) theory participates with the person or family in illuminating the meaning of situations, synchronizing the rhythms of connecting-separating, and moving beyond the struggle to what does not yet exist. The goal of nursing focuses on the quality of life as perceived by the person or family. The nurse guides changing health patterns that shape the quality of life, while recognizing the authority and decision-making power of the person or family.

Although Parse (1987) offers a practice methodology that flows directly from the ontological base of her theory, little has been published on the application of the theory to particular practice situations. The purpose of this article is to describe how Parse's theoretical framework altered the course of one family situation. Before illustrating how Parse's theory was used to mobilize a family's energies toward a changing health perspective, a brief review of the family situation follows.

THE FAMILY SITUATION

Mr. and Mrs. D., both in their seventies, lived together in a two-story home that had been their residence for more than 40 years. Since Mr. D had retired, he and his wife had established a pattern of doing most activities together, including paying the bills, shopping, or sitting on the porch. They enjoyed gardening, canning food, maintaining their home, and following their favorite college athletic teams. Mr. and Mrs. D were active in the lives of their two grown children and grandchildren. A daughter and her family had lived near them and visited frequently. A son, who lived and worked out of state, returned to his parents' household for visits every four to five months. At least twice each year, the couple traveled with their daughter's family to visit their son. Strong ties linked the entire family.

Mr. and Mrs. D had experienced relatively few illnesses in their lifetimes. They were content with their lifestyle and viewed themselves as well. Both had a medical diagnosis of arthritis, which they felt was a normal facet of aging. When Mrs. D lost the ability to write, she learned to type, and, when Mr. D felt stiff, he increased his self-prescribed exercise routine. They cherished their independence and overcame minor encumbrances.

Over a period of several months, Mr. D began experiencing loss of feeling in his fingers. Aching and weakness in his legs progressed to the point where he needed a cane for extended walking. Eventually, he secured a walker for occasional use when his legs felt especially weak. With passing time, Mr. D lost the ability to hold a pencil in his hands, and falling became a frequent occurrence. The family became concerned about Mr. D and encouraged him to visit his physician.

Medical evaluation revealed impingement on the spinal cord from calcified and arthritic vertebrae. Verification of the vertebral problem required hospitalization for diagnostic procedures. Mr. D's family encouraged the hospitalization in hopes that treatment would enable him to walk again safely. With this hope, Mr. D and his family agreed to rather tedious and risky diagnostic tests that combined myelograms with scanning procedures. Irritation from the dyes and manipulations used in these procedures rendered Mr. D unable to use his arms or legs. After two weeks of diagnostic procedures, Mr. D could not walk, feed himself, or perform most of the activities associated with daily living. At this point, Mr. D and his family decided with the physicians that a surgical decompression of the spinal cord was essential.

Two weeks of diagnostic evaluation had demonstrated that Mr. D could tolerate surgery. Indeed, his overall way of being was testimony to the benefits of a well rounded diet, daily practices of walking and riding a stationary bicycle, and comfortable interpersonal relationships. The only significant factors noted in his medical history included marked osteoarthritis and early stage Alzheimer's disease. Mr. D's history revealed few past hospitalizations other than two brief stays for removal of cataracts. A small basal cell carcinoma found on Mr. D's nose during his pre-operative diagnostic evaluation period was judged nonthreatening. It was determined that treatment of this growth could be postponed until the neurological problem was surgically corrected.

A decompression of the spinal cord at the third through sixth cervical vertebrae, with fusion of the vertebrae, was performed. Immediately after the surgery, Mr. D could raise both legs and grasp objects with either hand. After surgery, Mr. D was transferred to the hospital neurosurgical unit for recovery, where his neck was immobilized and he was placed on an air mattress. His intense pain was relieved by medication.

Although Mr. D's surgical incision healed nicely, his postoperative progress was limited. Severe spasticity developed in all extremities and showed no response to the medical treatment of antispasmodic agents or Valium. He also developed a spastic urinary bladder that required routine catheterization every 4 hours after removal of an indwelling catheter. Physical therapy was eventually initiated with Mr. D, but he could not stand independently. Exercises to facilitate purposeful arm movements were not effective. Several weeks after surgery, Mr. D still could not bathe or feed himself. He experienced weight loss and anorexia. A general low feeling permeated his being. He refused to attend physical therapy and, from a medical point of view, became confused with loss of orientation to place and time. Mr. D believed he was in a hotel being attended to by maids, and he perceived events and sounds in the environment differently from others. Unable to do otherwise, Mr. D just lay in bed until moved, fed, or bathed by other persons.

Throughout the several weeks of the post-operative period, care delivered to Mr. D by the nursing staff followed a traditional pattern. Mr. D was given a bath in bed each morning and placed in a chair while bed linens were changed. Fresh hospital gowns were provided as necessary. A special call bell that could be pressed without good finger movement was placed on Mr. D's chest when he was in bed. The nurses fed Mr. D his meals and provided him with ample liquid intake. Passive exercises were performed on his extremities, and sponge balls were given to him to improve his grip strength. When the nurses were with Mr. D, they focused on providing reality orientation, reminding him of his present location, day of the week, and time. Special care kept his skin intact. In addition, Mr. D was given his prescribed medications, and his respiratory, bowel, and bladder functions were carefully observed. He was given traditional custodial nursing care in an efficient manner. In spite of these efforts, Mr. D became more confused and irritable. He remained bedridden, unable to purposefully move his spastic legs.

During hospital visiting hours, Mr. D's wife, daughter, or son-in-law stayed at his bedside. The son who lived 350 miles away from the hospital arranged to spend several weekends with the family. Family members encouraged Mr. D's participation in prescribed therapies and tried to pacify his relentless requests to go home. Several weeks postoperatively, both the physicians and hospital social worker recommended transfer of Mr. D to a nursing home.

APPLICATION OF THE
MAN-LIVING-HEALTH THEORY

At this point, a nurse familiar with the theory of man-living-health developed by Parse (1981, 1987) began working with the D family. The different nursing approach that emerged created a dramatic change in the family's health process. Although the nursing activities occurred simultaneously, they can be separated to illustrate Parse's three dimensions of practice, illuminating meaning through explicating the event, synchronizing rhythms by moving with the flow of the family, and mobilizing transcendence by moving beyond the moment.

The initial dimension of practice focused on illuminating the meaning of the family's current situation. In sessions with the nurse, family members shared and discussed the emerging pattern of family health by describing their views of Mr. D's hospitalization, what was important to them, their plans and hopes for the future, how they lived day to day, and the importance of the environment. Nursing activities throughout the discussions focused on assisting members in articulating and clarifying their ideas. By encouraging the sharing of thoughts, the nurse helped family members gain a new perspective on the current situation.

This new perspective unfolded as the nurse guided the family in moving with Mr. D through his medically diagnosed confusion. The family explored the meaning of Mr. D's multidimensional reality with him and learned that he thought he was being punished. He viewed catheterization procedures as homosexual attacks and prescribed physical therapy activities, such as placing "round disks into round holes," as forced engagement in "childlike play within view of other adults who knew he should have been doing more meaningful tasks." Mr. D said that forced separation from his family, confinement to an unknown room, being told what to do, and the absence of his "work clothes" upset him greatly. He viewed taking pills and being fed as signs of illness. He said he resented not sharing daily living experiences with his wife and family. Mr. D concluded he was "protecting himself as best he could until he could get home."

Family members expressed frustration over Mr. D's entire situation. They were embarrassed by his confusion and feared the imminent loss of a cherished family member. Guilt surfaced as family members confronted their seeming inability to help Mr. D continue his usual pattern of daily living. Mrs. D wanted her husband to join her in decision making and daily events. She expressed loneliness and exhaustion as she experienced weight loss, sleeplessness, and a worsening of head and hand tremors.

As the nurse guided the D family through the process of explicating the meaning of their current situation, a new family view emerged. Family members believed that Mr. D's way of relating with others through confusion, and perhaps his entire way of being, were his way of announcing to others his view of a strange environment. They all recognized that the hospital routines were neither "fixing" Mr. D, nor helping him to get better and had, indeed, disrupted everything cherished by Mr. and Mrs. D. Simple values of sharing meals and making decisions together were part of their pattern of health, but the hospitalization had become a barrier to living these value priorities. The family sensed the importance of Mr. D's own decision making in relation to his health process.

Nursing activities related to explicating the situation and designed to help Mr. D's family illuminate the meaning of their current situation illustrate application of the principle that "structuring meaning multidimensionally is cocreating reality through the languaging of valuing and imaging" (Parsee, 1981, p. 42). By sharing feelings, values, and dreams the family arrived at a cocreated different view of the current situation. They were illuminating meaning, and in so doing, a consensus on new insights about the situation evolved.

The nursing dimension of illuminating meaning was processed by the nurse through posing questions that helped family members clarify and share thoughts and feelings. Their various viewpoints offered new insights for further exploration until themes arose and family consensus emerged. As nursing processes guided by Parse's theory were enacted, a sense of renewed connectedness among family members emerged along with a simultaneous desire to separate Mr. D from the hospital environment. The family's different view of the situation led to one immediate outcome, which was the request for extended visiting time with Mr. D along with supporting his refusals to attend physical therapy or follow the routines as prescribed by the institution. At this point, the nurse began directing energy toward planning for the newfound possibilities that Mr. D and his family envisioned.

The processes used by the nurse to help the D family find new meaning to their current situation illustrate a movement into the second practice dimension posed by Parse (1987), synchronizing rhythms. The family made a choice to "go with the flow" set by Mr. D and thus set a new rhythm. They wanted to reunite their family and began to discuss how this might occur. Ideas were shared with the nurses, who helped the family explore the merits and drawbacks of all projected possibilities.

A possibility came to fruition one Saturday morning when family members found Mr. D crying. He wanted to be out of the hospital, still viewed by him as a hotel, and refused physical therapy until he could do things "his way with his wife." The family began to actively explore the possibility of taking him home. Although Mrs. D expressed fear of being unable to care for her husband in their two-story home, she did want him out of the hospital. Their children wanted Mr. D to experience a familiar pattern of living, one to which he was accustomed, within his own environment.

While encouraging the family to act on their views, the nurse guided them in exploring how care could be provided for Mr. D. Family members struggled with responsibilities and options but devised a plan by Saturday evening that seemed comfortable for all family members. They were now strongly connected with Mr. D's own desires in a plan of action. Their plan was to restore Mr. D to his usual pattern of living within a familiar environment. The large family room in their daughter's home was to be converted into a bedroom furnished with Mr. and Mrs. D's pillows, bed linens, and cherished personal items. The plan consisted of bringing Mr. and Mrs. D together, enabling them to fall asleep and awaken together. A small table placed near the bed would allow Mrs. D to eat meals with Mr. D. Their son-in-law and grandson were committed to helping Mr. D into a bathroom that adjoined the newly devised bedroom. To enhance Mr. D's comfort, family members planned to spend evening hours watching the news and discussing daily events with Mr. and Mrs. D in their new quarters. The nurse would be available, as long as the family wished, to guide them and help Mrs. D learn to perform some tasks with Mr. D. In addition, their daughter and son-in-law felt they could take vacation days from their work for adequate periods of time to help begin a new family routine and assist with meals or other necessary tasks. Having made their plans, family members left the hospital Saturday evening, assuring Mr. D that they would be back to take him home the next day.

The D family set their own rhythm in devising their plan. Guiding them through making the plan to take Mr. D out of the hospital exemplifies how the nurse was synchronizing rhythms. The nurse neither advocated nor discredited the plan. Instead, nursing activities focused on going with the flow of the struggle to get Mr. D home. The nurse questioned, clarified answers, and suggested and explored options with family members as they struggled toward a harmonious solution.

Attempts by the nurse and Mr. D's family to cocreate a rhythmical pattern of living together, similar to the prehospitalization period, illustrate a different mode of synchronizing rhythms. Through their planning, the nurse, Mr. D, and his family were co-constituting desired ways of being with the world. In so doing, they were all living their value priorities. A major value priority for the family was Mr. D's comfort.

The nursing practice dimension of synchronizing rhythms flows from the principle that "cocreating rhythmical patterns of relating is living the paradoxical unity of revealing-concealing, enabling-limiting, while connecting-separating" (Parse, 1987, p. 164). Through self-disclosure, family members became more aware of each other's and of their own values. Their choices, evident in the plan developed with Mr. D, enabled their movement in some directions while limiting movement in others. Simultaneously, they were connecting with Mr. D in new ways while separating from other ways of being.

The plan devised by the D family that Saturday was in place and ready for implementation the next Sunday afternoon. During this time, part of the nursing care was devoted to facilitating the plan. At the family's request, the nurse met with Mr. D's physicians to discuss the family plan. The physicians supported the plan, knowing that the nurse would be with the family for several days. The physicians agreed to be available and further agreed to a cessation of Valium and other antispasmodic medications that may have been affecting Mr. D's orientation. The nurse secured the necessary supplies, dressed Mr. D in his blue jeans, sweat shirt, and tennis shoes, and arranged for ambulance transport to his new environment and anxiously waiting family. On Sunday afternoon, the family plan was initiated.

During the next 7 days, dramatic changes occurred. Mr. D could sit at the table with his wife and feed himself just a few hours after arriving at his new quarters. With the help of the nurse and his son-in-law, Mr. D awkwardly walked to the bathroom the first evening home. Within 2 days, Mr. D was walking with a walker and, after 1 week, he was climbing stairs. Although he could not remember much detail about his lengthy hospitalization, Mr. D's whole way of being changed. He knew exactly where he was and even engaged in discussions on current events. Helping his school-aged grandson with a homework assignment, Mr. D took a pen in his hand and wrote for the first time in months. In his desire to gain strength, Mr. D devised his own movement regime. He marched in time to his favorite band music, used a rope and a pulley system rigged to the ceiling by his son-in-law to exercise his shoulders, and lay in bed doing leg lifts. Sponge balls obtained in the hospital for hand exercises were replaced with small barbells and hand grips that Mr. D had used for exercise before his hospitalization. Mr. D was now pushing to get to his own home, helped by the recognition of his authority over activities within an environment that enabled the living of his valued lifestyle.

As soon as Mr. D was ambulating alone, he began to rebel against catheterizations, insisting that his bladder was fine. The nurse cooperated with him and changed the catheter routine to one of checking for residual. Soon after this, catheterizations were totally eliminated.

The entire family changed along with Mr. D. Mrs. D began eating, regaining the weight lost during Mr. D's hospitalization. Her head and hand tremors subsided to the more usual level, and she slept for extended periods of time. Other family members resumed their usual ways of debating issues with Mr. D and teasing him about the new ways he was learning to be. They also shared feelings about the changes in their lives by having Mr. and Mrs. D living with them. Their son-in-law wanted to be as helpful as possible, but he missed evenings alone with his wife. Their daughter was tired from trying to keep both her spouse and son contented while devoting so much time to her parents. She was concerned about her son's feelings in relation to having his grandparents living in his home, yet he expressed no discomfort. He was happy as long as his school and athletic activities remained on course. Both Mr. and Mrs. D expressed concern that they were creating problems and extra work for their daughter's family. Sharing and discussing these feelings and the changes in their lives with the nurse helped family members move on to a new way of being together.

Within 10 days, Mr. D was no longer taking any medications except vitamins, and he was walking totally unassisted. Convinced he was able, he announced his readiness to return to his own home. Once again the nurse guided the family through this proposed change, helping them find harmony in their varying feelings regarding the possible return of Mr. and Mrs. D to their own home. Mr. D, his son-in-law, and son were ready to make this second move. Mrs. D and her daughter were less comfortable with the prospect of Mr. and Mrs. D being alone in their own home. Reasoning with the nurse through these varying images of what might occur helped the family come to a harmonious plan with greater understanding of each other and themselves.

Changes were made in Mr. and Mrs. D's own home for Mr. D's safety. Secure handrails were installed in stairwells and along the bathtub, and furniture was relocated to ease Mr. D's mobility. Once these changes were made, Mr. and Mrs. D returned home alone with the understanding that the nurse would be visiting regularly. Quickly, Mr. and Mrs. D moved into a routine of being in their home and being together. The nurse accompanied Mr. and Mrs. D on follow-up visits to Mr. D's neurologist and neurosurgeon, who were amazed at his medical recovery. To take care of the basal cell carcinoma found on Mr. D's nose during his hospitalization, the nurse and Mr. D scheduled outpatient surgery with the dermatologist who had biopsied the growth in the hospital. However, the dermatologist could no longer find the growth. A second biopsy of the area, done to reconfirm the diagnosis, showed no malignant cells. As Mr. D left the dermatologist's office with the nurse, it was raining. He took the bandage off of his nose, picked his walker up in his arms, and quickly ran to the car.

To help Mr. and Mrs. D achieve the family's goal of returning to their own home, the nurse participated in illuminating their view of the emerging reality, synchronizing rhythms as they connected and separated in new ways, and mobilizing transcendence in cocreating new ways of being together. The nursing practice dimension of mobilizing transcendence (Parse, 1987) was evident in helping the D family achieve their desired way of life. This practice dimension entails moving beyond the meaning moment to the possibles, which occurred throughout the entire nurse-family process, but was particularly evident as the nurse helped Mr. and Mrs. D in preparing to go to their daughter's home and again in preparing to return to their own home. The nursing activities at these times illustrate application of the principle that "cotranscending with the possibles is powering unique ways of originating in the process of transforming" (Parse, 1987, p. 165). By moving beyond with the family at each level of their desire, the nurse participated in the family's powering new ways of being. Just being with and helping Mr. D and his family as they struggled with the unfamiliar and the familiar ways of being at the daughter's house was evidence of mobilizing transcendence.

In going to his own home, Mr. D did not return and engage in activities in the manner he had been accustomed to before his hospitalization. He learned new ways of accomplishing some tasks, such as getting out of bed and a chair, and he learned to accept help with some activities, such as dressing. Throughout this transitional period, the nurse directed energies toward helping the D family to be with the cherished familiar in different ways. By exploring options, listening to ideas, and analyzing viewpoints with the D family, the nurse guided them as they chose new ways of living. Throughout this process, the differing views of family members were aired, and they moved toward a clear understanding of the situation and each other. As the family members struggled with the meaning of Mr. D's situation, the nurse helped them explore new ways of being together. These new ways of being together helped Mr. D, his wife, and other family members to create a new emergence by inventing different ways of living their desired value priorities.

THEORETICAL STRUCTURES
OF MAN-LIVING-HEALTH

The concepts and principles of the theory of man-living-health give rise to theoretical structures that guide nursing practice. The three published theoretical structures are the following: "1) Powering is a way of revealing and concealing imaging, 2) originating is a manifestation of enabling and limiting valuing, and 3) transforming unfolds in the languaging of connecting and separating" (Parse, 1981, p. 72). These theoretical structures were evident in nursing practice with the D family through their changing health process.

Using Parse's (1981) first theoretical structure, "powering is a way of revealing and concealing imaging" (p. 89), the nurse focused on illuminating the D family's interpretation of Mr. D's illness and hospitalization. As family members revealed and concealed their feelings and hopes in different ways, new possibilities emerged that moved the family beyond the immediate situation to new struggles. Instead of concentrating on keeping Mr. D coherent and encouraging his involvement with hospital routines, the D family, after struggling with the meaning of the situation and envisioning different possibilities, began powering new ways of being with Mr. D. This powering changed from one of pushing Mr. D to cooperate with the hospital routine to pushing with Mr. D to design a plan to enhance familiar and desired patterns. Once encouraged by his family to achieve his goal, Mr. D's powering changed from resisting hospital routines to pushing to find the familiar in his new way of being. This pushing and resisting of powering evolved as the D family revealed new possibilities together. The value of creating a desired way of being for Mr. and Mrs. D became the family's focus.

Nursing practice relative to the theoretical structure, "originating is a manifestation of enabling and limiting valuing" (Parse, 1981, p. 90), embraced guiding the D family through unfolding prized values. As the D family worked to live the values of being together and of encouraging Mr. and Mrs. D to enjoy their life as they wanted, the nurse helped family members explore the enabling and limiting aspects of the evolving situation for themselves and each other. They understood that taking Mr. and Mrs. D to their daughter's home would enable them to realize select goals while limiting their involvement in other activities. Choices made would create changes for all family members and, though they were certain of the rightness of the decision, there was uncertainty related to the outcome. As the family members and Mr. and Mrs. D integrated values in a new way, they were enabling the process of originating. Simultaneously, family members were limiting themselves as they connected more fully with Mr. and Mrs. D and separated from usual activities and ways of being. Through enabling and limiting, choosing valued ways of living was originating.

The third theoretical structure of the theory of man-living-health, "transforming unfolds in the languaging of connecting and separating" (Parse, 1981, p. 90), was apparent in the way the D family members changed as they connected together while separating from hospital routines. By creating patterns of living with Mr. and Mrs. D, family members were sharing the familiar through their speech and movement. Eating together, sharing a bed, being together, and visiting with other family members were languaging values. These patterns were fostered by connecting Mr. D with a familiar environment while separating him from one viewed by him as hostile. As this connecting unfolded through languaging, the transforming process became more evident. At home, Mr. D changed in a manner that seemed impossible in the hospital. Other family members transformed as they cocreated new ways of being with themselves and Mr. and Mrs. D. With the aid of the nurse, new ways of viewing the familiar merged with languaged possibilities as the family struggled to help Mr. and Mrs. D and themselves in living their value priorities.

Another possible theoretical structure surfaced for the nurse as she worked with the D family. It appeared that their desire to move beyond the hospital and Mr. D's situation evolved as they discussed and elected the value of getting Mr. D home where he could more actively participate in governing his way of living. This common value, shared by all family members, seemed to connect the family, in a focused way, to achieving the value regardless of the limiting factors involved in taking Mr. D from the hospital. This focused connecting to one value seemed to energize the powering process. Powering changed from pushing in one way to collective pushing and resisting process in a different direction. Focused on a common goal, the D family became adamantly positive that they could succeed in returning Mr. and Mrs. D to their own home. Mr. D's spastic, immobile, incontinent, and confused medical condition seemed less threatening to the family than even the nurse imagined. Change in the family members' way of powering energized Mr. D as the family moved toward the common goal. Family members had made a collective choice and powered together to realize this choice. These data indicate that a fourth theoretical structure emanating from the concepts of the man-living-health theory could be that powering emerges through the connecting-separating of valuing.

Although this possible theoretical structure is not published in the theory of man-living-health, Parse (1987) states that other theoretical structures may be derived from the offered concepts and principles of the theory. The value of this theoretical structure is that it surfaced from practice guided by Parse's theory. The nurse was struck by the usefulness of attending to choosing and enacting values. As what was valued was collectively agreed upon by the D family, powering changed. It was the connecting-separating of valuing that seemed to energize and power the D family toward goals. As the nurse fostered the connecting-separating of valuing, the family's powering changed, enhancing the family's health.

CONCLUSION

The D family situation illustrates the value of using Parse's nursing theory to guide practice. Completing tasks to maintain hygiene, muscle tone, skin integrity, and orientation were not enhancing Mr. D's health. The values that shaped the quality of life for Mr. D and his family were unknown and absent from the traditional nursing care being provided.

The transformation of the D family occurred when a nurse began to focus on those health patterns that enhanced the quality of the family's life from their perspective. To this end, the concepts, principles, and theoretical structures of the theory of man-living-health seemed invaluable. The process of illuminating meaning guided the D family to a different understanding of the current situation and united the family in working toward a common goal. As the nurse worked with the D family to synchronize rhythms and mobilize transcendence, valued familiar ways of being became realities. By helping the D family live their value priority patterns, the family health unfolded. The change in the D family demonstrates the pragmatic value of the theory of man-living-health.

The nurse who practiced the theory of man-living-health to guide the D family's health process did not eliminate Mr. D's exercise, nourishment, or skin care. However, instead of focusing on these routine tasks, the nurse, through an intersubjective presence with the D family, moved them beyond the present to different insights and new hopes. The nurse went with the D family as they cocreated the lived experience of their value priorities. The nurse tuned into the D family's unfolding health process and guided them in choosing the quality of life they valued. This approach moved Mr. D and his family from what was to what could be.

REFERENCES

Fawcett, J. (1984). *Analysis and evaluation of conceptual models in nursing.* Philadelphia: Davis.

Fitzpatrick, J. J., & Whall, A. L. (Eds.). (1983). *Conceptual models of nursing: Analysis and application.* Bowie, MD: Brady.

Parse, R. R. (1981). *Man-living-health: A theory of nursing.* New York: Wiley & Sons.

Parse, R. R. (1987). Man-living-health theory of nursing. In R. R. Parse (Ed.), *Nursing science: Major paradigms, theories, and critiques* (pp. 159–180). Philadelphia: Saunders.

Stevens, B. J. (1979). *Nursing theory: Analysis, application, evaluation.* Boston: Little, Brown.

CHAPTER 9

Neuman's Systems Model for Nursing Practice as a Conceptual Framework for a Family Assessment

Charlotte A. Herrick, Lynne Goodykoontz

Neuman's Systems Model was used as a guide to the assessment and intervention for a dysfunctional family. The model gave direction to the selection of family therapy as the appropriate and successful intervention. The case example illustrates the application and use of Neuman's model in child and adolescent nursing practice.

Systems theory is a model for understanding family process and the foundation for Neuman's Systems Model to guide nursing practice. Nurses working with families in which there are emotionally disturbed children will find Neuman's Systems Model an excellent framework to develop plans of care for children and their families. Using Neuman's Model for a systematic assessment of the child and family, criteria may be identified to select appropriate interventions. Goldman-Graff and Graff (1982) reported that the model provides "a clear method for making diagnoses of family breakdown and for planning therapeutic approaches" (p. 217).

This article describes how Neuman's Model can be used as a guide for nurses working with disturbed children and families. A case study of the use of the model with a family is presented.

Neuman's Model provided the basis for assessment of a teenager and her family. Family therapy was chosen as the treatment modality based on criteria taken and defined from the model. The purpose of this article is to illustrate the application of Neuman's Systems Model to psychiatric nursing practice by case example.

Reprinted from *Journal of Child Adolescent Psychiatric Mental Health Nursing, Vol. 2* (No. 2), 1989, pp. 61–67. Used with permission of Nursecom, Inc.

NEUMAN'S MODEL RELATED TO
THE FAMILY SYSTEM

According to Neuman's Model (1982), a system consists of individual, family, group or community and has an inner core containing energy to achieve and maintain a balance—homeostasis (see Figure 1). The core contains the basic structures such as genetic structure, internal organ systems and personality structures common to organisms. The energy core perpetuates the system's existence and is essential to life. The energy core of the family system includes constitutional and genetic, individual and family traits as well as characteristics acquired through the process of socialization that enable an individual or family to maintain itself as well as to grow to higher levels of adaptation during the life cycle.

In families, past dynamics modeled by the family of origin are internalized and are frequently exhibited consciously and/or unconsciously in the family of procreation, for example, an abused child who becomes an abusive parent. The meshing of family traits, values and beliefs from the family of origin provides basic structures for the new family.

The inner energy core is surrounded by broken circles representing internal lines of resistance that serve to protect the energy core from internal and external stressors. The lines of resistance are the social and structural supports.

Reed (1982) identified these supports as values and beliefs which influence family relationships—both the ability of family members to relate and the degree of interdependency among family members. Environmental supports, particularly the family, provide physical and emotional support for the integrity of the individual family members. According to Flaskerud and van Servellen (1985), when the environmental stresses and supports are in balance, mental health exists. The severity of the symptoms experienced by an individual or family depend upon the strength and length of the stressful encounter, and the degree of the response, the strengths and the weaknesses of the core, as well as the strengths and weaknesses of the lines of resistance.

The solid circle which surrounds the inner lines of resistance represents the "normal line of defense" (Cross, 1985; Neuman, 1980). The normal line of defense symbolizes the degree of wellness or the state of adaptation a system has achieved. Coping mechanisms are acquired over time to achieve stability. These involve the family's ability to structure itself in terms of interpersonal relationships to meet both individual and family needs, including the needs for intimacy and affection. Communication and interactional patterns among family members to meet emotional and developmental needs require change and adaptation. Problem-solving skills are acquired over time, enabling family members to adapt as they evolve through the stages of growth and development.

The outer broken circle represents the "flexible line of defense," which is in a state of constant retraction and expansion to cope with rapid change. It is constantly changing in response to multiple stressors: biological, psychological, sociocultural and developmental (Cross, 1985). It, too, has structural variables such as rules, roles, task allocation and decision-making. Included in the flexible line of defense are mechanisms to resolve current internal and external conflicts. The flexible line of defense is the outer boundary between the family and the community. The degree of flexibility determines the amount of information and/or input available to the family and its individual members for

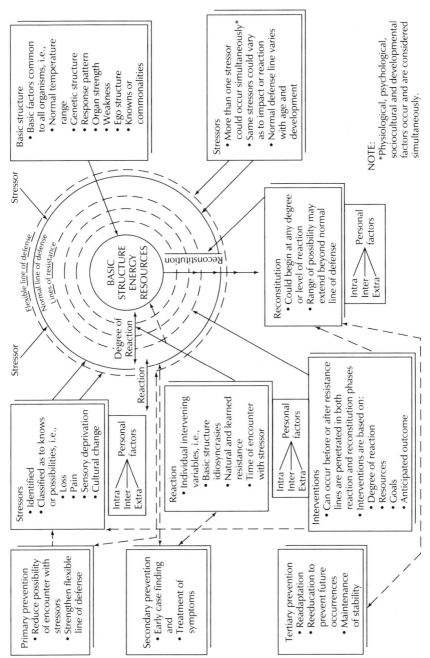

FIGURE 1. The Betty Newman Model: A Total Person Approach to Viewing Patient Problems. Copyright 1972 The American Journal of Nursing Company. Reprinted from original source: *Nursing Research*, May–June 1972. Vol 21, No 3. Used with permission. All rights reserved.

growth and development. The bond, or group identity, also provides family members with the motivation to meet family expectations as well as determine the degree of cohesiveness. The ability to open and close boundaries for feedback from the community assists the family with homeostasis and provides social support to maintain stability. It is common for dysfunctional families either to have inflexible and closed boundaries or boundaries that are so flexible that members are not only independent but are in fact disengaged.

The degree of flexibility of the outer line of defense, known as the "flexible line of defense," will determine the resistance versus motivation of the family to nursing interventions. If the boundary is either extremely rigid or disengaged, motivating the family toward reconstitution may be difficult.

Neuman's Model provides a guide to assess the following stressors: psychological, physiological, sociocultural or developmental, which are the result of intrasystem, intersystem or extrasystem stressors. Based upon the assessment of stressors, their source, the strength, the length of the encounter and the degree of penetration, the locus of treatment is determined. If the stressors are due to interfamily strife, the locus of treatment is the family. Intervention is needed in terms of levels of prevention. The goal of primary prevention is to protect the family's integrity, the secondary prevention goal is to shorten the length of the family disruption while the goal of tertiary prevention is to reduce the severity of defective family and individual functioning.

NEUMAN'S MODEL AS A FRAMEWORK FOR FAMILY THERAPY

Assumptions basic to both Neuman's Model and family systems theory are that family and individuals are open systems, which exchange energy by opening and closing boundaries, with the goal of achieving homeostasis while reaching for higher levels of adaptation. Each family member is an interdependent part of the whole family. A focus on an individual may overlook the interdependent roles and functions each individual plays as part of the family system (van Servellen, 1984). A symptom experienced by one family member may have significance not only for the individual but for the entire family. The interrelatedness of family members and the quality of their relationships are crucial factors in the survival of the family. Interfamilial relationships include patterns of communication, intimacy and bonding, decision-making and problem-solving, as well as values, beliefs and rules that determine members' roles. The pooling of individual family members' energies make the family system's energy greater than any one individual's. Consequently, the family as a whole may not only differ from an individual in terms of energy but its overall emotional needs may differ from the needs of the individual member. Balancing the needs of the individual and the family as a whole is a difficult task (Reed, 1982). Individual and family symptomatologies often are complex. A systems framework provides for effective assessment, planning and intervention.

Frequently, the family enters the mental health care delivery system complaining of the child's symptoms, either behavioral, affective or related to cognitive performance.

However, the child's symptoms may reflect the family's internal strife and conflict, or, to use Neuman's terminology, the child's symptoms are a result of "intersystem stressors." To focus on the child alone during the assessment phase of the nursing process means ignoring the family dynamics that either may have produced the symptom or maintained it. Any change that particularly affects the child affects the family, and vice versa (Reed, 1982).

THE MARENO FAMILY

The following is a case example that illustrates the application of Neuman's Model, particularly in the assessment and planning phases of the nursing process. It demonstrates, furthermore, how the model assisted in defining criteria for the selection of family therapy as a successful intervention.

The Mareno family were referred to the psychiatric outpatient clinic for assistance with a truant teenager. As the identified client was interviewed, it became apparent that other issues warranted inclusion of the whole family in therapeutic sessions.

The mother was currently seeing a psychiatrist for depression and was on medication. However, she was toxic one week or symptomatic the next week. Titrating the dose was difficult. Both parents had received individual and group counseling from a licensed professional counselor.

The father was currently attending Alcoholics Anonymous. The children had never been involved in counseling or any type of therapy.

Assessment

Assessment of the Mareno family included the types and sources of stressors on the family system. The taxonomy presented by Ziegler (1982) provided an outline of the major components of Neuman's Systems Model and was used in the nursing process with the Mareno family (see Figure 2).

Intrasystem Stressors

The targeted symptoms manifested in each individual member of the Mareno family and their psychological, genetic or physiological etiology are identified; the identified Intrasystem Stressors are:

Father: A recovering alcoholic who had a violent temper. At times, he was abusive toward the mother and the eldest daughter, Jody.

Mother: A chronically depressed woman who exhibited the vegetative signs of depression. She was tearful, withdrawn, fatigued, expressed feelings of hopelessness and helplessness; however, she was not suicidal. She had a sleep disturbance at night but frequently slept during the day, neglecting the children and depending upon Jody to provide child care. Her depression was poorly controlled by medication.

Jody: A slightly obese, sad-looking child who expressed a great deal of anger, particularly directed at her father. She left school because she was bored and hated the work. Consequently, she rarely studied. It was hard to study when her Dad was always

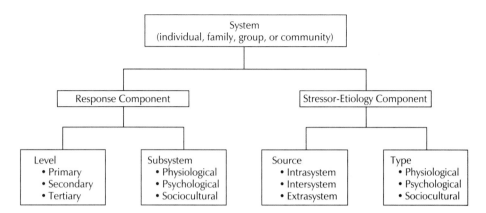

FIGURE 2. Major categories of the taxonomy. From "Taxonomy for Nursing Diagnosis Derived from Neuman Systems Model," by S. M. Ziegler. In B. Neuman (Ed.), *The Neuman Systems Model: Application to Nursing Education and Practice* (p. 58). Norwalk, CT: Appleton-Century-Crofts, 1982. Reprinted with permission.

angry and yelling at her and her siblings as well as at her mother. She felt that she and her mother took the brunt of his anger. Truancy was a way of getting back at her Dad for the abuse.

Carolyn: A slight, pretty child who did well in school. At first glance she appeared to be the "perfect child." She was the parents' pride and joy. However, during the family sessions, it became clear that she, too, was an angry child who expressed her anger by teasing her younger siblings.

Jake: A good-looking, well-built 7-year-old, who was often the family interpreter and catalyst for change. Jake was enuretic daily. He did well in school and was active in sports. He wanted Carolyn to play with him and like him but often his wish went unfulfilled.

Carrie: As the baby, she was often the family clown and distractor. She was a likeable child, whom everyone thought was "cute." She had orthopedic problems, requiring braces, which sometimes made her irritable and interfered with her sleep.

Intersystem Stressors

The family dynamics which affect each individual are examined as well as the impact of intrasystem stressors on the whole family. Indicators of family dynamics include: interpersonal communication, family climate (warmth versus distance and the degree of relatedness), the stage of growth and development of individuals, the family as a whole, coalitions or subgroups within the family and how they interface (e.g., a mother and son coalition, parental coalitions, and sibling coalitions), family rules, roles and role expectations (i.e., the "structure") all are assessed as part of the intersystem evaluation.

The identified Intersystem Stressors are:

(1) The new baby was an unplanned child who added financial and emotional stress to a family already having problems coping.

(2) Development stressors had to do with the new baby and Jody's entering puberty.

(3) Communication had broken down between parents. The interactional and transactional patterns were abusive behaviors by the father and withdrawal from father and family responsibilities by the mother.

(4) Communication had broken down between the father and the eldest daughter. The interactional and transactional patterns were paternal abusive behaviors towards Jody and her mother, resulting in an alliance between mother and Jody against father, plus Jody's acting-out behaviors. Truancy and school failure was Jody's mechanism for retaliation. Father perceived her school failure as a personal affront and always responded by restricting her to the house.

(5) Five out of six individual family members had symptoms indicating that the lines of resistance had been penetrated. Father: rage and abusive behavior; a recovering alcoholic; Mother: depression with some vegetative signs; Jody: school failure and truancy; Carolyn: hostile teasing of siblings; Jake: daily enuresis; Carrie: orthopedic problems.

(6) Both parents exhibited a sleep disorder. Father's sleep disturbance was part of the alcohol withdrawal. Mother's sleep disturbance was a result of the depression.

(7) Both parents were fatigued because of the baby's irritability due to the brace and Jake's enuresis, which interfered with their sleep.

Extrasystem Stressors

The environmental stressors, factors that influence the family as well as how open or closed are the family boundaries are assessed. Environmental stressors, for example, may be poverty, requiring a social or community as well as a psychological intervention. Unemployment may contribute to family violence and the closing of the flexible line of defense to outside influences.

The identified Extrasystem Stressors are:

(1) An expected inheritance due to a death in the family failed to materialize.

(2) Father did not receive an expected salary raise because of the financial difficulties of the company.

Assessment of the Flexible Line of Defense

Although the flexible line of defense was somewhat rigid, manifested by failure to enjoy each other and friends, the family was motivated to change and open to a family systems intervention.

Planning

Criteria Used to Select Family Therapy Intervention

(1) The family exhibited intersystem conflicts, both marital and family.

(2) Jody's truancy and school failure was a response to intersystem problems and a reflection of both marital and family interactional patterns.

(3) Jody was used as a scapegoat for the parents to avoid self-examination, although she was instrumental in getting some help for the family.

(4) There were hostile interfamily relationships between father and mother, between Jody and father and between Carolyn and her younger siblings.

(5) The family was enmeshed and the boundaries were rigid. No one did anything for fun, either with each other or outside the home with friends. Jody was constantly on restriction, so that autonomy was not supported and enmeshment was, interfering with the normal task of a teen to separate and individuate. The teenager was prohibited from separation/individuation because of the constant restriction to the house as punishment for poor grades, another example of the inflexible boundary.

(6) The family was disorganized to the point that household chores remained undone. In spite of their living in a middle class neighborhood, the nurse on a home visit noted their home was in poor condition. Household chores also stimulated arguments, with father getting angry and mother withdrawing, neglecting the work and getting more depressed. Expectations of the children to perform chores were inconsistent, except for Jody who was constantly expected to babysit. Role expectations were unclear.

(7) Other forms of treatment had been tried and had failed.

(8) Financial resources were limited. Five out of six of the family members exhibited symptoms that needed therapeutic intervention.

(9) The parents were committed to each other and to the family. They were motivated to solve their problems.

Considering the above criteria, a family therapy intervention was selected. The long-term goal was reconstitution for mother, father, and Jody. The short-term goals were to: (1) improve overall family functioning to decrease individual symptoms; (2) decrease father's projection of anger; (3) enhance the flexible line of defense to increase family activities with each other and the community; (4) enhance separation/individuation for Jody; (5) improve communication between parents so that Jody is no longer triangulated; (6) improve family climate to more warmth and less hostility; and (7) improve Jake's abilities for self-care.

Levels of Prevention

The primary, secondary and tertiary levels of prevention are based upon the severity of symptoms and response and the severity of the disruption of the individual or family homeostasis. The goal of a primary intervention is to maintain family stability. Developmental crises that are a normal part of growth and development are an example in which individual or family disruption is temporary and usually is manifested in transient anxiety. Interventions usually are educational or involve participation in self-help groups such as parenting classes.

Secondary prevention includes traumas that are acute, requiring immediate crisis intervention in order to prevent penetration of stressors beyond the lines of defense and resistance. High levels of anxiety usually result. The goal is to return the family to homeostasis as quickly as possible. Brief interventions usually contain the severity of the response. Grief work is an example of a secondary prevention intervention.

Tertiary prevention problems are chronic and have penetrated the lines of resistance so that the very core of the family or individual and its integrity is threatened. The goal is to reconstitute or rehabilitate the family and its members. Long-term interventions to achieve reconstitution and rehabilitation may be required to achieve homeostasis. Symptoms may involve both physical and psychological disabilities and, for some patients, symptoms may also involve cognitive functioning, frequently manifested by poor school performance in children and the inability to work and/or self-care deficits in adults.

The Level of Prevention—Mareno Family. Tertiary prevention was the identified level of intervention with this family because of the chronicity of the intersystem stress on all members of the family, requiring medication, AA, and family therapy.

Family therapy occurred once each week with all family members present for 60 minutes. If one member could not attend, the session was cancelled in order to emphasize the family focus. Treatment lasted one and one-half years. The co-therapists were a Psychiatric Resident and a Clinical Nurse Specialist at a University Out-patient Clinic.

During each family therapy session, members discussed current issues pertinent to the family. Initially, the focus was on Jody's truancy. Parent-therapists-teachers' conferences resulted in a behavioral contract for Jody regarding attendance and homework assignments. The son's enuresis was discussed and the parents were helped to handle the enuresis matter-of-factly and allow the child to take responsibility for his wet sheets. If he needed their help, the task was performed without emotion.

The father's explosiveness was explored, not only in terms of behavior but also as to the meaning behind the behavior. When examining his reaction to his daughter's poor grades, it became evident that he interpreted the poor grades as a personal affront. The feeling of loss experienced by the father over the grades replicated the loss he felt as a child when his mother attempted suicide. He felt the person he loved failed not only herself but him. His explosiveness also was a distancing behavior identified as a mechanism to deal with his covert sexual attraction to his daughter.

As the family began to understand their transactions with regard to the father's explosive behaviors, Jody's truancy and mother's withdrawal, the family climate improved. Mother and father were encouraged to expect Jody to be responsible for her schoolwork while mother assumed responsibility for the bulk of the child care.

After several sessions where the children sat between the parents, they were placed next to each other. This structural maneuver facilitated the parents' touching each other and enabled better eye contact while they were communicating and reestablished the parental coalition as the family's leadership team. The enhanced parental communication also intervened in the vicious cycle of anger and withdrawal. In order to achieve a more flexible line of defense, the parents established a time for them to be together without the children. When the parents gave themselves permission to have fun, the overall family climate improved.

Evaluation—Termination Summary

All members of the family participated. Upon discharge, father's abusive behaviors had ceased, as did Jody's truancy. Her grades had improved so that she was passed on to the next grade. She was no longer constantly restricted to the house and had started dating just prior to termination. Carolyn continued to tease her younger siblings but with less hostility. The parents were more aware of her teasing behaviors and were able to set limits. Mother's depression continued but was more intermittent. She expressed less helplessness and hopelessness. She was better regulated on the medication. She started to work part-time, which eased family finances and improved her self-esteem. The family participated in family outings, which they enjoyed, so that communication and the family climate were greatly improved. Jake only wet the bed occasionally and Carrie did not need the leg brace anymore. Father finally accepted that he was not going to be a wealthy man from the inheritance and that he needed to take control of his life and his career. He had stopped projecting his frustrations onto his wife and older daughter. Although mother continued to be plagued with depression, intrasystem problems or individual symptoms in other family members were relieved. Overall, the intersystem dynamics had greatly improved, allowing Jody to grow up and to participate in teen activities without the need to rebel against school and parents.

CONCLUSION

Neuman's Systems Model is a holistic framework for nursing practice which includes: (1) the identification of the type of stressors, the psychological, physiological, developmental or sociocultural stressors, as well as the response to determine the selection of specific interventions and modalities for treatment; (2) assessment of the source of the stressors, intra-, inter-, or extrasystem sources to determine the focus for treatment; (3) assessment of the level of the response, the severity of the stressful encounter and the symptoms. If the stressor is part of the normal growth process, then primary prevention is the selected intervention. If the encounter is acutely traumatic, then secondary prevention would be appropriate, using short-term interventions. However, if symptoms occur after a prolonged period of stress, then tertiary prevention is necessary, with the goal to reconstitute or restore the family and/or individual to health; and (4) assessment of the flexible line of defense or the flexibility or rigidity of the boundaries in terms of the family's motivation for intervention and change.

Neuman's Systems Model is a valuable tool to assist the child psychiatric nurse in assessing a child or adolescent and the family because of its holistic and systemic perspectives. Holistic and systemic perspectives were needed to assess the Mareno family because of the variety of problems and the scope of the symptoms. A family intervention was selected for this family because, although each member had intrasystem problems, many of the symptoms were a reflection of dysfunctional family dynamics, or intersystem stressors. Although mother's depression most likely had a psychophysiological etiology and father's alcoholism a genetic component, the children's symptoms, particularly Jody's, were a reflection of interpersonal stressors.

The Neuman model guided the assessment process and enabled the nurse to systematically assess a variety of variables. According to Reed (1982), the "Neuman Nursing Process Format then becomes a bridge between family theory and nursing practice" (p. 195). This bridge provides a conceptual framework to structure the assessment process for nurses working with disturbed children and their families to determine an appropriate plan of care.

REFERENCES

Cross, J. R. (1985). Betty Neuman. In J. B. Georgy (Ed.), *Nursing theories: The base for professional nursing* (pp. 258–286). Englewood Cliffs, NJ: Prentice Hall, Inc.

Flaskerud, J. H., & van Servellen, G. M. (1985). *Community mental health nursing theories and methods.* Norwalk, CT: Appleton-Century-Crofts.

Goldman-Graff, D., & Graff, H. (1982). The Neuman model adapted to family therapy. In B. Neuman (Ed.), *The Neuman systems model: Application to nursing education and practice* (pp. 217–222). Norwalk, CT: Appleton-Century-Crofts.

Neuman, Betty (Ed.). (1982). *The Neuman systems model: Application to nursing education and practice.* Norwalk, CT: Appleton-Century-Crofts.

Neuman, B. (1980). The Betty Neuman health-care systems model: A total person approach to patient problems. In J. P. Riehl & S. C. Roy (Eds.), *Conceptual models for nursing practice* (pp. 119–134). Norwalk, CT: Appleton-Century-Crofts.

Reed, K. (1982). The Neuman systems model: A basis for family psychosocial assessment and intervention. In B. Neuman (Ed.), *The Neuman systems model: Application to nursing education and practice* (pp. 188–195). Norwalk, CT: Appleton-Century-Crofts.

van Servellen, G. M. (1984). *Group and family therapy: A model for psychotherapeutic nursing practice.* St. Louis: Mosby.

Ziegler, S. M. (1982). Taxonomy for nursing diagnosis derived from Neuman systems model. In B. Neuman (Ed.), *The Neuman systems model: Application to nursing education and practice* (pp. 55–68). Norwalk, CT: Appleton-Century-Crofts.

CHAPTER 10

A Nursing Model for Addressing the Health Needs of Homeless Families

Andrea S. Berne, Candy Dato,
Diana J. Mason, Margaret Rafferty

Homelessness in the United States continues to be a major social problem directly affecting an estimated three million persons, of whom nearly 30 percent belong to families without permanent shelter. This paper reviews recent research concerning homeless families and conditions in which they live and outlines the significant health and mental health problems that these families experience. Effective nursing interventions for homeless families using Pesznecker's Model of Poverty are proposed. Nurses must advocate for changes in the social and political conditions that bring about homelessness since the resources to meet the needs of these families are either nonexistent or woefully inadequate.

Homelessness in the United States is a major social problem, directly affecting an estimated three million persons, of whom 30 percent are families. Of these families, 85 percent are headed by single women, a disproportionate number of whom are minorities. While families were the last subgroup to join the ranks of the homeless, they are now the fastest growing segment of that population. It is projected that in the near future a majority of the United States' homeless will be single mothers with children (City of New York Human Resources Administration, 1986a, 1986b; Institute of Medicine, 1988; Molnar, 1988).

Reprinted from *IMAGE: Journal of Nursing Scholarship, Vol.* 22 (No. 1), Spring 1990, pp. 8–13. Used with permission of the publisher.

ETIOLOGY OF FAMILY HOMELESSNESS

Homelessness is a relative condition that exists worldwide in both developed and underdeveloped countries, although it expresses itself differently in different parts of the world (Patton, 1988). It encompasses Britain's growing poor who are housed in the bread and breakfast rooms in London that have been described as the equivalent of third-world shantytowns (Clines, 1987). It includes the Ethiopian refugees in the Sudan and other countries where war and politics have uprooted entire communities (Smith, 1989). It can be seen in the increasing number of young adults sleeping in hostels and shelters in Denmark, Austria and Belgium (Hope & Young, 1987a; Tennison, 1983; Thomas, 1985). It is evident in the explosion of slums in the cities of developing nations such as the Philippines, Mexico and India (Busuttil, 1987). And it can be seen in the so-called hidden homeless in Hungary—the growing number of people who are doubled-up in the dwellings of friends or families who are living in decrepit housing (Hope & Young, 1987b). In 1985, the United Nations reported that 100 million people worldwide had no shelter, and it proclaimed 1987 as the International Year of Shelter for Homeless (Ramachandran, 1988).

Homelessness used to occur predominantly in third world countries where material resources were underdeveloped or scarce. Its rise in developed countries suggests a maldistribution of existing resources. Nowhere is this more evident than in the United States, where homelessness is primarily caused by the lack of affordable housing and increasing poverty.

The lack of affordable housing in the United States is the result of several factors:

- Gentrification, or a process in which low-income housing is replaced by middle-income and high-income housing.
- A freeze on the welfare shelter allowances in most states, resulting in an allowance that has not kept pace with the rising cost of renting an apartment.
- The Reagan Administration's decision to withdraw the federal government from its prior commitment to build and maintain low-income housing (Report of the Committee on Legal Problems of the Homeless, 1989; Institute of Medicine, 1988).

Since most of the homeless would not be without permanent housing if they could afford to pay the rents on the housing that is available, homelessness in the United States is largely a by-product of the increasing gap between the rich and poor. From 1980 to 1984, family income for the poorest 20 percent of the population declined by almost 8 percent, while that of the wealthiest 20 percent of families increased by almost 9 percent (United Auto Workers, 1985). The poorest three fifths of all families received only 32.7 percent of the total national income, while the wealthiest two fifths received 67.3 percent of the income; these were, respectively, the lowest and highest percentages recorded since 1947 (Bureau of the Census, 1985). The relative nature of poverty that is associated with homelessness is illustrated by data indicating that 35 percent of homeless mothers and fathers outside of New York City work, but their incomes are insufficient to pay for the rising cost of housing (Schmitt, 1988). Indeed, a recent study found that the poor are paying an increasing percentage of their income on housing—now 63 percent, as opposed to the standard of 30 percent that is deemed the "affordable" limit by the Department of Housing and Urban Development (Dionne, 1989).

FAMILY HOMELESSNESS AS POVERTY: A MODEL FOR NURSING

Pesznecker (1984) synthesized the literature on poverty and delineated an interactional, adaptational model of poverty (see Fig. 1). It postulates that one develops health-promoting or health-damaging responses to the stress of poverty, which are shaped by interactions between the individual/group and the environment—interactions that are further mediated by factors such as public policy. It presents the poor as individuals and groups who are continually faced with multiple and chronic stressors, including frustration over few employment options, inadequate and unsafe housing conditions, repeated exposure to violence and crime, inadequate child care assistance and insensitive attitudes and responses of social service and mental health agencies. The

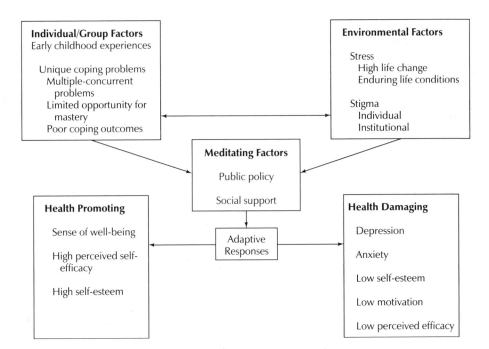

FIGURE 1. Adaptational model of poverty. From Betty L. Pesznecker, "The Poor: A Population at Risk," *Public Health Nursing, Vol. 1* (No. 4), December 1984, pp. 237–249. Reprinted by permission of Blackwell Scientific Publications, Inc.

coping abilities of the poor are strained by the unpredictable and unrelenting accumulation of these stressors. Mastery may be diminished so that a sense of helplessness develops with the resulting decrease in motivation as well as a sense of helplessness and hopelessness. The stigmatization of being poor in a society that measures one's worth by income only adds to the stress of poverty and makes it difficult to maintain any semblance of self-esteem or self-efficacy. Anxiety, depression and feelings of powerlessness are thus predictable concomitants of poverty.

The experience of homeless families can be described within this context. Pesznecker's (1984) model provides a basis for being particularly concerned about the children of these families and the bleak present and future they face. It incorporates the effect that the stigmas of poverty and homelessness can have on people who are often stigmatized also by their race and gender in a society that continues to contain covert and overt sexism and racism. It also provides a basis for nurses to incorporate social activism in their role as advocates and providers of care for homeless families.

HOMELESS CHILDREN

The research on homeless children is limited, but the data that are available suggest that homelessness is not an experience to which one can adapt positively. Wright and Weber (1987) reported that 16 percent of the homeless children have various chronic physical disorders, double the rate among patients in the general population. Asthma, anemia and malnutrition were among the most common. In the same study, many common acute pediatric problems were reported at inordinately high rates (upper respiratory infections, skin ailments, gastrointestinal problems, ear infections, eye disorders and dental problems). Data from Bellevue Hospital in New York City revealed that 50 percent of homeless children living in welfare hotels had immunization delays (Acker, Fierman & Dreyer, 1987).

Homeless infants living in welfare hotels in New York City had an infant mortality rate of 24.9 per 1000 live births in 1985. This was twice the overall city rate of 12.0/1000. Pregnant women living in welfare hotels in New York City were twice as likely to give birth to low-weight infants than were women living in the "city projects" (Chavkin, Kristal, Seabron & Guigli, 1987).

However, the effects of homelessness are even more profound on the mental health of the children. Bassuk and Rubin's (1987) study of children in Massachusetts shelters found that 47 percent of preschool children were delayed in at least one area of language, gross motor, fine motor and personal/social skills and development. One third of these children demonstrated problems in more than two areas. Almost half of the school-age children showed depression and anxiety, with the majority voicing suicidal ideation. The children were also noted to have sleep problems, shyness, withdrawal and aggression. Gewirtzman and Fodor (1987) reported that children in families left homeless after fires often exhibit these symptoms as well as isolation, disorientation, confusion, grief, psychosomatic complaints and regression. These problems are similar to those found in children of migrant workers and refugees and have been described as manifestations of posttraumatic stress disorder (PTSD) (Eth & Pynoos, 1985). PTSD is a reaction to some kind of psychological trauma and until recently was described mostly among war veterans. A psychologist in New York City reported that PTSD is the most common diagnosis among homeless children that she encounters (J. LeClair, personal communication; May 15, 1989).

Shelter life is stressful and shameful, compounding the children's problems. All school children are sensitive to dressing below peer standards, but homeless children may also face discriminatory remarks made by teachers and classmates, making them a "minority within a minority" (Gewirtzman & Fodor, 1987). Poor attendance and truancy are major problems for this population. School attendance among 10-year-olds to 16-year-olds at the Martinique Hotel, the largest welfare hotel in New York City, was less than 40 percent. In one study, 43 percent of the children had failed at least one grade; 24 percent were in special education classes; 50 percent were failing (Bassuk & Rubin, 1987).

Children without parents in New York City fare worse than do homeless children with parents. Instead of being placed in individual foster homes, these children increasingly are housed in congregate shelters—dormitory-like facilities—that have recently been critically exposed and condemned in a study by the Public Health Interest Consortium of New York City (Brooklyn Health Action Committee, 1989). Unsanitary conditions, spoiled food, blatant fire and safety hazards and inadequate staffing predominate in these facilities. The "orphans" are shuffled from shelter to shelter, their emotional needs are ignored and they endure conditions that are often debilitating and sometimes life-threatening. The study reports that in one review of childhood immunizations, only 22 percent of the children were adequately immunized. Some of the children were HIV-positive and are at great risk for communicable diseases that easily spread in the congregate facilities:

> The children in the shelters then are in profound psychological distress, and the custodial care they receive fails to lessen their pain. The harm to these children goes beyond their immediate suffering, however. It extends to their longterm emotional development. (p. 10)

The data on homeless children suggest that predominant responses of homeless children to their experience with poverty are ones that Pesznecker categorizes as health damaging. The future for these children may be short-lived and without much hope for a better life. Longitudinal studies are needed to examine the long-term effects of a childhood experience with homelessness and the extent to which homelessness is an experience that precludes health-promoting responses to poverty.

HOMELESS MOTHERS

There is a paucity of research on the health problems of homeless mothers. They are a neglected population. The experience of one of the authors (A. B.) is that the mothers wait for health care until they are so acutely ill that they need emergency treatment. They may not seek health care for themselves since they tend to view themselves as the least important person in the household. Their schedules may also preclude attendance at clinics.

When the homeless mothers are seen, as they were in the Health Care for the Homeless Demonstration Project from June 1985 to September 1987 (Wright & Weber, 1987), it was confirmed that they suffer from most physical disorders at higher rates than do the general population. In addition to numerous chronic illnesses, the rate of tuberculosis among the homeless exceeds that of the general population by a factor of 25 to perhaps several hundred. Anecdotal reports from public health nurses in New York City suggest that AIDS is increasingly prevalent among homeless families and progresses more rapidly in these poor women. The overcrowded conditions of shelters and welfare hotels clearly impact on the health of the homeless mothers, as does inadequate diet, substandard bathing facilities and multiple chronic stressors.

It is evident that these same stressors contribute to the mental health problems of homeless mothers, although there is little research in this area as well. The research that has been done coincides with studies of poverty that repeatedly describe an increase in mental health problems—particularly anxiety and depression—with increasing poverty (Belle, 1982; Dohrenwend & Dohrenwend, 1974; Hollingshead & Redlich, 1958). Bassuk's (1986) study of 82 families in 14 Massachusetts shelters reported that the majority of the mothers had a limited number of relationships, with 43 percent reporting no or minimal support, and 24 percent seeing their children as their major emotional support. Of the 82 families, 18 were being assessed for potential child abuse. As children, one third of the mothers had suffered physical abuse, while one in every nine were victims of sexual abuse. The mothers' histories showed a significant amount of major family disruption, loss of parents, lack of work skills and residential instability (Bassuk, Rubin & Lauriat, 1986). The data suggested intergenerational aspects of family disruption and emotional difficulties. Another study estimated that 24 percent of homeless families in New York City were victims of domestic violence (Victim Services Agency, 1989).

Homeless mothers need to be distinguished from another subgroup of the homeless, the homeless mentally ill. Homeless mothers are not psychotic any more frequently than is the general population, and the etiology of their homelessness lies in poverty rather than a combination of poverty and mental illness. Bassuk's (1986) study did find 71 percent of homeless mothers had personality disorders; however, both advocates for the homeless and Bassuk herself criticized this finding as being an exaggeration of the degree of psychopathology. The diagnostic labels do serve to indicate severe functional impairment and the need for help.

One of the health-damaging responses that some of these mothers may have to coping with homelessness is substance abuse, although documenting the prevalence of the problem and whether it is antecedent to or a product of homelessness is difficult. The study of the foster children in New York City (Brooklyn Health Action Committee, 1989) identified parental drug abuse as "the single biggest underlying factor in child abuse and neglect" (p. 34) that results in children being removed from their families. Bassuk (1986) found 10 percent of the mothers to be substance abusers, while New York City public health nurses have estimated that between 80 percent and 90 percent of the mothers in some shelters use crack. Crack has intensified the problem of drug abuse because of its high potency and rapidly addictive qualities. Crack has become a cause of homelessness in New York City, as addicts use money for the drug instead of housing.

Other health and mental health problems are expanded with substance abuse, and one would suspect that some of the character disorder problems seen in Bassuk's study were drug related.

As with homeless children, the data suggest that homelessness is a correlate of poverty that overwhelms the physical and emotional resources of homeless mothers. Pesznecker (1984) noted that poverty involves an interplay between environmental and individual factors. The poor encounter more stressors, especially surrounding money, social isolation, stigmatization and parenting, all of which can be exacerbated by homelessness. Coping positively with this multiplicity of persistent stressors becomes increasingly difficult, particularly if one is repetitively unable to change them. Depression, anxiety and feelings of powerlessness readily ensue. Under Pesznecker's model, the mental health problems of homeless mothers are most appropriately viewed as health-damaging responses to harsh environmental conditions that breed demoralization, hopelessness and despair. The model also suggests points of intervention that can foster health-promoting responses to homelessness.

HEALTH CARE SERVICES
FOR HOMELESS FAMILIES

Access to health care has been a major problem for homeless families (Institute of Medicine, 1988). For example, a survey of sheltered children in Seattle revealed that 59 percent of the children had no regular care provider. The same group used emergency rooms at a rate of two to three times the rate of the general pediatric population in the United States (Miller & Lin, 1988). Although substance abuse appears to be a growing problem among homeless mothers, there is a paucity of drug treatment programs in the United States, particularly those that provide long-term treatment with a family focus.

Three traditional approaches that have been used to provide health care services to homeless families are the traditional out-patient department (OPD) or clinics, onsite services and comprehensive outreach.

The Clinics

Ambulatory care for the poor is generally delivered in "clinics." While funding from the national government and a nationwide grant from a private foundation have resulted in some outreach services to homeless families, most continue to lack access to anything except emergency room care. This has resulted in a woeful lack of prenatal care for homeless women who then present at the emergency room in labor and are at greater risk for maternal and infant morbidity and mortality (Chavkin et al., 1987).

Even homeless people who do have access to routine health care services often have difficulty negotiating the system. Families are usually sheltered outside their neighborhood of origin so that they are unfamiliar with and apprehensive about new health care providers. For families that are moved multiple times, it is difficult, if not impossible, to establish a stable relationship with a primary provider. Many hospital clinics have long waits for appointments, lack continuity of care and often are under-staffed. There have been many reports of families with "hotel addresses" being treated poorly. The clinic staff may blame the homeless for lack of immunizations and records and missed appointments, labeling them "noncompliant." In addition, families often do not keep appointments because of fear of being reported to the Child Welfare Bureau for neglect and/or abuse related to being homeless. For these reasons, the clinic system increases the stressors and stigma with which homeless families must cope and fosters health-damaging responses such as anxiety, low self-esteem and low motivation.

On-Site Services

In some settings, visiting health teams have set up shop. The goal of many of these projects is to mainstream the families into existing clinics. While this is conceptually pleasing and congruent with the goal of establishing coordinated comprehensive care for all, this approach has limitations. The efforts of two or three health providers on site are inadequate to offset the stress and stigma of this extreme level of poverty. On-site providers have become frustrated by some of the same problems that the families are up against with the system as it presently exists, as they try to refer the families to existing services. There are transportation problems, delays in getting appointments and inad-equate care. "Homeless providers" fall victim to the same discrimination that the home-less themselves face. The level of effort is inadequate to make a significant difference, but it is often used by politicians to demonstrate that they are "doing something" when, in fact, they are not. On-site services are too often a bandaid approach to the health problems of homeless families.

Comprehensive Mobile Outreach Services

One model program has enough resources to mitigate some of the effects of the poverty that underlies homelessness. The New York Children's Health Project has expanded on the concept of on-site services by providing comprehensive pediatric care with mobile medical units to children living in hotels and shelters in New York City. This project works collaboratively with the public health nurses and city social workers who are on-site at the hotels five days a week doing intake and casefinding. The public health nurses visit the families as they enter the system and take an initial health assessment. They identify children in need of immunizations, mothers in need of prenatal care and a wide variety of other acute and chronic health care needs. By knocking on doors, they attempt to cross the impenetrable boundary that exists between the family and the outside world.

Acute and chronic medical problems are diagnosed and treated by nurse practi-tioners and physicians. School, day care and camp forms and Women, Infants and Children certifications are frequently completed by the nurses, which has made an enormous impact on enrollment in such programs. In addition, nurses discuss routine health maintenance issues such as growth and development and nutrition as well as strategies for hotel living.

IMAGINE YOU ARE HOMELESS . . .

Imagine you are a 33-year-old woman with three children. Your apartment burned down six months ago. You and your children had been living with your sister in her cramped apartment until she had another baby, and now there simply was not enough room for everyone.

You sleep in your car at night. During the day, you walk the streets with your children trying to find an apartment you can afford. Finally, you go to the department of social services to try to find shelter for the night and are told that your children may have to be placed in foster care if a place cannot be found for all of you. Knowing that the foster care system in this city is unreliable and sometimes unsafe, you agree to spend the first night in an overcrowded warehouse-type shelter, where you end up sleeping on the floor.

You and your children have no privacy here. Many of the children and adults have colds and you hear that tuberculosis has been an increasing problem among the homeless. When the opportunity arises, you agree to move into one of the single-room occupancy hotels that the city is using to house homeless families "temporarily." That temporary shelter becomes your home for 13 months.

The temporary shelter consists of one 10 by 10 ft. room. You have no kitchen, no refrigerator, no stove or cooking facilities. There is one bed for you and your three children.

You pull the mattress off the bed at night to make room for all of you to sleep and then pull the sheets off the bed in the day to eat on the floor.

You use running water to keep your baby's milk cool and you do the dishes in the tub where you bathe and store things.

There is no place for your children to play, no place to sit, no place to do homework. When they try to play in the hall, they are approached by drug dealers and sometimes even pimps.

This is what life is like for you and your children. Imagine the gradual dissipation of your own and your children's self-esteem and the isolation and depression that eventually overwhelm you. Imagine having a future without space, without privacy, without hope.

This project essentially provides "middle-class" pediatric health care to the poorest of the poor. Because of the intensive supports built into the program, there is a 70 percent to 80 percent compliance rate, which is comparable to middle-class compliance. The project demonstrates the mitigating effects that public policy and social support—the mediating factors in Pesznecker's model—can have on the ongoing stressors confronting homeless families.

DESIGNING EFFECTIVE INTERVENTIONS
FOR HOMELESS FAMILIES

This is not to suggest that comprehensive health services for the homeless are the magic tonic for the problems of homelessness. These families have an enormous number of problems of which health problems are only one small part. Indeed, nursing interventions with homeless families must reflect an understanding of the connections between health and other life and societal conditions. Pesznecker's Adaptation Model of Poverty reflects this understanding. It also is distinguished from most poverty frameworks that actually "blame the victim"—an approach that is contrary to nursing's view of health as a human-environment interaction (Mason, 1981). Her model provides direction for interventions with homeless families that address both the individuals and families and the environment and society.

Pesznecker's model suggests that homeless families can best be assisted through strategies that empower them to develop the skills and self-esteem to recognize and act on opportunities for moving out of homelessness and poverty as well as to cope more positively when those opportunities are not present. Approaching the homeless mothers and children with caring and respect is prerequisite to countering the stigmatizing attitudes that they face in other encounters with society. Additionally, homeless families need tangible and intangible support to cope with the multiple stressors in their lives. Such supports range from adequate public assistance and shelter subsidies to having a network of friends and professionals who will provide both mental and material support during times of crisis. In many communities, homeless families are removed from their community of origin and may be moved through a variety of communities during their experience with homelessness. Maintaining relationships with friends or providers becomes almost impossible. Policies that required each community to have a plan for maintaining families who need emergency housing would enable the maintenance and development of such support systems.

There has been a tendency for health care providers to view psychotherapy as a necessary intervention for homeless families, particularly given the mental health problems outlined earlier. Pesznecker's model suggests that stress management training may be an instrumental intervention. Support for this proposition is evident in two stress reduction projects with women in the United States and Canada who were on public assistance (Resnick, 1984; Tableman, Feis, Marciniak & Howard, 1985). Unfortunately, these approaches are seldom included in the health and social services that are available to homeless families.

Several model projects such as the Henry Street Settlement House in New York City and Trevor's Place in Philadelphia provide safe, clean shelter and supportive on-site services to families. These supportive services include 24-hour on-site staff, day care, after-school tutoring, job training for mothers, assistance with entitlement, and assistance with relocation. These projects have found that the mental outlook of both parents and children improves dramatically under these stable conditions. Children start attending school again; grades and behavior improve. This approach to homelessness both increases coping options and provides some stability so that referrals for self-help groups, stress reduction techniques or traditional psychotherapy services for the homeless who have major functional psychiatric disorders can have some hope for success.

Most health care services for the homeless are really secondary and tertiary prevention. True primary prevention of homelessness demands social policies that call for:

- Affordable housing
- Education and job training
- Meaningful work at an adequate wage
- Adequate levels of public assistance for families that cannot sustain themselves including adequate shelter allowances
- Accessible and adequate child care
- Access to health prevention and promotion including education about preventing pregnancy and substance abuse and coping with stress
- Drug treatment on demand

And if homelessness on an international level is considered, nursing's advocacy for primary prevention of homelessness would include efforts to promote world peace and improved means for resolving intranational and international political disputes.

Nurses can influence and shape policies that deal with homeless families through political advocacy. The American Nurses' Association has included homelessness among the issues it advocates in Washington, D.C., and many other state nurses' associations have done likewise. In New York City, the local district nurses' association adopted a position on homelessness that calls for affordable housing, adequate temporary shelter and accessible health care services.

If the nursing community is committed to primary prevention for homeless women and children, then we must participate in the debate regarding whether or not housing is a human right (Burns, 1988) and recognize the connections between the health of homeless women and children and the broader social, economic and political issues of our times. Such a perspective demands that we also understand that we truly are one world community and that these connections extend beyond geographic boundaries. We challenge the nursing community worldwide to join together in calling for conditions and policies that are health sustaining instead of health damaging, that are supportive and nurturing of families and that make housing a basic human right, without which one cannot ensure health.

REFERENCES

Acker, P., Fierman, A. H., & Dreyer, B. P. (1987). Health: An assessment of parameters of health-care and nutrition in homeless children (abstract). *American Journal of Diseases of Children, 141,* 388.

Bassuk, E. (1986). Homeless families: Single mothers and their children in Boston shelters. In E. Bassuk (Ed.), *The mental health needs of homeless persons: New directions for mental health services.* San Francisco: Jossey-Bass.

Bassuk, E., & Rubin, L. (1987). Homeless children: A neglected population. *American Journal of Orthopsychiatry, 57*(2), 279–286.

Bassuk, E., Rubin, L., & Lauriat, A. (1986). Characteristics of sheltered homeless families. *American Journal of Public Health, 76,* 1097–1101.

Belle, D. (1982). *Lives in stress: Women and depression.* Beverly Hills: Sage.

Brooklyn Health Action Committee. (1989). *Inexcusable harm: The effect of institutionalization on young foster children in New York City.* New York: Public Interest Health Consortium of New York City.

United Auto Workers of America. (1985). *Building America's future.* Detroit: UAW.

Bureau of the Census. (1985). *Money income and poverty status of families and persons in the United States: 1984.* Washington, DC: The U.S. Government Printing Office.

Burns, L. S. (1988). Hope for the homeless in the U.S.: Lessons from the Third World. *Cities, 5,* 33–40.

Busuttil, S. (1987). Houselessness and the training problem. *Cities, 4,* 152–158.

Chavkin, W., Kristal, A., Seabron, C., & Guigli, P. (1987). The reproductive experience of women living in hotels for the homeless in NYC. *New York State Journal of Medicine, 371,* 10–13.

City of New York Human Resources Administration. (1986a, October). *A one-day "snapshot" of homeless families at the Forbell Street Shelter and the Martinique Hotel.* New York: The Administration.

City of New York Human Resources Administration. (1986b, October). *Characteristics and housing histories of families seeking shelter from HRA.* NY: The Administration.

Clines, F. X. (1987). For poor, bed and breakfast at $34 million a year. *The New York Times,* October 22, 3.

Dionne, E. J. (1989). Poor paying more for their shelter. *The New York Times,* April 17, A18.

Dohrenwend, B.S., & Dohrenwend, B. P. (1974). *Stressful life events: Their nature and effects.* New York: John Wiley and Sons.

Eth, S., & Pynoos, R. (1985). *Post-traumatic stress disorder in children.* Washington, D.C.: American Psychiatric Association.

Gewirtzman, R., & Fodor, I. (1987). The homeless child at school: From welfare hotel to classroom. *Child Welfare, 66*(3), 237–245.

Hollingshead, A. B., & Redlich, F. C. (1958). *Social class and mental illness: A community study.* New York: John Wiley and Sons.

Hope, M., & Young, J. (1987a, August). Homelessness in Austria rising, although social programs help. *Safety Network, 4*(12), 2.

Hope, M., & Young, J. (1987b, December). Housing privatization in Hungary—Will it cause more homelessness? *Safety Network, 5*(3), 2.

Institute of Medicine. (1988). *Homelessness, health, and human needs.* Washington, D.C.: National Academy Press.

Mason, D. (1981). Perspectives on poverty. *IMAGE, 13,* 82–85.

Miller, D. S., & Lin, E. H. B. (1988). Children in sheltered homeless families: Reported health status and use of health services. *Pediatrics, 81*(5), 668–673.

Molnar, J. (1988). *Home is where the heart is: The crisis of homeless children and families in New York City.* New York: Bank Street College of Education.

Patton, C. V. (1988). *Spontaneous shelter: International perspectives and prospects.* Philadelphia: Temple University Press.

Pesznecker, B. (1984). The poor: A population at risk. *Public Health Nursing, 1*(4), 237–249.

Ramachandran, A. (1988). International Year of Shelter for the Homeless. *Cities, 5,* 144–162.

Report of the Committee on Legal Problems of the Homeless. (1989). *The record of the Association of the Bar of the City of New York, 44*(1), 33–88.

Resnick, G. (1984). The short and long-term impact of a competency-based program for disadvantaged women. *Journal of Social Service Research, 7*(4), 37–49.

Schmitt, E. (1988, December 26). Suburbs cope with the steep rise in the homeless. *The New York Times,* 1.

Smith, S. (1989). People without land. *American Journal of Nursing, 89*(2), 208–209.

Tableman, B., Feis, C. L., Marciniak, D., & Howard, D. (1985). Stress management training for low-income women. *Prevention in Human Services, 3*(4), 71–85.

Tennison, D. C. (1983). Homeless people grow numerous in Europe, despite welfare states. *The Wall Street Journal, 80,* April 25, 1 +.

Thomas, J. (1985). The homeless of Europe: A scourge of our time. *The New York Times,* October 7.

Victim Services Agency. (1989). *The screening and diversion of battered women in the New York City emergency housing system.* New York: The Agency.

Wright, J. D., & Weber, E. (1987). *Homelessness and health.* New York: McGraw-Hill.

CHAPTER 11

Family Paradigm Theory and Family Rituals: Implications for Child and Family Health

Doris W. Campbell

ABSTRACT

Family paradigm theory explains variations in families that are based on their shared beliefs about the social world and their family's place within it. Key concepts of the theory and some of the supporting research are presented. Family rituals provide a window for viewing the family's efforts to maintain this shared concept of family identity. Suggestions for evaluating ritual use in families during times of stress and/or transition are provided. Ritual evaluation may give clues to difficulties families face in maintaining a shared identity during challenging periods of change or conflict.

The focus of this article is a theoretical model of the family developed by Reiss.[1] The model distinguishes among families based on their shared family identity and their perceptions of the family's interaction with its social world. Family rituals provide a window for viewing the family's efforts to maintain this shared concept of family identity. Ritual evaluation may give clues to difficulties families face in maintaining a shared identity during times of family stress or family transition.

Increasingly, the value of a family perspective in the primary care of children and adolescents is recognized. Since the family is one of the most important influences on the development of children, this model may be a useful guide for primary health care providers who work with children and their families.

FAMILY PARADIGM THEORY

A paradigm represents an overall image or world view. Each family develops its own style of dealing with issues of everyday living based on its concept of family and the place of the family in its social world. Reiss uses the abstract term "family paradigm" to describe the fundamental beliefs, convictions or core assumptions shared by family members about the nature of the social environment and the family's place within it.[1] The family's paradigm—or world view—emerges in the course of family development and serves to guide family organization and problem-solving. Family paradigms are abstract and are translated into observable behavior processes through regimes or regulating mechanisms. Family rituals are examples of regulating mechanisms. The interrelationship between the concepts of paradigm, regime and process is shown in Figure 1.

When a family's image is successfully translated into process, the family succeeds at being itself. A family may, however, be guided by a concept of family that cannot be put into practice because the family's actual organization cannot produce the desired behaviors.[2] For example, a remarried family may experience difficulty arranging for a child to celebrate his or her birthday because of conflicts in the child's schedule or conflicts between the child's two sets of parents.

Family paradigm theory assumes that the family's basic beliefs guide its interpretation of and responses to a variety of social situations; the paradigm subtly regulates a family's everyday interactions and provides a stable form of reference for when the family must interpret and respond as a group to unfamiliar or challenging social situations or settings.[1-2] Though the family paradigm can undergo radical change during periods of severe family disorganization, it usually persists for years and even generations.

Extensive work by Reiss and a team of researchers identified four family paradigms that are based on distinct approaches used by families to problem-solve:

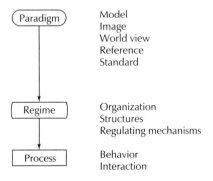

FIGURE 1. Paradigm, Regime and Process: Three Levels of Analysis.[2]

Consensus-Sensitive (Closed) Families

These families need agreement and rapid closure of issues without dissent. Little information is taken from the social world, which is perceived as threatening, chaotic and unknowable. Children growing up in such families are expected to be obedient and dependent. Clinically, these families appear doggedly united, often maintaining marriages in the face of severe adversity and conflict.[1-3]

Achievement-Sensitive (Random) Families

Such families have a high tolerance for uncertainty, tend to delay closure on solutions to problems, and reward inventive, competitive, individualistic behaviors in family members. Clinically, the families are cynical, hostile and angry, with a dog-eat-dog view of the motivation of others. Children are reared in a permissive environment in which parents fail to set limits and provide lax or little supervision.[1-3]

Environment-Sensitive (Open) Families

These families also have a high investment in change and a high tolerance for uncertainty. However, they practice optimal integration of old and new solutions to problems, and they merge individual and group needs. The environment is viewed as surmountable and trustworthy. Clinically, they are involved, direct and honest in confronting problems and confident in their ability to master them. Children in these families learn to be autonomous, cooperative and responsible.[1-3]

Distance-Sensitive (Synchronous) Families

These families tend to have a low investment in closure but also a low tolerance for uncertainty. Consequently, they move toward early closure and automatic, effortless solutions to problems. Information is taken from outside the family, but each individual is expected to master the information on his or her own. Sharing information is seen as a sign of weakness. Distance-sensitive families are described as disengaged but not chaotic. Clinically, such families appear to be perplexed and overwhelmed. Parents have been described as incompetent and literal-minded.[1-3]

Each of the four basic family types can form the basis for successful family functioning, but real families rarely exhibit "pure" paradigms. For example, some families will operate under mixed paradigms developed by incorporating beliefs from their various cultural and ethnic families of origin. Families guided by different paradigms tend to use specific approaches to problem-solving and may be prone to distinct types of difficulties.

FAMILY RITUALS

Reiss suggests that the health of a family depends on the protection of its basic world view or paradigm.[1-2,4] Family rituals are composed of certain ordinary and routine family-interaction behaviors. They are used by families to maintain family identity over time, sometimes from generation to generation (e.g., the bar mitzvah signifies a developmental milestone in Jewish families). Ritual disruption has been associated with breakdown of the family paradigm in cases of serious family disorder, such as parental alcoholism.[5-6] "Rituals stabilize identity throughout family life by clarifying expected roles, delineating boundaries within and without the family, and defining rules so that all members know that 'this is the way our family is' " (Wolin and Bennett, p. 401).[7]

The three categories of rituals include family celebrations, family traditions and patterned family interactions.[7-8] Family celebrations are holidays and occasions that are widely practiced throughout a culture and are special in the mind of the family. Rites of passage such as weddings, baptisms and bar mitzvahs; annual religious celebrations such as Christmas and Easter; and secular holiday observances such as Thanksgiving and New Year's are examples of celebration rituals. These standardized observances are usually specific to the subculture in which they are observed and are characterized by the use of symbols that pertain to the ritual (e.g., candles and the menorah during Hanukkah). Family celebrations offer family members an opportunity to share special occasions with family and friends. They assert the family's identity to the larger culture, and through repetition over time, contribute to the family's stability.[7-8]

Family traditions, as a ritual group, are less culture-specific and more individualized for each family than family celebrations. They include such rituals as vacations, visits to extended family members, birthday and anniversary parties. Family traditions may occur with less regularity in some families than in others. They also vary in level of organization from family to family. Although the culture at large makes a contribution to shaping family traditions (e.g., birthday cards), the family has considerable freedom in choosing the traditions it will emphasize.[7-8]

Of all rituals, patterned family interactions are enacted most frequently, but involve the least amount of conscious planning by participants. Examples of patterned family interactions include such routines as regular dinner time, bedtime rituals for children, the customary treatment of guests in the home or weekend leisure activities. Everyday greetings and goodbyes are rituals in some families. Regardless of the pattern, these interactions help to define the roles and responsibilities of family members and serve to organize daily life.[7-8]

While family rituals appear to be commonplace activities, they are an important mechanism through which families express their shared concept of family.

CLINICAL APPLICATIONS

Reiss' family paradigm theory and the function of rituals in maintaining a healthy family concept provide a useful framework for assessing threats to a family's sense of identity. The health care provider/clinician who is sensitive to the significance of family rituals for family health pays close attention to the place of ritual in the life of the family when family assessments are conducted.

Suggestions for evaluating family rituals include an assessment of the following:[8]

- Does the family underutilize rituals? Families who do not celebrate or mark family changes, or who do not join in larger social rituals may be left without some of the benefits of rituals, such as group cohesion and support for role shifts.
- Does the family follow rigid patterns of ritual? In families with inflexible rituals things are always done the same way, at the same time, with the same people.
- Are family rituals skewed? A family with skewed rituals tends to emphasize one aspect of family life (e.g., ethnicity, religion, etc.) or favors a particular set of relatives, neglecting essential elements of the family's composition. For example, the family always gets together with the mother's side of the family for Christmas and other events, ignoring the father's side of the family.
- Has the ritual process been interrupted or not experienced? For example, prejudices in the larger society may prevent families of children with AIDS from experiencing some of the traditional cultural rituals that support transitions. Homelessness may also interrupt the ability of a family to maintain its identity through the use of rituals.
- Are the rituals hollow? Hollow rituals are celebrated out of a sense of obligation, with little meaning found in either the process or the event. Rituals that have lost their vitality or that end up creating more stress for family members are examples of hollow rituals.
- Is the family flexible in adapting its rituals? For example, are the routines and rituals for bedtime the same for the 10-year-old as for the 4-year-old?

Examples of clinical problems that may severely threaten a family's identity include AIDS, family violence, child abuse and neglect, substance abuse and adolescent pregnancy. Birth of a handicapped child, death, or injury of a child that results in permanent disability may also threaten family identity and disrupt ritual performance. Ritual assessment can examine the extent to which a family believes it has had to give up certain rituals because of a clinical problem. Wolin et al. and Bennett et al. studied the family's most widely practiced rituals and observed how these were affected by parental alcohol abuse. Children in ritual-protected families fared better during the transition to adulthood than did children growing up in ritual-disrupted families. Extreme ritual disruption was significantly related to the transmission of alcoholism to the children's generation, whereas ritual-protection was associated with less transmission.[5-6]

Imber-Black, Roberts and Whiting[8] suggest using orienting and reflexive questions when assessing rituals. These questioning techniques permit the practitioner/clinician to evaluate the family's level of ritualization and to introduce the family to information about its use of ritual. Orienting questions help familiarize the practitioner/clinician with the family's life experiences and also make the family aware of its problems. Examples of orienting questions include the following (see Case Study 1): What was the last family event that you celebrated? How did you celebrate Thanksgiving,

CASE STUDY 1

Aspects of a Family's World View Influence Its Response to a Disabling Accident

The Martin family, basically a "closed" family type, functioned well until two years ago when their son Chad, now 14, was struck by a car. Chad sustained serious head injuries, resulting in intellectual, emotional, sensory and physical dysfunction. Mr. Martin silently blames Mrs. Martin for Chad's accident. When the accident happened, Chad was walking home from Little League practice because his mom was working late and was unable to pick him up from the ballfield. Following the accident, Mr. Martin started to drink heavily. He has become abusive and violent toward his wife and impatient with their 7-year-old daughter Karen. He has been unable to adjust to Chad's new identity. Chad's inability to share his thoughts in a logical manner embarrasses Mr. Martin, who avoids conversations with Chad and never takes him on outings. Mr. Martin works sporadically as a computer technician but loses jobs frequently because he fails to show up for work. Mrs. Martin worked as an executive secretary before Chad was hurt. She now stays at home as his primary caregiver.

Mr. Martin believes that a woman's place is in the home and had always resented the fact that his wife worked. Since Chad's accident, Mrs. Martin has come to believe that perhaps she should have waited until the children were "grown and gone" before going to work. She remembers, with regret, that women in her family of origin never worked outside of the home. The extra income she earned, however, allowed her family to go on camping trips several times a year and to get away as a couple every once in a while. Since Chad's accident, the Martins have not celebrated any significant family events, including Christmas and the children's birthdays.

Karen is beginning to have problems at school. She rarely completes assignments and frequently visits the school clinic complaining of a stomachache. She cherishes a birthday card that she received two months ago from a teacher. She has not shared the card with her parents, although she feels sad that they forgot her birthday again this year. She was invited by Mrs. Jones, the next-door neighbor, to stop by after school for cookies and to see her collection of dolls. Although Karen was interested in visiting Mrs. Jones, she is aware of the rule made explicit by her father when they moved to the neighborhood a few months ago: "Don't go snooping around the neighborhood talking to people. The less the neighbors know about us, the better."

The family nurse practitioner who visits the Martins as case manager for Chad suggested the family seek help at the counseling center. This idea was flatly rejected by Mr. Martin, who felt it would be a sign of weakness for the family to take their problems to outsiders. Mrs. Martin and the children quickly agreed. Chad stated, "We're not kooks." The nurse practitioner then explored ritual use for additional clues to the family's world view, both before and after the accident.

Christmas (or other cultural traditions) before Chad was hurt? How do you celebrate these occasions now? How often did you get together with others in your family for family gatherings before the accident? How often do you get together with others in your family now? Do you think you get together with family more or less than other families you know? Who is most comfortable with how you currently celebrate events?

Reflexive questions encourage family members to observe their own ritual behaviors and give clues to where the family might want to make some changes. Sample reflexive questions include the following: If you were to get together more often as a family to share and celebrate events, who would be the most likely to enjoy it? Who would probably initiate events? Responses to these questions can help the practitioner decide whether or not all or some members of the family see themselves as underritualized. They also provide information about the family's access to and use of larger societal rituals for support (e.g., Christmas, community and school activities).[8-9]

Children who grow up in consensus-sensitive (closed) families may be learning to view their world as chaotic and unknowable. Adolescent patients from such families are described as happy-go-lucky, but they are often covertly manipulative and hostile.[3]

Maturational crises may also challenge the identity of some families, e.g., the birth of a child, children leaving for school or marriage, and other family transitions such as divorce and remarriage.

The remarried family's identity may come to include rituals centered around the transition of young children between homes and summer vacations with stepparents and biological parents. Customs surrounding family celebrations such as birthdays, graduations and weddings become important as children move from childhood, to adolescence and into adulthood.[10] The practitioner/clinician can help remarried families consider creative possibilities for the success of these important events, thereby decreasing family tension and awkwardness.

Orienting questions that might be asked of Melody and Jim (see Case Study 2) during an assessment of rituals include the following: How have bedtime rituals changed for the children? How have birthday parties changed? Are the same people involved in the nighttime rituals? How have their roles changed? Examples of reflexive questions include the following: What would need to change in planning for an event (family celebration, tradition) in order for it to be more meaningful? When might these changes be made? What new rituals has the family created?[8]

Flexibility in adapting rituals is essential in families with children. In remarried families, ritual performance provides opportunities for families to define family identity as it pertains to the immediate stepfamily, binuclear family and remarried family suprasystem.[10]

CONCLUSION

Family paradigm theory has been shown to be clinically useful for practitioners interested in theory-based practice. Assessing the impact of family stress on ritual use and adaptation may provide clues about a family's need to either maintain or change

---

CASE STUDY 2

**Counseling Helps Remarried Family
Confront Tension**

Melody and Jim were referred for family counseling by the nurse practitioner who manages their son's asthma. The couple describe the disruptive effects of their ongoing battle with Jim's former wife Sandra over care of 4-year-old Donna and 6-year-old Timothy—Jim's children from his marriage to Sandra. Timothy has asthma, and Sandra claims his attacks always increase in frequency after he spends time with Melody and Jim. Donna enjoys a special bedtime ritual with Melody and Jim, but Timothy refuses to participate in any activity involving Melody. Melody and Jim planned a birthday party at McDonald's for Timothy and invited Sandra and both sets of grandparents. Jim's parents attended, but neither Sandra nor her parents attended. Timothy was sullen and acted out during the party, which ended abruptly when he had a severe episode of wheezing.

At the counseling center, the family participates cooperatively in sessions. Though currently functioning as a disabled family, they are confronting their problems openly. Over the past few weeks, Timothy has had fewer asthma attacks and is beginning to share his feelings during family counseling sessions.

---

its paradigm. A breakdown in a family's paradigm can lead to two possibilities: continued family disintegration, or qualitative changes within the family that promote self-healing. At this stage, families are particularly open to new and outside influences.[2,9] Though filled with risk, a family crisis can serve a positive function in the life of its members. Ultimately, it can open the family to new experiences and the possibility of altering its sense of self and the outside world, thereby transforming a paradigm that may have guided the family for years or even generations.

REFERENCES

1. Reiss, D. *The family's construction of reality,* Cambridge, MA: Harvard University Press, 1981.
2. Constantine, L. *Family paradigms: The practice of theory in family therapy,* New York: Guilford Press, 1986.
3. Costell, R. and Reiss, D. "The family meets the hospital: Clinical presentation of a laboratory based family typology," *Archives of General Psychiatry, 39,* 1982, pp. 433–88.
4. Reiss, D. "The working family: A researcher's view of health in the household," *American Journal of Psychiatry, 139,* 1982, pp. 1412–20.
5. Wolin, S., et al. "Disrupted family rituals: A factor in the intergenerational transmission of alcoholism," *Journal of Studies of Alcohol, 41,* 1980, pp. 199–214.
6. Bennett, L., et al. "Couples at risk for transmission of alcoholism: Protective influences," *Family Process, 26,* 1987, pp. 111–29.
7. Wolin, S. J., and Bennett, L.A. "Family Rituals," *Family Process, 23,* 1984, pp. 401–20.

8. Imber-Black, E., Roberts, J. and Whiting, R. *Rituals in families and family therapy,* New York: Norton and Co., 1988.
 9. Oliveri, M. E. and Reiss, D. "Families Schemata of Social Relationships," *Family Process, 21,* 1982, pp. 295–311.
10. Whiteside, M. "Family rituals as a key to kinship connections in remarried amilies," *Family Relations, 38,* 1989, pp. 34–9.

CHAPTER 12

A Framework for Planning Public Health Nursing Services to Families

Rosemary K. Vahldieck, Sharon R. Reeves, Margaret Schmelzer

ABSTRACT

We designed a model to assist public health nurses and nursing supervisory staff in planning, delivering, and evaluating their services to families. Specifically, the intent was to assist nurses to estimate the numbers and types of services required. The model includes a gradient of family health characteristics, an original delineation of nine basic public health nursing services, a coping index and scoring guidelines, and a methodology for integrating assessment of health needs and coping abilities.

A theoretical model was designed to promote a systematic approach for planning and evaluating family-directed public health nursing services. Components of the model include a classification of family health characteristics into five levels; definitions and primary approaches for nine specific public health nursing (PHN) services; the family health-specific coping index (FHSCI) made up of nine domains of coping with scoring guidelines (Christensen, Josten, & Choi, 1983); and a methodology for integrating assessments of family health characteristics and family coping abilities to delineate estimates for nursing services by types and numbers of PHN-family contacts.

"A Framework for Planning Public Health Nursing Services to Families," by Rosemary K. Vahldieck. From *Public Health Nursing, Vol. 6* (No. 2), 1989, pp. 102–107. Reprinted by permission of Blackwell Scientific Publications, Inc.

PURPOSE

It is essential to document the effectiveness of PHN services if the profession is to maintain a prescribed role in today's health care system. The demand for accountability is clear; additional work is needed to specify essential practice areas so that the services can be evaluated with confidence and consistency. Analyses of research in public health nursing (Highriter, 1977, 1984; Feetham, 1984; Coombs-Orme, Reis, & Ward, 1985; Sullivan, 1984) describe a broad range of interests studied, but highlight need for theory development to "clarify conceptual underpinnings of the profession and increase the efficacy of the practice" (Sullivan, 1984, p. 177). A prerequisite to establishing theories that explain and predict the relationship between the content and process of PHN service and the health outcomes of the population served is a descriptive model that identifies the basic elements of PHN practice, namely, the characteristics of client health states, the determinants of client nursing needs, and definitions for a specified set of nursing services.

Although the clientele of the PHN includes groups, families, and individuals selected for service because of expected benefit to the health of a total community or population group (American Public Health Association, 1980), the proposed model focuses primarily on the family. Well recognized as an important precept, the process of achieving family-directed services that supersedes the usual orientation to the health state of an individual family member is fraught with difficulties, both practical and conceptual (Highriter, 1983; Feetham, 1984; Speer & Sachs, 1985). Guidelines to clarify and facilitate that process could be helpful in making assessments of family progress toward attaining desired health goals, the contribution of the practitioner, and the effectiveness of the profession.

The ultimate value of any theoretical model must be evaluated with scientific rigor (Giovannetti, 1979). The HSFCI, an adaptation of the Richmond-Hopkins family coping index (Freeman & Lowe, 1963), has been subjected to reliability and validity testing (Choi, Josten, & Christensen, 1983). Reality testing of the proposed model that integrates the HSFCI with a gradient of health characteristics to form a scale of intensity of need for nursing service is essential for evaluating its usefulness to PHN practice. Until that can be achieved, anticipated benefits from immediate use of the planning framework include the following:

1. Improved facility in planning family-directed PHN services
2. Increased effectiveness in supervising caseload planning
3. Integration of uniform procedures in family case management for tracking and recording the nursing process, consisting of components of assessment, planning, implementation, and evaluation
4. Practicability in assessing the quality and impact of PHN services to families
5. Generation of data for monitoring caseloads, projecting workloads, allocating staff effort, and evaluating programs

MODEL DEVELOPMENT

A desire to improve agency procedures for assessing quality of services, shared by nursing administrative personnel of two Wisconsin local public health agencies and a state consultant, prompted initial collaborative efforts. Published descriptions of practice frameworks developed or used by other agencies (Visiting Nurse Service of Metropolitan Detroit, 1982; Daubert, 1979; Christensen, Josten, & Choi, 1983; Simmons, 1980) were reviewed, and gaps and overlaps were identified. The authors then developed an instrument that includes two unique components: a set of nine specific public health nursing services, and a five-level classification of family health characteristics. Use of the added components in combination with the FHSCI is expected to promote accuracy and consistency in nursing assessments of family need and response to services provided.

The instrument was introduced in a pilot test to supervisory and staff nurses employed by 14 local public health agencies in the Wisconsin Division of Health Southern Region. Represented were both city and county agencies, some providing home health services in addition to preventive public health care, and several visiting nurse agencies. The tool was intended to have utility in planning all family-focused nursing services provided in the home setting.

Positive response dominated both verbal and written feedback obtained from the nurses involved in the pilot test. Favorably highlighted were the family focus, nursing process framework, case management procedures, and perceptions about the impact of nursing intervention. Problem areas centered on categorizing families according to their health status and coping abilities. It was recommended that the instrument be refined and that forms used for recording be improved.

The interdependency of the sources of family health and nursing needs has long been recognized. Health circumstances, social-cultural milieu, environment, and family behavior patterns are so intertwined that each must be considered in relation to the others to capture the true essence of family health status (Freeman, 1963). Insight gained from the pilot test feedback emphasized that a total view of family health is most accurate when it includes each related health determinant through the application of unidimensional scales that facilitate consistent measurement (Highriter, 1983).

Subsequent revisions of the instrument were directed toward an original formulation of definitions for five levels of health characteristics with examples exclusive of individual health states. Directions for rating family coping abilities were modified to incorporate a database format for recording initial and subsequent assessment rating scores with observations. Guidelines for using the framework in case management were specified, and a one-page record form, master plan was created for summarizing nursing assessments, goals, services, and progress to provide an overview of nurse-family joint efforts.

TABLE 1
Family Health Characteristics

Level	Definition	Examples
1	Alteration in normal health state, self-limiting or correctable; low potential for sequelae.	Acute communicable disease-enterics; amblyopia; developmental delay; emotional disorders; hearing loss; low-risk pregnancy
2	Clinically demonstrable condition abnormality/laboratory test that identifies higher than average risk for future development of disease.	Exposure to teratogens and mutagens; family history of genetic disease; gravida 19–35 yrs; hypertension; iron deficiency; Mantoux converter; obesity
3	Acute, reversible, or chronic disease, genetic/developmental deviation, with therapeutic potential for regaining optimum functioning and controlling/minimizing probable sequelae.	Anemias; cerebral palsy; childhood chronic illness; chronic mental illness; congestive heart failure; developmental disability; diabetes; failure to thrive; hepatitis; meningitis; multiple sclerosis; prematurity; sudden infant death syndrome; sexually transmitted disease; stroke
4	Irreversible disease/disability with therapeutic potential for minimizing physical and emotional suffering.	Advanced emphysema; AIDS; amyotrophic lateral sclerosis; Alzheimer's disease; end-stage renal; end-stage cancer
5	Undiagnosed/untreated condition with high potential for life-threatening sequelae and unpredictable potential for reversing or controlling complications.	Abuse/neglect; signs of acute communicable disease with outbreak/epidemic potential; potential suicide

FAMILY HEALTH CHARACTERISTICS

Table 1 gives definitions of and examples for five levels of health conditions, abnormalities, and diseases. The groupings offer a severity index for projecting need for public health nursing services, level 1 being low, to incorporate the full continuum of health states that can characterize the PHN caseload. Level 2, consisting of high-risk factors for which preventive measures are advisable, addresses National Institutes of Health recommendations for further differentiation of primary and secondary disease prevention (Gordon, 1983). Criteria applied to the designation of the five levels include (1) existing and potential effects of the health problem on quality and length of life; (2) anticipated impact of the health problem on family resources and functioning to manage the cost and personal care, provide emotional support, and respond to other demands for adaptation; (3) likely impact of nursing intervention to assist the family promote, maintain, or restore health, prevent illness, effect rehabilitation, and control sequelae, pain, and discomfort; and (4) social and health implications to the community of the problem, its extension or exacerbation.

Such a classification provides an objective instrument for (1) initiating and discontinuing services to families according to agency-designated priorities; (2) organizing services according to an established approach for a total caseload made up of families representing several levels of health characteristics; and (3) emphasizing the interrelationships among health conditions, family health, and potential impact of nursing.

PHN SERVICES TO FAMILIES

Prescribing a specified set of public health nursing services may seem restrictive to some practitioners who favor a freer approach in service definition, creatively framed in a response to each situation encountered. Potential benefits from a structured approach are significant. Adopting the particular scope of professional activity applicable to family work can produce positive effects on conducting and supervising case planning, forecasting time and effort, and facilitating communication about the role of nursing in this important endeavor.

DEFINITIONS AND APPROACHES

Public health nursing is defined as an intervention directed to achieving a positive health outcome. The following original set of nine services, fundamental to PHN practice, are directed toward achieving a positive impact on a family's coping abilities, and preventing harmful consequences of inadequate coping that can cause permanent incapacity or death to a family member and have a negative impact on the community.

1. Assessment and evaluation of requirements for services
   a. Definition: the initial appraisal of the family health characteristics and ability effectively to manage their health care requirements related to the dimensions of physical independence, therapeutic competence, knowledge

of health condition, application of principles of general hygiene, health attitudes, emotional competence, family living patterns, physical environment, use of resources.

  b. Primary approaches: review of records and reports, health history of family, application of the FHSCI.

2. Assessment and evaluation of estimated progress
  a. Definition: the process of determining the impact of family or nurse actions on the status of family abilities and health care requirements by appraising progress in attaining established goals.
  b. Primary approaches: interview, observation, physical appraisal.

3. Planning to establish health goals and outcomes
  a. Definition: the design, by nurse with family participation, of specific and coordinated strategies directed toward strengthening family abilities and reducing family health care requirements.
  b. Primary approaches: assign family-nurse priorities to problems according to existing or potential risk and preventive measures; identify family strengths and resources; delineate goals, family-nurse actions, and time frames (contracting).

4. Provide information
  a. Definition: give factual data about single-focused, uncomplicated issues to increase knowledge and understanding, and supply a background for decision making.
  b. Primary approaches: present facts, answer questions and clarify misunderstandings, interpret medical terminology, offer selected written material and resources for family review and consideration.

5. Health counseling
  a. Definition: the process of facilitating self-directed learning toward adaptation and positive change in family health capabilities and care requirements.
  b. Primary approaches, provided as appropriate within the framework of nurse-family collaborative relationship: consultation, guidance, instruction, support.

6. Administration of physical procedures
  a. Definition: application of specific measures, tests, techniques to prevent disease, identify unrecognized illness or defect and promote diagnostic approaches, treat or stabilize illness or disability, ensure maintenance of an optimal state of health.
  b. Primary approaches: immunization, screening tests, therapeutic rehabilitative techniques, assistance with activities of daily living.

7. Advocacy
  a. Definition: locating and coordinating formal and informal resources, or other helping activity in behalf of those who cannot, or perceive themselves as unable to, solve their dilemmas on their own. Goals for helping are established with client participation and directed at both client and organization system levels.

   b. Primary approaches: assertive action to protect client rights, facilitating delivery of services to family in crisis, case management to coordinate multi-provider services.
8. Emotional support
   a. Definition: providing acceptance, encouragement and assistance to family/individuals to initiate or persevere in taking a positive health action.
   b. Primary approaches: communicate reassurance while client is practicing a new skill or making a decision, demonstrate acceptance and empathy during crisis.
9. Referral
   a. Definition: the exchange of pertinent information with other service providers in order to introduce client and resource, and facilitate coordination of services to be provided.
   b. Primary approaches: written or verbal transmittal or appropriate information, feedback to ensure referral completion and promote coordinated effort.

PLANNING SERVICES

Table 2 presents a method for anticipating specific public health nursing services and an average number of PHN-family contacts based on family health characteristics (FHC) level and family health characteristics (HSFCI) score.

FHC and PHN Services

Family health characteristics provide the basis for initiating PHN services, singly or in any combination, that appropriately fit the immediate situation. The level of FHC does not determine the specific services to be used, but differentiates the plan for their delivery, the timing and frequency of PHN-family contacts. Families with numerous health problems of different or similar severity or level need services that respond to those complexities. Table 2 portrays the increased number of PHN-family contacts generally anticipated from level 1 (2 to 5) to subsequent levels; 2, 2 to 6; 3, 4 to 10; 4 and 5, 4 to 10 or more.

Family Coping Abilities and PHN Services

Family health characteristics are central to achieving positive health behavioral outcomes through PHN intervention. Family coping abilities (FCA) determine the specific nursing services to be used. Table 2 identifies specific services that may be useful for families with low, moderate, and high coping scores, as they are expected to require different groupings or public health nursing services. For families with low FCA scores, all services but health counseling are indicated. For those with moderate scores, all services but advocacy are identified. The PHN services identified for families with high

TABLE 2

Anticipated PHN Services and Average Number of PHN-Family Contacts by Family Health Characteristics (FHC) and Family Coping Abilities (FCA)

	PHN Services*			PHN-Family Contacts† (average number)		
	FCA HSFCI Score			FCA HSFCI Score		
FHC Level	Low 9–13	Moderate 22–32	High 40–45	Low 9–13	Moderate 22–32	High 40–45
1	1, 2, 3, 4, 6, 7, 8, 9	1, 2, 3, 4, 5, 6, 8, 9	1, 4, 6	5	3	2
2	1, 2, 3, 4, 6, 7, 8, 9	1, 2, 3, 4, 5, 6, 8, 9	1, 4, 6	6	4	2
3	1, 2, 3, 4, 6, 7, 8, 9	1, 2, 3, 4, 5, 6, 8, 9	1, 4, 6	10	7	4
4	1, 2, 3, 4, 6, 7, 8, 9	1, 2, 3, 4, 5, 6, 8, 9	1, 4, 6	10 or more	7	4
5	1, 2, 3, 4, 6, 7, 8, 9	1, 2, 3, 4, 5, 6, 8, 9	1, 4, 6	10 or more	7	4

*PHN services: 1 Assess/evaluate requirements for service; 2 Assess/evaluate to estimate progress; 3 Plan to establish health goals/outcomes; 4 Provide information; 5 Health counseling; 6 Administer physical procedures; 7 Advocacy; 8 Emotional support; 9 Referral.
†PHN-family contact includes all interactions for the provision of service(s) regardless of place performed or method used.

coping scores are limited to numbers 1, 4, and 6. Services for families with coping scores that rank between the low to moderate and moderate to high have to be individualized to reflect these variations.

Family coping abilities determine the timing and frequency of PHN services. Higher FHC scores suggest that the optimum impact of services can be realized with fewer contacts concentrated within a short time. Lower FCA scores suggest the advantage of a greater number of contacts distributed over a longer time period. Generally many PHN services are provided in combination within a specific contact. Whereas service 4 (provide information) can be accomplished within a single contact, to be effective, health counseling is given during a series of contacts over a period of time (e.g., 3 months). The total number of contacts anticipated in any given situation is directly dependent on family progress expected or demonstrated. Lack of expected progress should prompt a critical review of the FCA and estimate of change/goal, or the PHN services provided. Exceptions to recommended services and contacts include specification of physician's orders and agency policy or program priority.

QUESTIONS REMAINING

Despite a real sense of accomplishment from our efforts that stem in part from the positive reports from agency staffs who are in various stages of implementing the model, we are keenly aware of the complex questions remaining to be answered. Are the indexes proposed for family health characteristics and PHN services appropriate, relevant, and useful? Does the suggested juxtaposition of these practice variables and family coping abilities contribute to the determination of quality and impact of services? The task ahead is arduous, the benefits are far reaching.

ACKNOWLEDGMENTS

The authors acknowledge the significant contribution of the directors of nursing, supervisors, and staff nurses from the public health agencies in the Wisconsin Division of Health Southern Region who supported this project with their encouragement and suggestions, and participated in the pilot test.

REFERENCES

American Public Health Association, Public Health Nursing Section. (1980). *The definition and role of public health nursing in the delivery of health care.* Washington, DC: Author.

Choi, T., Josten, L., & Christensen, M. L. (1983, November). Health-specific family coping index for noninstitutional care. *American Journal of Public Health, 73,* 1275–1277.

Christensen, M. L., Josten, L., & Choi, T. (1983, November). *Health-specific family coping index.* St. Paul, MN: Ramsey County Public Health Nursing Section.

Coombs-Orme, T., Reis, J., & Ward, L. D. (1985, September-October). Effectiveness of home visits by public health nurses in maternal and child health. *Public Health Reports, 100,* 490–499.

Daubert, E. A. (1979, July). Patient classification system and outcome criteria. *Nursing Outlook, 27,* 450–454.

Feetham, S. L., (1984). Family research: Issues and directions for nursing. In H. H. Werley and J. J. Fitzpatrick (Eds.), *Annual Review of Nursing Research,* Vol. 2 (pp. 3–25). New York: Springer.

Freeman, R. B. (1963). *Public Health Nursing Practice,* ed. 3. Philadelphia: W. B. Saunders.

Freeman, R. B., & Lowe, M. (1963, January). A method for appraising family public health nursing needs. *American Journal of Public Health, 53,* 47–52.

Giovannetti, P. (1979, February). Understanding patient classification system. *Journal of Nursing Administration, 9,* 4–9.

Gordon, R.S. (1983, March-April). An operational classification of disease prevention. *Public Health Reports, 98,* 107–109.

Highriter, M. E. (1977, May-June). The status of community health nursing research. *Nursing Research, 26,* 183–192.

Highriter, M. E. (1983, November). Measurement of family progress in coping with health problems. *American Journal of Public Health, 73,* 1248–1250.

Highriter, M. E. (1984). Public health nursing evaluation, education, and professional issues: 1977 to 1981. In H. H. Werley and J. J. Fitzpatrick (Eds.), *Annual Review of Nursing Research,* Vol. 2 (pp. 165–189). New York: Springer.

Simmons, D. A. (1980, June). *A classification scheme for client problems in community health nursing.* (DHHS Publication No. HRA 80–16). Hyattsville, MD: Division of Nursing.

Speer, J. J., & Sachs, B. (1985, September-October). Selecting the appropriate family assessment tool. *Pediatric Nursing, 11,* 349–355.

Sullivan, J. A. (1984). Overview of community health nursing research and evaluation. In J. A. Sullivan (Ed.), *Directions in community health nursing* (pp. 175–206). Boston: Blackwell.

Visiting Nurse Association of Metropolitan Detroit. (1982). *Nursing diagnosis and expected outcome statements.* Detroit: Author.

CHAPTER 13

A Family Perspective on Aging and Health

Nancy L. Wilson, Rosanne Trost

Improved health care for older Americans will be one of the great challenges of the next several decades. By the year 2030, approximately 21% of the population will be 65 and older. Families with more than one generation over age 65 are growing in number, resulting in an increased focus on the demographic and social trends affecting family relationships in later life: retirement, health care, economic stability, altered social networks, and coping with the challenges of normal aging.

In recent years, community agencies and institutions have begun to recognize and respond to the needs of the elderly and their family members. Yet, an increased understanding of normal aging and the diseases common to later life is needed, as well as more information about how older people maintain their functioning. In addition, there is more to learn about multi-generational families and what strategies support them in their caregiving efforts on behalf of aging members.

The demographics of an aging society are having a profound effect on every institution in American life, including the health care system. One of the great health care challenges of the next several decades will be improved health care for older Americans, especially the growing number of "old-old," those 75 years and older, who are at greatest risk of impairment due to disease.[1]

The number of people 65 to 74 years of age will increase 20% by the end of this century. There will be a 50% increase in the 75 to 84 age group and the 85 year and older

Reprinted from *Health Values, Vol II* (No. 2), March/April 1987, pp. 52–57. Used with permission.

group will increase by 80%. By the year 2030, approximately 21% of the population will be in the 65 and older age group. The significant increase among the very old has resulted in growth in the number of families with four or more generations. Families with more than one generation over age 65 are growing in number. Beyond the sheer increase in number are the other demographic and social trends affecting family relationships in later life and the provision of family care and support to aging members with health problems. The increase in geographic mobility, the growing percentage of women in the workplace, and the high rate of divorce are among these trends.

The aging process and the role of the family in later life are areas plagued with popular mythology that hinders individual lifestyles and the formation of informed social policy. Among the myths on aging are the notions that all old people are frail, depressed, and unable to remember things or exercise good judgment in managing their lives.[2] In fact, the majority of older persons do adapt well to changes they encounter with aging. Although 75% of the elderly have a chronic condition such as arthritis or cardiovascular disease, they do continue to live productive lives. Another myth is that older people are isolated from their families and are "dumped" into nursing homes when they need care. Most older Americans maintain regular contact with their families, although they prefer to live apart from their children.[3] At any one time, only 5% of those over age 65 are institutionalized; however, the longer one lives, the greater the likelihood of being institutionalized and 25% of that age group spend some time in a nursing home at some point in their lifetime. The majority of older people with impaired functioning are able to remain at home because the family rather than the formal service system is the major provider of care.[4]

NORMAL AGING

The aging process does not begin at age 65 or 75; it is a lifelong process from birth until death. Furthermore, aging is multidimensional, consisting of interacting biological, psychological, and social processes. There is often confusion between normal aging and the effects of disease that occur more frequently in later life. Normal aging refers to biological processes that are time-related and not a function of stress, injury, or chronic disease. Pathological aging refers to a decrease in functioning due to an abnormality. Valuable studies of aging and health have produced much useful data; however, more research is needed—particularly on persons over the age of 85—to help distinguish the effects of normal aging from other biological processes, especially disease.

With the aging process, some physical changes are inevitable; however, no two people age in the same manner. After 40, vision and hearing begin a gradual deterioration and in some instances this deterioration may be quite noticeable over the next three decades of life. The immune system and the nervous system often show a great degree of change, and recuperation from minor illnesses may be prolonged. Other changes such as behavioral slowing or reduced lung capacity may have only limited impact on the daily functioning of an individual.

Aging successfully depends on health, not just absence of disease. According to Fries, the onset of disability in the elderly may be postponed and the period of deterioration may be compressed into a shorter time span, closer to the end of life.[5] For example, cardiovascular disease is the most frequent cause of death in persons over age 65; however, some cardiovascular disease in older persons is preventable, or it may be possible to postpone its occurrence by modifying certain risk factors. Maintaining health and well-being may also play a role in cancer prevention. Although one out of ten persons will develop cancer by the age of 70, current research suggests the possibility that the stimuli causing it may be independent of the aging process.

Changes in memory, learning, and problem-solving have been found in some but not all aged individuals and are accelerated after age 70. These changes are often a result of the increased prevalence of disease in advanced years. There is a documented decrease in reaction time, but older people are still able to acquire new skills.[6] Practice significantly improves the performance of older persons, especially if a task is unfamiliar. Visual imagery has been shown to enhance performance and could be an important component of a health education program.

Coping techniques do not seem to change with age. Basic social and emotional coping styles may persist for over 70 years and these mechanisms are determined more by the person than by age.[7] Coping with stress, however, requires a great deal of energy and can upset the equilibrium of an older person, particularly if there are multiple stressors.

Family roles are in a constant state of change. In young families, the parent assumes the independent role while the child is dependent on the parent for care.[8] As the child enters adolescence, much of the dependency is discarded and family conflicts may occur. When some parents age and require assistance due to disability or loss, they may become more dependent on their adult children. In addition to changing family roles, individuals may face new challenges specific to their own development. Female adult children may be facing menopause; the male may be experiencing his own crisis of midlife; these events can cause major transitions in their own social roles and functioning.

Recent studies of family interaction at different ages have shown some continuity of patterns in later years. For example, parents and children who visit frequently in later life tended to do so in the early years.[9] Likewise, research has documented the mutual aid that occurs in later years, with many older adults contributing money and services to younger generations and receiving emotional support and help from the family during times of illness.[10]

COPING WITH CHALLENGES OF AGING

There are different types of stresses and losses that may challenge an older person's ability to maintain a sense of well-being and control over life, including declines in health status, loss of loved ones, etc. Because aging occurs within a family context, adult children also need to cope with the changes they see in their parents and focus on the balance of strengths and weaknesses displayed by the older person.

In anticipating some of these changes, older adults and other family members can optimize well-being through careful planning and communication. In addition to making adaptations within the family, the elderly and family members may find it most helpful to explore what options for new activities or services are available in the community prior to having a pressing need for this information. A growing number of communities have information and referral services or case management programs to assist older people and families with locating community resources, including opportunities for employment, help at home, health care, and social activities.

RETIREMENT

Retirement is inevitable for the majority of workers if one remains in the work force long enough; however, mandatory retirement may be unpleasant, particularly if it comes earlier than expected. Whether voluntary or mandatory, retirement may pose problems for couples, particularly if both spouses have been working outside the home. The retirement of either spouse necessitates an adjustment in their relationship in much the same way as when children were born. Problems may be minimized by planning for this particular transition and realizing that the adjustment to retirement takes some time. Self-esteem is often linked with a person's job and new sources of self-fulfillment may need to be explored. In some instances, having a part-time or volunteer job is helpful. If there are grandchildren, the retiree may assume a more active grandparent role. If the older person takes the time prior to retirement to explore these options, then the adjustment to retirement, whenever it occurs, may be easier and less traumatic.

ECONOMIC CHANGES

Change in financial status often accompanies retirement, or may result from reduced household income due to death or prolonged illness. Preparation may be made through a savings plan, as well as by discussing ways to minimize expenses if and when the need arises. Older people and their family members are often unfamiliar with existing entitlement programs such as Social Security and Medicare. An important aspect of assuring health and minimizing financial problems involves gaining an understanding of available public benefits and securing supplemental coverage for medical and long-term care.

ALTERED SOCIAL NETWORKS

Social ties are often altered as people age. Friends or family members may move away or illness and death may strike a number of them, leaving the older person with fewer sources of friendship and support.

Death of a spouse is a profound loss affecting all family members, particularly the surviving spouse. Usually the survivor is a woman; however, when the husband is the survivor, his adjustment may be even more difficult because death of a wife is less expected in our culture and sources of help are geared more to the women. Age has no effect on the grieving process, which is similar no matter when it is experienced over the life cycle. The expression of grief, however, is individualized. The widowed may face an identity crisis, along with loneliness and a sense of emptiness and isolation, even though family and friends may be in close proximity. Grief is a normal process; it should not be hastened by well-meaning family members. Major decisions should be postponed during this time to allow the spouse to become emotionally stable and independent. Adult children who have lost a parent need to be aware that they are adjusting to their own loss, but may also be called on to give support to the parent. This dual process can be very exhausting and the children need to recognize their limitations. At times, it may be worthwhile for family members to seek professional help to adjust to the loss.

Planning for death is quite difficult, but some preparations are beneficial to the family members. The use of a "Living Will" instructs physicians and family members about one's wishes regarding the use of life support systems in the event of a terminal illness.[11] Planning allows an individual to make responsible decisions and lessens the burden for other family members. As marriages become more like partnerships and responsibilities are shared, there may be fewer household adjustments when the death occurs.

Sometimes an older family member may need to relocate geographically due to changes in social, financial, or health status. Whether the relocation of the aging parent(s) occurs in crisis or has been planned, there are ramifications for the entire family. Older people often do not wish to change their lifestyle or give up privacy to move in with adult children, even though there is a high degree of interaction between the generations. Any change in living arrangements needs to be carefully thought out and discussed by all family members.

CHANGING HEALTH STATUS

Continuing gerontological research has found that disease and disability, not the aging process, pose the greatest threat to health in the later years. There are some steps the older person can take to promote good health. Exercise benefits the cardiovascular system, promotes well-being, and often helps with normal weight maintenance. Proper nutrition also plays an important role in the health of the elderly. Medications, chronic conditions, improperly fitted dentures, and dislike of eating alone often have an effect on an individual's nutritional status. There is ample justification to encourage older persons to discontinue cigarette smoking because of the many risks it poses to chronic disease such as emphysema, lung cancer, and cardiovascular disease.

Health care planning is essential for all family members. The goals of health care for the elderly must be to maintain health and independent functioning and to treat illnesses, both acute and chronic, with the best medical knowledge. Regular medical and dental checkups are important, as early detection can prevent the progression of serious disease. In addition, older people with a specific health condition should obtain information about that illness and its prescribed treatment. Hospitals and community agencies frequently offer prevention and treatment programs that focus on specific health conditions such as osteoporosis and cardiovascular disease.

Often, the adult child may need to play an active role in helping the aging parent to maintain good health. In some cases, the parent may resist seeking health care due to fear of learning that a serious condition exists. The child may also be experiencing those same fears; however, both their fears may be alleviated by a joint visit to the physician's office.[12]

In some cases the adult child (usually a woman) needs to assume an active care-giving role on behalf of an older parent who has limited functioning due to one or more chronic illnesses, physical or mental. The type of assistance an impaired elder requires may vary significantly and rarely remains static.

Some adult children may accept willingly the new role of caregiver; others, how-ever, may feel resentment toward the parent who is becoming dependent. This resent-ment may be a result of many factors. These include lack of time, a desire to be free from extra responsibility, and a possible negative effect on one's own family life. Even more important, the adult children may be facing the parent's mortality—as well as their own—for the first time.

Whether or not they assume an active role in caregiving, individual family mem-bers will have their own unique responses to an older parent or loved one who becomes impaired due to a chronic illness or condition. They may react with anger or guilt or may be overly solicitous and protective. Some of the factors influencing these responses include the role the impaired elder has played in the family previously; family patterns; the individual's coping skills; competing demands such as work or child rearing; and available resources. These responses do not remain static, however, and often change when family situations are in a state of transition.

It is important to recognize that caregivers have their own special needs. In his work with caregivers of dementia patients, Zarit has identified the following major needs:

> 1) Receive information about the nature and prognosis of the patient's disorder; 2) be given permission to attend to their own needs; 3) engage in problem-solving about coping with the patient's behavioral problems; 4) develop strategies for maximizing the patient's level of functioning; and 5) be connected to supportive social and health services.[13]

In recent years, community agencies and institutions providing health and social services have begun to recognize the needs of both the elderly with chronic disabilities and their family members. There are now specialized publications, caregiver hand-books, programs such as family support groups and counseling, and other resources to assist individuals in need as well as professionals concerned with the aging individual and the family (Table 1).

The future health and well-being of a growing aging population rests on many variables. An increased understanding of normal aging and the diseases common to later life is needed as well as more information about what factors help older people maintain their functioning. There is also more to learn about the complexity of multi-generation families and what strategies support families in their caregiving efforts on behalf of aging members.

TABLE 1
Selected Resources on Aging, Health, and Caregiving

National Council on Aging
Family Caregivers Program
Health Promotion and Aging Program
600 Maryland Avenue, SW
West Wing 100
Washington, D.C. 20024
(202) 479-1200
(publications, national guides)

National Support Center for Families of the Aging
P.O. Box 245
Swarthmore, PA 19081
(printed and audiovisual materials)

As Parents Grow Older: A Manual for Program Replication
Aida G. Silverman, Carl I. Bronce, and Carol Zielinski
P.O. Box 548
Brighton, MI 48116

Consumer Materials
Cohen SZ, Gans BM: *The Other Generation Gap: You and Your Aging Parents.*
New York, Warner Books, 1980.

Mace NL, Rabins PV: *The 36-Hour Day: A Family Guide to Caring for Persons with Alzheimer's Disease, Related Dementing Illness and Memory Loss in Later Life.*
Baltimore, The Johns Hopkins University Press, 1982.

Otten J, Shelley FD: *When Your Parents Grow Old.* New York, Funk and Wagnalls, 1978.

Silverstone B, Hyman HK: *You and Your Aging Parent.* New York, Pantheon Books, 1976.

Help Yourself to Good Health.
Expand Associates/PFP
7923 Eastern Avenue
Suite 400
Silver Springs, MD 20910
(free single copies)

Procino J: *Growing Older, Getting Better: A Handbook for Women in the Second Half of Life.* Reading, MA, Addison-Wesley, 1983.

REFERENCES

1. Neugarten, B. L. Age groups in American society and the rise of the young old. *Annals of the American Academy of Political and Social Science* 1974; 415:187–198.
2. Fruge, E., & Niederehe, G: Family dimensions of health care for the aged, in Henao, S., Grose, N. P. (eds.); *Principles of family systems in family medicine,* New York: Brunner/Mazel, 1985.

3. Kaplan, J. The family in aging (Editorial), *Gerontologist* 1975: 15:385.
4. Brody, E. The informal support system and health of the future aged, in Gaitz, C., Niederehe, G., Wilson, N. (eds): *Aging 2000: Our health care destiny.* New York: Springer-Verlag, 1985.
5. Fries, J. F. The biological constraints on human aging: Implications for health policy. Health Care for the Elderly: *Regional Responses to National Policy Issues.* April 17-18, 1985.
6. Lawton, M. P.: Geropsychological knowledge as a background for psychotherapy with older people. *J Geriatr Psychiatry* 1976; 9:221–234.
7. Andres, R., Bierman, E. L., Hazzard, W. R., et al. *Principles of geriatric medicine.* New York: McGraw-Hill, 1985.
8. Silverstone, B., & Hyman, H. K. *You and your aging parent.* New York: Pantheon Books, 1976.
9. Leigh, G. K. Kinship interaction over the family life span. *Journal of Marriage and the Family,* 1982; 44(1):197–208.
10. Troll, L. E. Parents and children in later life. *Generations—Quarterly Journal of the American Society on Aging* 1986; 10(4):23–25.
11. Aranson, S., & Sadin, S. Legal and financial planning for incapacity, in *Support for family caregivers of the elderly: Proceedings of a national symposium.* Washington, DC: National Council on Aging, 1984, pp. 43–54.
12. McRoberts, A. Interview, *Houston Chronicle,* April 11, 1976, p. 21.
13. Zarit, S. H. The organic brain syndromes and family relationships, in Ragan, P. K. (ed): *Aging parents,* Los Angeles: University of Southern California, 1979.

UNIT 2

FAMILY HEALTH NURSING RESEARCH

Nurses need to stay current in many changing areas of health care. The application of nursing research is vital to the profession. The articles selected for this section provide insights into family nursing issues, trends, and evolving theory-based research. In addition, future directions in family nursing research are exemplified. The articles also contain relevant findings that will help move family nursing toward a theoretical body of knowledge that will guide practice. All of the articles were written by authors with expertise in particular areas.

CHAPTER 14

Issues Related to the Unit of Analysis in Family Nursing Research[1]

Constance R. Uphold, Ora L. Strickland

The family has become an important focus of nursing research (Feetham, 1984); however, the nursing literature provides only a few guidelines on the family research process (Barnard, 1984; Gilliss, 1983). Although family research methods have characteristics that are similar to those of studies on individuals, the distinctive features of families pose unique challenges to nurse researchers. Families represent more than a set of discrete individuals. Family members interact with each other as well as observing and internalizing the actions of other members (Laing, 1971). Because the family is more than the sum of its individual members, a major issue facing nurse researchers who study families is the choice and use of the appropriate unit of analysis.

The purpose of this article is to discuss factors that should be considered by nurse researchers when deciding to use one informant versus several informants in family research. Next, several strategies for combining individual family member data into scores that reflect the family as a unit will be considered as well as related assumptions, benefits, and limitations of each approach.

THE ONE INDIVIDUAL INFORMANT

Traditionally, family researchers in nursing as well as other disciplines have relied on one family member, primarily the wife or a college student, for information about

From *Western Journal of Nursing Research, Vol. 11* (No. 4), 1989, pp. 405–417. Copyright © 1989 by Sage Publications, Inc. Reprinted by permission of Sage Publications, Inc.

family phenomena (Olson, 1977). Recently, the use of only one family member as an informant has been devalued because this approach is believed to result in a biased perspective of family phenomena (Straus, 1964). However, the use of one informant in family study may be preferable. The choice of who and how many family respondents should be included in a study depends on the theory underlying the study and the research question. The individual informant may provide important data on the relational properties between family members. For example, the individual respondent may be asked to make two reports, one on his or her individual characteristics and one on the perceived individual characteristics of other persons in the family. Information on the family relationship can be obtained by deriving a score of association between the informant's two reports and delineating a pattern (Thompson & Walker, 1982). An example of a research question using this approach is, How similar are wives' health beliefs to their perceptions of their husbands' health beliefs?

Rather than statistically deriving an association, the researcher may ask the informant to estimate the congruency between various members' individual characteristics. The question then becomes, Do wives perceive similarity between their health beliefs and those of their husband or child? If the researcher simply asks the respondent to comment on a family attribute, the question is, What do women perceive the health beliefs of their families to be?

The major assumption underlying the examples presented above is that the individual family member's perspective is a valuable source of information about family phenomena. Thus personal constructions of family experience are accorded the highest priority. Such constructions are accorded primacy by theories such as symbolic interaction, attribution, and crisis theory. These theories assume that it is the individual's perceptions that shape his or beliefs, values, and behaviors and those of others. Because one's perceptions are assumed to be the guiding force behind behavior within the family, it becomes most logical for the individual to become the unit of analysis for the study.

In a similar vein, one family member may be the most appropriate source for data collection when the study is based on ecological theory and the family is viewed as the context for individual growth, development, and well-being. Several nursing research studies have been reported that viewed the family as the environment of the individual (Feetham, 1984; MacCarthy & Morison, 1972). For example, a nurse researcher would be justified in using one family member as the informant when his or her perceptions of the family's influence on his or her health, well-being, or treatment were the focus of study. The single-informant approach also may enable a family member openly to express feelings, perceptions, and family secrets that would not be divulged if the whole family were questioned together (Thomas, 1987).

Only one informant may be used in studies in which the researcher assumes that one individual in the family is the most accurate and knowledgeable member. For example, the family member who manages the family's domestic affairs or who is the primary care provider for an ill member may be more attuned to family events and perceptions important to the research than other less involved family members. The member who stays at home daily would be acceptable as the sole informant on topics such as family accident proneness and family dietary practices.

The weak-link model is a good example of how the researcher's theoretical perspective can justify and guide the selection of a single family informant's scores for addressing a research question. In this approach, data are collected from all relevant family members but *only* the extreme or deviant family member's score is used to reflect the family variable of interest. The ultimate outcome is that one family member becomes the informant, but the choice is based on the deviance of his or her scores. The assumption of this approach is that a family can function only to the level of the least-functioning individual member. For instance, it can be convincingly argued that a couple is likely to have marital difficulties when one spouse is dissatisfied (Baucom & Mehlman, 1984). Another example is that family conflict is likely to occur if any member of the family is unwilling to make changes or is blind to the problems of the family.

Choosing the most deviant score to represent the family unit has the greatest potential use when there are extreme scores and a wide range of variance among family members (Fisher, Kokes, Ransom, Phillips, & Rudd, 1985). On the other hand, it can be argued that researchers using this approach will be losing valuable information by discarding all but the most extreme member's score. It is possible that the deviant member's score reflects a high portion of measurement error. In this case, the researcher would be replacing valid information from the majority of family members with less valid data from one deviant member.

On a pragmatic note, collecting data from one source is less costly and creates fewer statistical analysis problems than collecting data from many family members. However, the one-informant approach limits the generalizability of conclusions because data derived from such studies cannot automatically be related to findings from studies using multiple respondents. The one-informant approach provides only one person's "reality." It may be convincingly argued that the family has dynamic and emergent properties that cannot be sufficiently studied by asking one respondent to describe the family experience.

MULTIPLE FAMILY MEMBERS AS INFORMANTS

It has been suggested that researchers will gain greater insight into family phenomena by measuring the responses of multiple family members (Szinovacz, 1983). This is particularly the case in situations in which studies are based on conceptual frameworks, such as family systems theory or structural-functionalism, that may necessitate obtaining information from the perspective of several family members. However, using several family members as respondents does not guarantee that more reliable and valid family data will be obtained. Combining the responses or scores of several family members can present problems. Researchers working with multiple scores on the same variable from various family members struggle with problems arising from correlated measures, particularly at the data analysis stage. Another concern is related to the bias that may be created when the researcher cannot obtain data from the entire family unit because one or more family members choose not to participate. Extensive efforts to recruit and retain all family members as participants in a study are often required to decrease the likelihood of bias.

When data from multiple family members are used, problems with scoring arise. In a study using combined scores from multiple family members, measurement error is likely to be increased. Every score on a measure is composed of a true score and error. The composite family score thus reflects the addition of true scores as well as error from the various members' scores. Certain constructs may be appropriate for study at the level of the individual but may be meaningless at the level of the family. For example, summing the scores of individual family members' physical health status and calling the resultant score a measure of family health would be inappropriate (White, 1984).

An additional problem in family measurement is that most instruments are designed for one informant. If an instrument was designed to be used by one family member, it is best to employ it in the way it was intended. Because family members are in different stages of development, it may be inappropriate to use a single instrument for all members.

Researchers can benefit from using multiple family respondents for triangulation. In this approach data are obtained from several sources on the same variable to assess convergent validity (Mitchell, 1986). Gathering data on the same phenomenon from different family members can provide the investigator with evidence regarding the validity of data obtained and instruments used. It also is lucrative to employ data from several family members to reflect the family as a whole. There are several approaches to combining the scores of individual family members. These are discussed below.

The Summative Approach

One way of handling data from multiple family respondents is to add all the individual scores to obtain a summative score. This approach assumes that each member of the family has an equal and important role in describing family experiences. There is not a differential weighting based on age, developmental level, position, or sex (Fisher et al., 1985). The summative approach, then, does not reflect the inherent differences in power and authority that reside in most families. It does not recognize that some family members, such as the mother or father, by virtue of their position and history may have a more comprehensive view of the family than the children.

The summative approach also assumes that familial relationships are such that low scores of one family member can be directly counterbalanced by the other family members' high scores (Baucom & Mehlman, 1984). Thus a family that has a score of 120 on a family stress response measure could have one member who is highly stressed with a score of 80 and two members who have low stress levels with scores of 20 each. Another family that has a score of 120 may have three members who each rate their stress level moderately with scores of 40. Although most clinicians and researchers would probably agree that the two families are fundamentally different in terms of stress, the summative score approach fails to reveal these differences.

The derivation of the summative family score has the advantage of being simple and easily replicable from study to study, and it increases the range and variance of family scores. This increase in variance may be beneficial in detecting statistical differences among families in subsequent analyses.

A major weakness of the summative approach is that summative score comparisons cannot be made between families of different sizes. Therefore, the researcher would have to sample families with the same number of members or exclude certain members of larger families.

As Fisher et al. (1985) note, the interpretation of a summative score may be problematic when the "family" score exceeds the upper limit of the scale measuring the family phenomenon. For instance, a family score of 120 lacks theoretical meaning if the actual instrument has a maximum of 80 points.

When using the summative approach, important information concerning the patterns within the family are lost. For instance, a high composite score on family cohesion suggests that the family is functioning well. However, this high score may be mainly a function of one member's perception of near perfection in the family.

The Family Mean Score

In the family mean score approach individual members' scores are added and then averaged. An advantage is that the upper limit of the scale measuring the family phenomenon will never be exceeded. Thus the family's relative position on psychometric instruments can be interpreted. Averaging individuals' scores enables the researcher to make comparisons among families with different numbers of members. The mean score also may portray the family unit in ways other scores cannot by reflecting everyday family living that often involves compromises (Olson & McCubbin, 1983). For example, a researcher interested in studying division of labor in households that provide care to an elderly parent may assume that the siblings' behaviors reflect a compromise that has evolved through negotiation.

The mean score approach has the drawback of reducing score variance. The mean score of several family members will be less varied than the original individual scores. Reducing the variance can affect statistical conclusion validity when subsequent analyses are undertaken. The scores of family members who have extremely high or low ratings may be hidden when a family average is used, particularly in large families. There is a relationship between family size and the influence of deviant individuals on the final mean score (Fisher et al., 1985).

The Maximized Family Score

The assumption underlying this approach is that an event happening to one family member will have an impact on all other members and thereby affect the family as a unit. This approach is consistent with theories, such as family systems theory, that focus on the interrelatedness of family members. To obtain a maximized family score, family members are questioned and if any member notes an event as occurring it is included in scoring as a "family" event. A single score for the family variable measured is derived that represents all involved family members' views. Olson and McCubbin (1983) used this approach in their family stress and coping study. If either the wife or husband indicated a stressful occurrence, it was rated as a stressor for the couple. When both individuals checked the event as distressing, it still was counted as only one occurrence.

There are other areas in which the maximized family score approach may be applicable, such as health care visits, conflicts, and complaints (Fisher et al., 1985). This approach may be useful when studying discrete situational events or when there are so many events occurring that accurate recall by a single person is impossible. However, it is questionable whether minor stressors that occur outside the home—for example, at school or work—have a notable impact on the whole family.

The maximized family score approach has the advantage of representing all family members' perceptions in a single score, but this strength can also be considered a limitation. If one family member's perceptions are biased or incorrect, they are included in the overall score, which inflates measurement error and reduced the validity of the score.

The Difference Approach

In this approach, differences between family members' responses are of central concern. Whereas summative and mean scores conceal discrepancies, the difference approach highlights the incongruity of responses. An assumption is that each individual has a unique perception of the family and by focusing on the divergence of the members' perceptions, greater knowledge of family dynamics can be obtained. Lending credence to the conceptual importance of studying family member differences are studies that show that discrepancies are related to certain negative outcomes, such as conflict (Billings, 1979); stress (McCubbin et al., 1980); and relationship dissatisfaction (Birchler & Webb, 1977).

There are several conceptual problems in using the difference model. Typically, a discrepancy index that involves computing the difference between family members' responses is used. This index can be obtained either by subtracting one member's total score from another member's score and converting this to an absolute value (Olson & McCubbin, 1983) or by calculating differences for each item. A discrepancy score demonstrates the degree of divergence between the members' responses; it does not reveal the location of a family along a scale continuum, nor does it reveal the direction of the difference (Tiggle, Peters, Kelley, & Vincent, 1982). For instance, Family A and Family B both have discrepancy scores of 5. However, in Family A the two members have scores of 45 and 50, whereas the two members of Family B have scores of 5 and 10. It is probable that Family A functions quite differently from Family B although their discrepancy scores are equal. Therefore, simple discrepancy scores may be conceptually misleading (Baucom & Mehlman, 1984; Fisher et al., 1985).

Discrepancy scores contain less variance than the original family members' scores; this tends to reduce the power of subsequent statistical analyses. To circumvent this problem, score transformations or weights can be used (Cohen & Cohen, 1983; Fisher et al., 1985). In addition, differences between family members may simply reflect measurement error rather than true perceptual differences (Douglas & Wind, 1978; Quarm, 1981; Schumm, 1982). Thus interpreting differences as theoretically important must be done cautiously.

There is controversy about how to calculate differences between family members. As previously noted, a discrepancy score may be calculated by subtracting one member's score from another, by counting the number of items all family members agree upon, or by using a percentage to represent the item agreement. Both sums and percentages provide valuable descriptive data but have restricted use for most statistical analyses (Olson & McCubbin, 1983).

Correlations between the responses of family members have often been used to examine discrepancies. A low correlation between the responses of family members would reflect that differences exist. However, the results of correlational analysis may be misleading. A correlation coefficient demonstrates the extent to which family members' scores rise and fall together, but it does not demonstrate distance between the scores (Schumm, 1982).

Olson and McCubbin (1983), in their stress study, calculated couple ratio scores by dividing the score for each spouse by the sum of scores of both individuals. In addition to detecting spousal differences, the ratio score indicates the relative balance in the relationship on the dimension of concern. However, the ratio does not provide an indication of the location of the couple on a scale continuum.

Others have investigated discrepancies via aggregate-level analyses. In this approach, the mean responses of husbands and wives or children and parents are compared. For instance, when individual family members' scores are not highly correlated, group t-tests, one-way analysis of variance, and discriminant analysis for multiple dependent variables are appropriate statistical procedures (Schumm, Barnes, Ballman, Jurich, & Milliken, 1985). Although this type of analysis provides important information on how groups of people differ across families, it must not be considered intra- or within-family analysis (Thompson & Walker, 1982; Troll & Bengtson, 1979). To actually investigate differences between family members paired t-tests, agreement coefficients (Robinson, 1957) or repeated measures designs (Ball, McKenry, & Price-Bonham, 1983) should be used because they provide statistical indices of differences between family members' scores.

Combined Approaches

Baucom and Mehlman (1984) suggest that a sum plus difference model may be used when the researcher is interested in the overall level of the family score as well as the discrepancies in scores. The researcher can simply add both summative and discrepancy scores together. Alternatively, one can weight the mean couple score by the discrepancy score or vice versa (Fisher et al., 1985). The combined approaches are easy to calculate and have pragmatic appeal. However, the assumptions and conceptual underpinnings of the summative and difference approaches are not congruent. Therefore, combining two conceptually different approaches to derive a score may create problems in interpreting results.

Typological Analysis Approach

In this approach psychometric measures with different categories are used to classify families into various types, based upon theory. The researcher can compare family types (used as a nominal measure) on one or more dependent variables with chi-square, analysis of variance, or discriminant analysis. Furthermore, the use of typologies may be useful in reducing data to a manageable level with complicated models in which two or more family members provide responses regarding several independent and dependent variables (Olson, 1981; Schumm et al., 1985). Examples of types of nursing studies in which such typologies might be derived are those that deal with married couples' responses to spousal illnesses, and parental or family responses to the illness or death of a child.

Multivariate Approaches for Dealing with Multiple Family Data

Multiple regression procedures for analysis of family data offer the researcher the opportunity to insert the level, discrepancy, and order scores into an equation to predict a dependent variable (Fisher et al., 1985). For example, the researcher could include a family's summed cohesion score, a score based on the differences in family members' perceptions of cohesion, and information concerning the member who had the highest cohesion score to predict the family's level of stress. One danger of this procedure is that the three independent variables are likely to be highly correlated. Multicollinearity results in unstable beta coefficients and difficulty interpreting results.

A covariance-based scoring technique is another possible way to use responses of several family members (Schumm & Kirn, 1982). Covariance-based weights can be obtained via factor analysis, canonical correlation, multiple regression, discriminant analysis, or simple correlation. The derivation of the weights, however, requires the use of a large sample of families (Walters, Pittman, & Norrell, 1984).

In commonality analysis (Walters et al., 1984) the original scores of family members are weighted in various ways, depending on the theoretical orientation of the researcher. By combining family members' scores, commonality analysis can be used to partition the resulting pool of variance. The pooled variance can be partitioned by focusing on the variance common to all family members, by using the variance shared by at least two members, or by taking the variance that is unique to each family member.

A major limitation of using multivariate weighting for the analysis of family data is that it makes the comparison of results across studies virtually impossible. Data from each family member in a particular study determines the way the final family profile evolves. Therefore, unless other studies use the same combination of family members and the same weights for each family member's score, comparisons between studies would be meaningless.

Cluster analysis has also been used to analyze family data (Douglas & Wind, 1978; Filsinger, McAvoy, & Lewis, 1982) to find family patterns. Similar families are grouped together depending on the pattern or relationship among their scores. The groupings result in empirical family classifications that may then be useful in clinical practice to help identify family styles. The focus in cluster analysis is on describing families and generating theory rather than on exploring relationships among variables or testing theory (Fisher et al., 1985; Miller, Rollins, & Thomas, 1982). Cluster analysis requires a large sample. The resultant classifications may be conceptually meaningless (Fisher et al., 1985). Cluster analysis uses the data from various instruments that measure several dependent and/or independent variables to derive empirical classifications based on patterns of scores, whereas in the typological analysis approach described above, psychometric measures are designed specifically to classify family data based upon theory.

Confirmatory factor analysis and structural modeling (Fisher et al., 1985) also may be used for analysis of data from multiple family members. These approaches are designed to allow for measures that are correlated (Jöreskog & Sörbom, 1986). The researcher can identify and analyze the measures that share common method variance, and the correlated measures of family members can be included and analyzed accordingly (Miller, Rollins, & Thomas, 1982). A limitation of this strategy is the complexity of the statistical procedures.

CONCLUSION

The advantages and disadvantages of several strategies for obtaining family relational data have been presented. Using one individual member as an informant for the family can provide valuable information. Likewise, the combining of multiple family members' scores into a unit or composite score can offer a different perspective on families.

All the strategies described have unique strengths and weaknesses. Before making a decision, the researcher should carefully evaluate the assumptions underlying each approach. The choice of who should be the source of data collection must be based on the purpose of the study, the research question, the theoretical basis of the study, and the specific unit about whom the researcher intends to generalize. When data are obtained from multiple family members, it also is incumbent upon the researcher to become thoroughly familiar with the characteristics of the data. A better decision can then be made regarding appropriate manipulation of data to represent family phenomena. A researcher may use several approaches together for handling multiple family data given his or her purposes, research questions, conceptual framework, and the nature of the data.

NOTE

The authors gratefully acknowledge Dr. Elizabeth R. Lenz for her suggestions regarding this manuscript.

REFERENCES

Ball, D., McKenry, P. C., & Price-Bonham, S. (1983). Use of repeated measures in family research. *Journal of Marriage and the Family, 45*, 885–896.

Barnard, K. E. (1984). The family as a unit of measurement. *Maternal Child Nursing, 9*, 21.

Baucom, D. H., & Mehlman, S. K. (1984). Predicting marital status following behavioral marital therapy: A comparison of models of marital relationships. In K. Hahlweg & N. S. Jacobson (Eds.), *Marital interaction analysis and modification* (pp. 89–104). New York: Guilford Press.

Billings, A. (1979). Conflict resolution in distressed and non-distressed married couples. *Journal of Consulting and Clinical Psychology, 47*, 368–376.

Birchler, G. R., & Webb, L. J. (1977). Discriminating interaction behaviors in happy and unhappy marriages. *Journal of Consulting and Clinical Psychology, 45,* 341–343.

Cohen, J., & Cohen, P. (1983). *Applied multiple regression/correlation analysis for the behavioral sciences.* Hillsdale, NJ: Lawrence Erlbaum.

Douglas, S. P., & Wind, Y. (1978). Examining family role and authority patterns: Two methodological issues. *Journal of Marriage and the Family, 40,* 35–47.

Feetham, S. L. (1984). Family research: Issues and directions for nursing. In H. Werley, & J. J. Fitzpatrick (Eds.), *Annual review of nursing research* (Vol. 2, pp. 3–25). New York: Springer.

Filsinger, E. E., McAvoy, P., & Lewis, R. A. (1982). An empirical typology of dyadic formation. *Family Process, 21,* 321–325.

Fisher, L., Kokes, R. F., Ransom, D. C., Phillips, S. L., & Rudd, P. (1985). Alternative strategies for creating "relational" family data. *Family Process, 24,* 213–224.

Gilliss, C. L. (1983). The family as a unit of analysis: Strategies for the nurse researcher. *Advances in Nursing Science, 5,* 50–59.

Jöreskog, K. G., & Sörbom, D. (1986). *LISREL VI: Analysis of linear structural relationships by maximum likelihood, instrumental variables, and least squares methods.* Sweden: University of Uppsala, Department of Statistics.

Laing, R. D. (1971). *The politics of the family and other essays.* New York: Pantheon Books.

MacCarthy, J., & Morison, J. (1972). An explanatory test of a method of studying illness among preschool children. *Nursing Research, 21,* 319–326.

McCubbin, H. I., Joy, C. B., Cauble, A. E., Compeau, J. K., Patterson, J. M., & Needle, R. H. (1980). Family stress and coping: A decade review. *Journal of Marriage and the Family, 42,* 855–871.

Miller, B. C., Rollins, B. C., & Thomas, D. L. (1982). On methods of studying marriages and families. *Journal of Marriage and the Family, 44,* 851–872.

Mitchell, E. F. (1986). Multiple-triangulation: A methodology for nursing science. *Advances in Nursing Science, 8,* 18–26.

Olson, D. H. (1977). Insiders' and outsiders' views of relationships: Research studies. In G. Levinger & H. L. Raush (Eds.), *Close relationships: Perspectives on the meaning of intimacy* (pp. 115–135). Amherst: University of Massachusetts Press.

Olson, D. H. (1981). Family typologies: Bridging family research and family therapy. In E. E. Filsinger & R. A. Lewis (Eds.). *Assessing marriage: New behavioral approaches* (pp. 74–89). Beverly Hills, CA: Sage.

Olson, D. H., & McCubbin, H. I. (1983). *Families: What makes them work?* Beverly Hills, CA: Sage.

Quarm, D. (1981). Random measurement error as a source of discrepancies between the reports of wives and husbands concerning marital power and task allocation. *Journal of Marriage and the Family, 43,* 521–535.

Robinson, W. S. (1957). The statistical measurement of agreement. *American Sociological Review, 22,* 17–25.

Schumm, W. R. (1982). Integrating theory, measurement and data analysis in family studies survey research. *Journal of Marriage and the Family, 44,* 983–998.

Schumm, W. R., Barnes, H. L., Ballman, S. R., Jurich, A. P., & Milliken, G. A. (1985). Approaches to statistical analysis of family data. *Home Economics Research Journal, 14,* 112–122.

Schumm, W. R., & Kirn, J. E. (1982). Evaluating equity in the marital relationship. *Psychological Reports, 51,* 759–762.

Straus, M. A. (1964). Measuring families. In H. T. Christensen (Ed.), *Handbook of marriage and the family* (pp. 335–398). Skokie, IL: Rand McNally.

Szinovacz, M. E. (1983). Using couple data as a methodological tool: The case of marital violence. *Journal of Marriage and the Family, 45,* 633–644.

Thomas, R. B. (1987). Methodological issues and problems in family health care research. *Journal of Marriage and the Family, 49,* 65–70.

Thompson, L., & Walker, A. J. (1982). The dyad as the unit of analysis: Conceptual and methodological issues. *Journal of Marriage and the Family, 44,* 889–900.

Tiggle, R. B., Peters, M. D., Kelley, H. H., & Vincent, J. (1982). Correlational and discrepancy indices of understanding and their relation to marital satisfaction. *Journal of Marriage and the Family, 44,* 209–215.

Troll, L., & Bengtson, V. (1979). Generations in the family. In W. R. Burr, R. Hill, F. I. Nye, & I. L. Reiss (Eds.), *Contemporary theories about the family* (Vol. 1, pp. 127–161). New York: Free Press.

Walters, L. H., Pittman, J. F., & Norrell, J. E. (1984). Development of a quantitative measure of a family from self-reports of family members. *Journal of Family Issues, 5,* 497–513.

White, J. M. (1984). Not the sum of its parts. *Journal of Family Issues, 5,* 515–518.

CHAPTER 15

Health Promotion in the Family: Current Findings and Directives for Nursing Research

Mary E. Duffy

This paper reviews the current nursing research findings on health promotion within the family and provides directives for future research. The concept of health promotion—the overall enhancement of well-being—is contrasted with primary or disease prevention, the specific protection from a health threat. The conceptual parameters of health promotion were used to search the nursing research journals for studies of health promotion in the family. The four major nursing research journals were reviewed and yielded five articles in 105 issues which addressed this phenomenon. The findings from these studies as well as other research literature are used to develop future directives. The directives are presented for both the internal environment of the family and its external environment. Areas for study related to the internal environment include definitions of health and health promotion, descriptions of current health promotion behaviours and those practised over time, decision making, fathering, and methods of intervention. Research of the external environment includes the societal norms, societal interventions, and the effects of societal institutions. This discussion of health promotion in the family describes an agenda for nursing research which is necessary to support nursing practice with families if 'health for all' is to be reached by the year 2000.

Reprinted from *Journal of Advanced Nursing, Vol. 13*, 1988, pp. 109–117. Used with permission of Blackwell Scientific Publications, Ltd., and the author.

THE FAMILY

The family influences the lifestyles—health and non-health behaviours—and health status of its members. As the basic unit of health care management, the family assumes responsibility for at least 75% of all health care provided to its members— health promotion, disease prevention, early intervention, and rehabilitation. Nursing research is contributing to the development of a knowledge base which describes the interaction beween family dynamics and the prevention and treatment of diseases. However, researchers have neglected to study with comparable zeal the health promotion activities of the family. Although the family is a client of nursing (American Nurses' Association 1980, World Health Organization 1985) the majority of health promotion research reported in the nursing research journals are studies of individuals. The purposes of this paper are to review the current nursing research findings on health promotion within the family and to provide directives for future research.

HEALTH PROMOTION

According to Pender (1982) health promotion is those 'activities directed toward *sustaining* or *increasing* the level of well-being, self-actualization, and personal fulfillment.' In contrast to disease or primary prevention—the specific protection from a health threat—the purpose of health promotion is a generalized enhancement of well-being. The generalized nature of health promotion suggests it is or should be an integrated component of the lifestyle of individuals and families and of the environment created by the social structure. Health promotion behaviours are used to increase the level of adaptive health for an individual or group and not to remove a specific threat to health. This latter health goal defines disease or primary prevention behaviours. For example, an individual may begin a health programme of jogging and weight loss. If the goal is primary prevention, the health behaviours might be undertaken specifically to decrease the risk of heart disease. However, if the goal is health promotion, the same health behaviours could lead to an enhancement in overall healthiness: emotional, feelings of exuberance; physical, increased strength and stamina; and social, improvements in the quantity and quality of relationships. Similarly, the family that applies the principles of health promotion to its lifestyle may prioritize family recreational time since it is an opportunity for the individuals to spend time in an activity that is enjoyable for them and brings them closer together physically and emotionally.

At the environmental level, health promotion is the development of an environment which is conducive to overall healthiness. These conditions are more than the essential characteristics of an environment designed to eliminate specific health problems such as smallpox, lead poisoning, adolescent suicide, or smoking behaviours. Instead, health promotion alters the underlying social structure which creates the stressors that lead, eventually, to specific health problems. These stressors include economic and social policies which affect the distribution of basic resources including food, shelter, sanitation and safety. 'Current assessment of world health policy indicates that lack of basic needs is the primary barrier to wellness' (McFarlane 1985).

While health promotion and disease prevention behaviours are not mutually exclusive activities, it is important to differentiate between the two concepts. Since health promotion has a broader focus than primary prevention, the definition of health changes in the health promotion framework. Health is not merely the absence of disease or the risks of disease but it is 'a dynamic state of being in which the developmental and behavioural potential of an individual is realized to the fullest extent possible' (ANA 1980). When these conceptual distinctions are applied to research, the ensuing directives for health promotion research and those for primary or disease prevention research are quite varied (Merritt 1986). Health promotion research addresses the general health of the population and the development of that population to its fullest potential. Disease prevention research investigates factors specific to a particular illness, disability or condition and the interventions necessary to prevent the problem.

Lifestyles

In practice and in research, the study of health promotion is inseparable from the study of lifestyles, typical ways of life. The behaviours associated with health promotion are the components of the family's lifestyle. Exercise, good nutrition, stress reduction, hygiene, and rest become part of the family's daily routine, a lifestyle shaped by a philosophy of health. This integration between a philosophy of health and the family's lifestyle does not develop in isolation within the family. Societal factors influence the health perceptions of family members and the emotional, physical and material ability of the family to incorporate health promotion into its lifestyle.

According to Milio (1985), health instruction works; that is, behaviour change results, when individual or family education is reinforced by a social and political climate which supports a healthy environment. Issues of concern at this level include media portrayals of violence, alcohol use, and smoking; the distribution of material resources; access to health care; and the provision of basic human needs; housing, food, employment, etc. Individuals, families, and societies that practice health promotion behaviours are concerned with the impact of all their activities—from individual decisions to societal policies—on the health of individuals, families and the community. Therefore, a research agenda on family health promotion must look at the effects of the internal and external environments of the family on their health promotion behaviours.

NURSING AND HEALTH PROMOTION

The conceptual distinction between health promotion and primary prevention is very important in nursing since nurses provide a large part of health care, not medical care, in most countries (WHO 1985). Health promotion guides the nurse and client away from a definition of health as the absence of disease and towards a concern with generalized well-being. This latter concern directs the focus of care and research to the lifestyle and environment of the client. The enhancement of well-being in the presence or absence of disease becomes a legitimate arena for nursing practice, research and education.

The following examples describe health promotion issues that are concerns of nursing at the local, national and international levels. For example, in western countries lifestyle contributes over 50% to the development of chronic illnesses (Dever 1980) and for many children these lifestyle patterns have led to the development of at least one risk factor for cardiovascular disease before the age of 12 years (William *et al.* 1981). The affluence which leads to the diseases of excess in the developed countries overshadows the grave conditions of the poor in these same countries. In the United States there are 35 million poor Americans and 13.3 million of those poor are children. The State of Maine Child Death Survey estimated that 10,000 American children die each year from poverty (Children's Defense Fund 1985). The report indicates that each year poor children are three times more likely to die than non-poor children. More specifically, poverty in American children is concentrated in certain ethnic groups: 48% of the poor children are black, and 38% are hispanic, compared to 17% who are caucasian.

These same contrasting patterns of excess and impoverishment seen in the United States are present between developed and developing countries. Lifestyle patterns and the environment threaten well-being throughout the world. In developing countries insufficient environmental resources perpetuate lifestyles characterized by inadequate nutrition, unsanitary conditions, mobility, and other factors which prevent families from realizing their potential well-being. These families can only be concerned with survival in environments which perpetuate malnutrition and disease.

The international arena becomes a significant environment for families in poor countries. The willingness of resource rich countries like the United States to contribute to the development of poorer countries is a political decision. Yet it is the financial and people power assistance that many countries need to supplement their own plans and actions. In a recent issue of *The Nations Health*, a newsletter of the American Public Health Association, Ruth Roemer (1986), the association's president, reported on the health promotion outcome in a poor, developing country of Asia when money from the community and central government was combined with multilateral and bilateral foreign aid. The result was the construction of structures which make available safe water and ventilated pit-latrines for each household. This example of international co-operation describes health promotion at its most rudimentary level in a developing country.

Nursing is in a position to have an impact on the decisions made in each of the preceding situations. Through research focused on health and health promotion, nurses can create an improvement in the well-being of individuals, families and communities. Since the family is the basic unit of health care, the study of health promotion activities in the family should be a critical area of concern for nurse researchers. If 'health for all' is to be reached by the year 2000 (WHO 1979), health promotion in the family must be prioritized on the nursing research agendas.

HEALTH PROMOTION RESEARCH: THE NURSING RESEARCH JOURNALS

Current findings indicate that research of health promotion in the family is, for all essential purposes, non-existent in the nursing research journals. Four nursing research journals—*Nursing Research, Research in Nursing and Health, Western Journal of Nursing Research* and *International Journal of Nursing Studies*—were reviewed to identify the number and types of studies related to health promotion in the family which were published between January 1980 and June 1986. Health promotion in the family was defined as follows: those health activities undertaken by a unit consisting of at least one adult caretaker and one child for the purposes of sustaining or enhancing the level of physical, emotional, and social well-being of the family and its individual members. This research analysis included studies of societal and family factors which influence the practice of health promotion in the family.

The review was done by the articles' titles and abstracts. First, each article title was reviewed. If a title indicated even a remote relationship between the study purpose and health promotion in the family, the abstract was read. If further clarification was needed the article was read.

The results of this review of 105 issues of the journals yielded five articles (4.8%) which addressed health promotion activities in the family. One article was instrument development, one looked at the provision of child care services through the types of day care the children attended, and three articles were family studies. These latter articles investigated aspects of family dynamics and the practise of health promotion behaviours. For example, O'Brien (1980) researched the relationships between mother-child communication and the child's exploratory behaviour and self-differentiation. She found a positive and significant correlation between the overall pattern of parental acknowledgement of the child and the child's differentiation of self. Among the non-significant findings reported by O'Brien (1980) was a trend which indicated differing expectations by mothers for boys and girls.

A study of one-parent families headed by women found the general lifestyle patterns of the mother influenced the practice of health promotion behaviours in the family (Duffy 1986). The more psychological growth experienced by the woman as an outcome of her status as a solo parent, the more the family tried new health promotion behaviours for the purpose of enhancing personal well-being.

Other studies of health promotion reported in these journals focused on individuals. In fact, the overwhelming majority of the studies used the individual as the research participant and studied either disease prevention or intervention behaviours. These findings were not unexpected since it has been reported elsewhere that despite the practice emphasis on families, nursing research has continued its individual orientation (Murphy 1986) and, until recently, its selection of families from populations identified as pathological or abnormal (Feetham 1984).

Without further nursing research on health promotion in the family, practitioners will not have a sufficient body of knowledge to influence public and health policy and to work with individuals and families in the promotion of their health. According to O'Brien (1980):

> The literature abounds with speculation as to the kind of parental behaviours that facilitate the child's developmental progress. Yet, there is a paucity of research on parent-child communication and its relation to child development using subjects

drawn from populations of 'healthy' parents and children. Such research is needed in order to build a substantive body of knowledge for health promotion.

Fortunately the empirical knowledge on health promotion in the family is not limited to what exists in the nursing research journals. The range of health promotion studies is rather extensive since health promotion is concerned with lifestyle behaviours and the family's environment. These studies include, but are not limited to, the development of health promotion attitudes and behaviours in family members; the influence of the media, especially television, on viewers; the impact of social policies; nutrition; and parent-child communication. In the next section of this paper some of the current findings on health promotion in the family will be used to provide directives for future nursing research.

DIRECTIVES FOR STUDYING
HEALTH PROMOTION IN THE FAMILY

Health promotion in the family is the result of an interaction between the internal environment of the family and the external environment which impinges upon it. Family dynamics, the interrelationships among the family members, are the internal conditions which affect health promotion behaviours. The external environment consists of several influences: kinship network, neighbourhood, community, and the larger society. The research directives which follow will be discussed in two categories: family dynamics and the external environment.

Family Dynamics

The study of health promotion in the family begins with family dynamics. The influence of the mother—specifically her level of education, her health attitudes, and her health practices—has been documented in several studies to be a significant influence on the health practices of her children. For example, in a follow-up study of childhood symptomatology, Mechanic (1979) found that young adults who reported fewer symptoms remembered their parents emphasizing self-care and health promotion. In a study of Chilean children (McFarlane 1985), the researcher found that children with one or more infections, when compared to healthy children, were more likely to have a mother who was healthy, educated, and older—at least 35 years of age. For these children, characteristics of the mother directly influenced their health status.

The family's influences on the development of health promotion practices is both direct and indirect. While the family is the major socializer of preschool and school-aged children, their influence goes beyond the obvious promotion of health—food choices, exercise, hygiene, sleep, etc. The family establishes a norm which directs the decision-making of its members in areas of friendships, media, recreation, work, school, etc. (Mullen 1983). For example, parents can either encourage, tolerate, discourage, or forbid children from watching television violence. Research indicates that television does influence its viewers and appears to be related to increased aggressive behaviour (Pearl *et al.* 1982), socialization toward an active consumer role, and perceptions of the 'real' world that parallel the television stereotypes (Rubinstein & Brown 1985). On the other hand, television can be used as a positive influence on health (Milio 1985). Parents are in a position to differentiate between these various effects of television and to decide for themselves and their children the type of viewing that is permissible. Yet, parents and the family are not the sole influencers on the child. At varying degrees of intensity through the child's life, age, peers, school, television, and medical care temper the family's influence (Mullen 1983).

Decision-making or problem-solving is another dimension of parenting that contributes to health promotion practices of children. Lewis & Lewis (1982) found that children with poor health-related decision-making skills had difficulty making decisions in other areas of their lives. This same decision-making pattern was seen in a study of one-parent families headed by women (Duffy 1984). The women who made general lifestyle decisions which were growth oriented and motivated towards change, practised and encouraged health promotion behaviours for themselves and their children. Women who made decisions by default—letting what happens happen—or maintained routine behaviours, used the same pattern in their health practices. These women did not seek new health information or attempt to change their behaviour patterns. For example, the latter group of women and their children may have brushed their teeth or practised good hygiene because it was an established routine but they did not attempt to learn new health promoting behaviours that could enhance their well-being.

Parenting style itself can enhance health practices. The use of autonomy, reward and reason had a positive influence on the health practices of children (Pratt 1973, 1976). A study by Laskey & Eichelberger (1985) found that children whose parents transferred health self-care decision-making to them in a progressive and developmentally appropriate manner did practise self-care behaviours and could relate the reasons for practising these behaviours. Much more research is needed on these patterns of decision-making and their transfer from parents to children.

Directives for Future Research

There are several directives for future research on health promotion in the family which concern the family's internal dynamics. Table 1 lists the major research questions. To begin with, research which describes the health promotion behaviours in families is needed. This type of study could identify patterns of behaviours occurring in families. The richness of these data would be enhanced if the family studies were longitudinal so that changes in parental and child behaviours could be studied together and over time. Some research questions are: What are the health promotion practises and patterns in the family as a unit? What happens to the group interaction—the influence of the members on each other—and health promotion practices over time?

There are several research questions which investigate the family's perceptions of health and health promotion behaviours. The family's definition of health and health promotion, their perceptions of health promotion practices, and the value placed on health and health promotion behaviours are three areas of study. It is important to

TABLE 1

Health Promotion: Directives for Family Research

1. What are the family health promotion behaviours?
2. What changes occur, over time, in the family's health promotion behaviours?
3. What are the family's definitions of health and health promotion behaviours?
4. What is the value placed on health and health promotion behaviours? How does that value compare to other values in the family's life?
5. What is the influence of parenting style on the development of health promotion behaviours by children?
6. What is the influence of fathers on the health promotion behaviours of children?
7. What is the effect, if any, of various family characteristics on the family's health promotion behaviours?
8. What methods of intervention are most effective in encouraging health promotion in the family?

understand the family's definition of health promotion behaviours, otherwise the behaviours studied will be those identified by professionals only. In Duffy's (1986) study the families included washing clothes, hygiene, nutritional supplements, praying for health, and dressing for the weather in their lists of health promotion behaviours. This approach requires the researcher to ask families what they do to feel good and to improve their health rather than limit the inquiry to a list of behaviours for the family to respond to.

The value of health and health promotion behaviours within the context of the family environment needs study. An understanding is needed of the various stressors in families which distract families, even those with a commitment to health promotion, away from health promotion practices. Coeytaux (1984) recommended that researchers ask why some parents are more concerned about prevention (health promotion) than other parents and what accounts for the difference.

Parenting is a major research area in health promotion research. Areas for study include parenting styles which facilitate or prevent health promotion behaviours, parental methods for teaching health promotion to children, and parental decision-making styles and their relationship to health promotion behaviours. These areas of research can build upon works previously cited. For example, the relationships between decision making, in general and in specific, for health need further study. How do the parents' general patterns of decision making influence the child's pattern and what are the effects of health behaviour decision making? Does the use of autonomy in the parent-child relationship encourage health promotion practices throughout childhood or is it developmentally specific?

While the mother continues to be an important part of family health care, many fathers have become involved in this role. A dearth of knowledge exists regarding the relationships between characteristics of fathers and the practice of health promotion behaviours in families.

The findings from each of these research areas will, most likely, be affected by the characteristics of the family and in order to assist families in practice, knowledge about the influence of various family characteristics on their health promotion behaviours must be understood. These characteristics include family type (single or two parent); age of the family members; numbers of children; income; employment status; education; place (country) of residence; and so forth. An example of the dearth of information on family type and health is evident when the literature on single-parent families and health is reviewed. Despite the fact that 23% of all children in the United States are living with one parent and 90% of those children are living with their mothers, studies of female headed, single-parent families are virtually non-existent in the literature on family and health (Loveland-Cherry 1986).

Psychological Characteristics

In addition to demographic characteristics, an understanding is needed of the family's psychological characteristics. Do the family members believe they can impact their health by practising health promotion behaviours? How much control do family members believe they have over their own lives and how effective, do they believe, are their attempts to make changes in their lives?

Once a rich descriptive data base is available, research on interventions to encourage the practice of health promotion behaviours in families should occur. These interventions need to be tailored to the families and not reflect a Western, middle-class bias. For example, Butrin & Newman (1986) looked at time orientation and hemispheric dominance to assess the type of health promotion teaching programmes appropriate for a rural population in Zaire. In Haiti, a study was conducted of visual literacy among non-literates (Gustafson 1986). Both studies provide knowledge that can be used in the development of health promotion education programmes for families that are less likely to be responsive to didactic teaching. The research questions should investigate methods of transmitting health knowledge that build upon but are not limited to conventional health education approaches.

Other intervention studies can build on the family's role as a natural support group since support groups can encourage health promotion behaviours. Related research questions are: How does the family function as a support group in the promotion of health among its members? What types of support are needed by the members?

As stated earlier, the family exists in a larger social environment and is not immune from the influences of that environment. Therefore, it is necessary to study the family-environment interaction in order to understand the practice of health promotion behaviours in families.

External Environment

However influential the family is on the practices of health promotion by its members, the family cannot be studied in a vacuum. The influence of the larger society is pervasive in all countries regardless of the country's level of economic development.

As the options for health promotion available to the family decrease, the focus on society as the unit of intervention increases. For example, in countries in which the majority of people suffer from malnutrition, the family has few opportunities for health promotion since their struggle is to meet a basic human need (Maslow 1962). Society has the responsibility to help these children to meet their basic needs.

> However over-burdened or inefficient the individual parent, the health of the children is society's responsibility: it should not be *possible,* whatever the circumstances, for children to remain unimmunised (without conscientious objections) or to suffer the unnecessary worsening of chronic conditions (Blaxter and Patterson 1983).

In an intergenerational study of mothers and daughters, these same researchers reported that environment of poverty rather than the health behaviours and attitudes of mothers contributed to the accidents in the families. Poverty is the greatest threat to health promotion since it decreases the family's options, thus contributing to many of the health problems faced by the poor (Sidel 1986). However, societal interventions can facilitate health promotion in low-income families by providing needed services. A study in Bogotá, Colombia, found that a state run pre-school enhanced the well-being of the mothers and the children (de Ramos 1984). The mothers felt the benefits of this quality day-care programme were: (1) the possibility of improved income since the mother could look for employment while the child was at daycare, (2) socialization for mothers who were primarily isolated because of their demanding schedules, and (3) the alleviation of guilt experienced by mothers who leave their children at day-care.

Regardless of economic level, society establishes norms which facilitate or impede health promotion (Dwore & Kreuter 1980). For example, in the United States, there has been a noticeable decrease in smoking on television (Rubinstein & Brown 1985), a decrease which parallels the general decline in smoking among the population. Yet the commitment to prohibit smoking in the United States remains tenuous and as a result, smoking continues to be a problem within certain segments. Finland has demonstrated the effectiveness of a societal commitment to end smoking through governmental regulation in combination with health education and media intervention (Milio 1985).

Regulation and media are only two variables of the environment which impact family health promotion behaviours. The empirical study of the relationships between health promotion in the family and environmental conditions is fertile since little work has occurred in this area. Most health promotion research and practice targets the individual and the individual's responsibility to maintain her or his health. Yet it is difficult to separate the lifestyle behaviours of the individual from the environmental factors which shape those behaviours.

A few of the research questions to be asked are listed in Table 2. These questions include: How do the norms of society facilitate or impede the practice of health promotion behaviours in families? How does society define health? What support—financial, emotional, practical—does society offer for families to encourage health promotion? What are the effects of the societal institutions—political climate, religious tolerance, economic wealth—on the practice of health promotion behaviours in families? What role does health policy play?

TABLE 2
Health Promotion: Directives for Research of the External Environment

1. What role is society able and willing to play in the promotion of health in families?
2. What societal interventions can decrease the impact of poverty in families?
3. What are the societal norms regarding health promotion behaviours?
4. What are the effects of societal institutions on the practice of health promotion behaviours in families?

Answers to these questions will help us to understand the role of society in the practice of health promotion behaviours in families. Abdicating the responsibility for health promotion to families and individuals has not worked. 'Until the perceptions and values and norms of the larger society change, we cannot rationally expect individual behaviour to alter significantly' (Sidel 1986).

CONCLUSION

Nursing practice has recognized the importance of health promotion in the family to the improvement in individual and community health. However, there is a dearth of nursing research to guide these practitioners. The review of four nursing research journals provided the evidence of this dearth of knowledge. The advancement of family health promotion to the forefront of the nursing research agenda is needed.

Health promotion in the family is the study of the enhancement of well-being. Internal family dynamics and external environmental factors interrelate to affect the health and health promotion behaviours of families. In this paper directives were discussed for the study of the relationships between the family's internal and external environments and their practise of health promotion behaviours.

REFERENCES

American Nurses' Association (1980). *A Social Policy Statement.* American Nurses' Association, Kansas City.

Blaxter, M., & Patterson, E. (1983). The health behaviour of mothers and daughters. In *Families at risk* (Madge, N., ed.), London: Heinemann, pp. 174–196.

Butrin, J., & Newman, M. A. (1986). Health promotion in Zaire: Time perspective and cerebral hemispheric dominance as relevant factors. *Public Health Nursing* 3(3), 183–191.

Children's Defense Fund (1985). *A children's defense budget: An analysis of the president's FY 1986 budget and children.* Washington, DC: Children's Defense Fund.

Coeytaux, F. (1984). *The role of the family in health: Appropriate research methods.* Geneva: WHO.

de Ramos, E. B. (1984). Working mothers of pre-school children in an underdeveloped society. *Women's Studies International Forum,* 7(6), 415–422.

Dever, G. E. A. (1980). *Community health analysis: A holistic approach.* Germantown, MD: Aspen.

Duffy, M. E. (1984). Transcending options: Creating a milieu for practicing high level wellness. *Health Care for Women International,* 5, 145–161.

Duffy, M. E. (1986). Primary prevention behaviors: The female-headed, one-parent family. *Research in Nursing and Health,* 9, 115–122.

Dwore, R. B., & Kreuter, M. W. (1980). Reinforcing the case for health promotion. *Family and Community Health, 2,* 103–119.

Feetham, S. (1984). Family research in nursing. In *Annual review of nursing research,* Volume 2 (Wesley, H. H. & Fitzpatrick, J. J., eds). New York: Springer.

Gustafson, M. B. (1986). Research among Haitian village women: Implications for the nurse's role in health evaluation. *Public Health Nursing, 3*(4), 250–256.

Laskey, P. A., & Eichelberger, K. M. (1985). Health-related views and self-care behaviors in young children. *Family Relations, 34,* 13–18.

Lewis, C. E., & Lewis, M. A. (1982). Determinants of children's health-related beliefs and behaviors. *Family and Community Health, 4*(4), 85–97.

Loveland-Cherry, C. J. (1986). Personal health practices in single parent and two parent families. *Family Relations, 35,* 133–139.

Maslow, A. H. (1962). *Toward a psychology of being.* Princeton, NJ: Van Nostrand.

McFarlane, J. (1985). Use of an ecologic model to identify children at risk for infection and to quantify the expected impact of the risk factors. *Public Health Nursing 2*(1), 2–22.

Mechanic, D. (1979). Correlates of psychological distress among young adults. A theoretical hypothesis and results from a 16 year follow-up study. *Archives of General Psychiatry 36,* 1233–1239.

Merrit, D. (1986). The national center for nursing research. *Image: Journal of Nursing Scholarship 18*(3), 84–85.

Milio, N. (1985). Health education = health instruction + health news: Media experiences in the United States, Finland, Australia, and England. In *The media, social science, and social policy for children* (Rubinstein, E. A., & Brown, J. D., eds). Norwood, NJ: Ablex Publishing.

Mullen, P. D. (1983). Promoting child health: Channels of socialization. *Family and Community Health 5,* 52–68.

Murphy, S. (1986). Family study and nursing research. *Image 18*(4), 170–174.

O'Brien, R. A. (1980). Relationship of parent-child communication to child's exploratory behavior and self-differentiation. *Nursing Research 29*(3), 150–156.

Pearl, D., Bouthilet, L., & Lazar, J. (1982). *Television and behavior: Ten years of scientific process and implications for the eighties* (Volume 1). Washington, DC: US Government Printing Office.

Pender, N. J. (1982). *Health promotion in nursing practice.* Norwalk, CT: Appleton-Century-Crofts.

Pratt, L. (1973). Child rearing methods and children's health behavior. *Journal of Health and Social Behavior 14,* 61–69.

Pratt, L. (1976). *Family structure and effective health behavior.* Boston: Houghton Mifflin.

Roemer, R. (1986). APHA members support more international health work. *The Nation's Health 16*(12), 2.

Rubinstein, E. A., & Brown, J. D. (1985). Television and children: A public policy dilemma. In *The media, social science, and social policy for children.* (Rubinstein, E.A., & Brown, J. D., eds). Norwood, NJ: Ablex Publishing.

Sidel, R. (1986). *Women and children last: The plight of poor women in affluent America.* New York: Viking Penguin.

William, C., Carter, B., & Wynder, E. (1981). Prevalence of selected cardiovascular and cancer risk factors in a pediatric population. *Preventive Medicine 10,* 121–132.

World Health Organization (1979). *Formulating strategies for health for all by the year 2000.* Geneva: World Health Organization.

World Health Organization (1985). *A guide to curriculum review for basic nursing education: Orientation to primary health care and community health.* Geneva: World Health Organization.

CHAPTER 16

A Psychometric Analysis of the Family Environment Scale

Carol J. Loveland-Cherry, JoAnne M. Youngblut, Nancy W. Kline Leidy

Psychometric properties of the Moos (1979) Family Environment Scale (FES) were studied in a sample of 73 two-parent and 19 single-parent families. Mothers and fathers completed the FES questionnaire while the child in the family closest to 11 years old was administered the FES in an interview. Moos reported initial internal consistency estimates (Kuder-Richardson 20s) between .64 and .79. In this study, KR20s ranged from .24 to .75 for the entire sample, and differences among mothers, fathers, and children in the KR20s calculated for each group were found. Although Moos hypothesized three dimensions into which the 10 subscales fall, confirmatory factor analysis using LISREL VI did not support this assertion.

Historically, nursing has identified the family as both an important environment related to the health of individuals and as a client unit. Early research centered primarily on dyadic relationships within the family rather than on the family system. The shift to a focus on the family as the unit of analysis necessarily requires nurse researchers to attend to the measurement of family system variables. This article presents a psychometric analysis of Moos' Family Environment Scale (FES), a tool that is used extensively in family research.

THE FAMILY ENVIRONMENT SCALE

The FES was developed within a social-ecological framework that focused on interactions between individuals and their environments and implications of these interactions for human functioning, including health and health behaviors (Moos, 1979; Moos, Insel, & Humphrey, 1974). The 90-item questionnaire was designed to explore three major dimensions of the family environment: interpersonal relationships among family members, directions of personal growth emphasized in the family, and the basic organizational structure of the group. Ten subscales are subsumed within these dimensions. The Relationship dimension is made up of three subscales: Cohesion, Expressiveness, and Conflict. The Personal Growth dimension includes the Independence, Achievement Orientation, Intellectual-Cultural Orientation, Active-Recreational Orientation, and Moral-Religious Emphasis subscales. The Organization and Control subscales comprise the System Maintenance dimension (Moos & Moos, 1986). The 10 subscales are hypothesized to measure conceptually distinct, but related, dimensions of the family environment.

A true–false format is used for the individual items. Respondents are directed to decide if the statements are primarily false or true of their family. If the respondent believes the statements are true for some family members and false for others, they are to select the option characteristic of most members. Using the template provided, a summative score is derived for each subscale. Standard score equivalents are available for raw scores. Either individual or family mean scores may be used in the analyses.

Although numerous studies have used the FES as a measure of family environment, information concerning reliability of the measure has been minimal or absent. Moos and Moos (1986) reported psychometric properties of the FES based on responses from individuals in 1, 067 families. Internal consistencies for each of the subscales, using the Kuder-Richardson 20, ranged from .61 to .78. Item-to-subscale correlations ranged from .27 to .44. Intercorrelations among the 10 subscales ranged from .41 to .53. Test–retest reliabilities were reported as ranging from .68 to .86 for a 2-month interval, .54 to .86 for a 4-month interval, and .52 to .89 for a 12-month interval.

Some gender differences have been noted for individual subscales. A comparison of wives' and husbands' perceptions indicated that the former tended to view their family settings more positively than their husbands on Moral-Religious Emphasis, Organization, Intellectual-Cultural, and Active-Recreational Orientation. Male children viewed their families as more achievement oriented than female children (Moos & Moos, 1986). A second study of adolescents found that females reported significantly more Expressiveness in their families than males did and males reported significantly more Achievement Orientation than females (Enos & Handal, 1985).

METHOD

Sample: Analyses were based on data from a convenience sample of 257 individuals from 92 nonclinical families who participated in a study on health and health behaviors in families. The parents and one child from each family participated. There were 19 (20.1%) female-headed single-parent families and 73 (79.3%) two-parent families. Ninety-two children (50 males and 42 females), 92 mothers, and 73 fathers participated. Mean age for the children was 11.5 years. For mothers the mean age was 39 years and for fathers, 41 years. Families ranged in size from 2 to 7 with a mean of 4.33 members. The sample was largely white (90.3%) with 16 (6.2%) blacks, 3 Asians (1.2%), and 6 other (2.3%). Mean income for two-parent families fell in the $40,000 to $45,999 category and for single-parent families in the $12,000 to $14,999 category. SES scores, measured by Green's (1970) three-factor index, were negatively skewed, indicating the sample consisted primarily of middle- and upper-class families.

Data collection took place in the home. Each parent completed the FES questionnaire. The child in the family closest to 11 years old was administered the FES in an interview format.

RESULTS

Psychometric analysis of the FES subscales was conducted in three parts, (a) reliability estimation, (b) item analysis, and (c) factor analysis. Because data were collected from two or three members of each family, the sample was divided into three groups—mothers, fathers, and children—for the analyses. Results for each of these groups and for the entire sample are presented.

Means and standard deviations for the 10 FES subscales for the total sample were compared with values reported by Moos and Moos (1986), using two sample t tests (Table 1). Means for the current sample were significantly higher for five subscales.

Scores of family members were compared using paired t tests. The first set of analyses focused on two-parent families. For these families, there were no significant differences in means for mothers and fathers. Children's Expressiveness (mother/child

TABLE 1
Comparison of Means Between Moos and Moos' Sample (1986) and the Current Sample

Subscales	Moos and Moos Sample (N = 1,125)		Study Sample (N = 257)		t Value
	M	SD	M	SD	
Cohesion	6.61	(1.36)	7.50	(1.72)	8.99*
Expressive	5.45	(1.55)	5.56	(1.88)	1.00
Conflict	3.31	(1.85)	3.74	(2.17)	3.31*
Independence	6.61	(1.19)	6.61	(1.28)	0.00
Achievement	5.47	(1.61)	5.49	(1.86)	0.18
Intellectual-Cultural	5.63	(1.72)	7.49	(1.65)	16.30*
Active Recreational	5.35	(1.87)	7.02	(1.69)	13.15*
Moral-Religious	4.72	(1.98)	4.80	(2.47)	0.57
Organization	5.41	(1.83)	5.48	(2.21)	0.54
Control	4.34	(1.81)	5.02	(1.95)	5.38*

*$p < .001$

$t = 7.28$ and father/child $t = 7.33$, $df = 73$, $p < .0005$), Conflict (mother/child $t = 3.45$ and father/child $t = 3.42$, $df = 73$, $p < .002$), and Independence (mother/child $t = 3.15$ and father/child $t = 2.68$, $df = 73$, $p < .01$) subscale scores were significantly lower than those of either of their parents. Children's scores were also significantly lower than their mothers' scores on the Intellectual-Cultural scale, $t = 2.18$, $df = 73$, $p < .05$. When single-parent mothers and their children were added to the sample of married mothers and their children, the difference for the Intellectual-Cultural subscale was no longer statistically significant.

Reliability Estimation: Internal consistency estimates were calculated for each subscale using the Kuder-Richardson 20 (KR20) due to the FES's dichotomous response format (Carmines & Zeller, 1979; Nunnally, 1978). Negatively worded items were reverse scored. Moos and Moos (1986) reported KR20s between .61 for Independence and .78 for Cohesion, Intellectual-Cultural, and Moral-Religious Emphasis. The range of internal consistencies for the total sample in the current study was from .23 for Independence to .75 for Moral-Religious Emphasis. Each of these KR20s was below that reported by Moos and Moos. Direct comparison between mothers, fathers, and children in this study and those in the study by Moos and Moos was not possible because they reported internal consistencies for only the total sample.

For parents as a group in the current study, KR20s ranged from .22 for Independence to .78 for Moral-Religious Emphasis. Internal consistency estimates ranged from .13 for Independence to .80 for Intellectual-Cultural Orientation for fathers, from .28 for Independence to .80 for Moral-Religious Emphasis for mothers, and from .22 for Independence to .71 for Moral-Religious Emphasis for children.

Comparison of reliability estimates across family subgroups provides additional insight into the instrument's performance. In this study, children's reliabilities were consistently lower than those of their parents. Although the difference for four of these scales was less than .06, children were considerably lower (from .15 to .29 points) for Expressiveness, Achievement, and Active-Recreational. During the interviews, children frequently asked questions about the meaning of the items or expressed their difficulty in answering due to the dichotomous format, saying that sometimes the item was true but that sometimes it was false. Their indecision and difficulty with interpretation may have accounted for the low KR20s obtained for this group, reflecting high measurement error.

There was little difference between mothers and fathers in their KR20s for five subscales: Cohesion, Conflict, Moral-Religious, Control, and Organization. Fathers' scores had much higher reliability (from .09 to .26 points) than mothers for four subscales: Expressiveness, Achievement, Intellectual-Cultural, and Active-Recreational. Mothers' KR20s were much higher for only one subscale, Independence, which had very low KR20s for all three groups.

Item Analysis: An item analysis was conducted to identify poorly functioning items, because deletion of these items could result in higher subscale internal consistencies and less attenuation in other analyses (Nunnally, 1978). Criteria used to identify poorly functioning items were (a) an increase in the KR20 if the item was deleted and (b) a correlation of less than .30 between an item and the subscale score computed without that item (the corrected item to total correlation) (Nunnally). Subscales with lower

KR20s had more poorly functioning items than stronger scales; however, the poorly functioning items were not consistent across groups.

Factor Analysis: Because factor analysis is often used as an indicator of scale validity, it would have been helpful to examine the factor structure of the items for each subscale. However, a factor analysis of all 90 items was not possible with this sample because of its size. Using the total sample would have yielded a case-to-variable ratio of 3 to 1 which does not meet Nunnally's (1978) criterion of 10 cases for each variable analyzed.

Moos (1979) identified three larger dimensions into which the 10 subscales fall. Therefore, a test of the hypothesis that his factor model adequately represents the factor structure for each of the groups in this study was conducted. Several confirmatory factor analyses using *LISREL VI* (Joreskog & Sorbom, 1986) were performed. Standardized family scores for each subscale were derived using Moos' (1979) recommendation and were used to construct the first correlation matrix to be analyzed.

Fit of the model to the data was tested with the chi-square statistic. If the model fits well, the chi square will be low and nonsignificant, indicating little statistical difference between the observed correlation matrix and the matrix predicted by the model (Long, 1983). However, in this study, the chi square obtained was very large and highly significant, $\chi^2 = 195.8, df = 32, p < .00005$. Because chi square is influenced by the sample size, inspection of the parameters obtained provides additional information about the fit of the model. Five factor loadings were lower than acceptable (less than .50) and one was larger than 1.0. Improbable values were also obtained for the variance of the error terms. Based on the high chi square, the low factor loadings, and the improbable values obtained, the fit of the model to the data was poor (Figure 1).

Individual raw summative scores were then analyzed separately for mothers, fathers, and children. For each group the fit of the model to the data was poor. The chi square for each group was large and highly significant (children, $\chi^2 = 83.47$; mothers, $\chi^2 = 91.53$; and fathers, $\chi^2 = 98.71$; for each group, $p < .00005, df = 32$). The problems encountered with low loadings for the family scores were apparent in the results obtained for each group also.

These results could be related to the differences noted between the means for this sample and the means Moos and Moos (1986) reported. However, when their published correlation matrix was analyzed, the same results were obtained. The chi square was large and highly significant, $\chi^2 = 81.17, df = 32, p < .00005$. Five factor loadings were below .50, one was greater than 1.0, and one was negative. Error variances were very high (greater than .70) for six subscales, indicating that the three underlying factors explained very little of the variance in the subscale scores, and one was negative, an impossible value. Therefore, none of the confirmatory factor analyses conducted using *LISREL VI,* including the analysis of the correlation matrix published by Moos and Moos (1986), supported the hypothesized factor structure (Moos, 1979).

Because Moos' model did not fit the data, an exploratory factor analysis using principal components extraction and oblique rotation was performed using subscale scores as the variables to be analyzed. Use of an oblique rotation is consistent with Moos' conceptualization which allows for some correlation between subscales. Kaiser's criterion of retaining factors having eigenvalues greater than 1 (Kim & Mueller, 1978) was

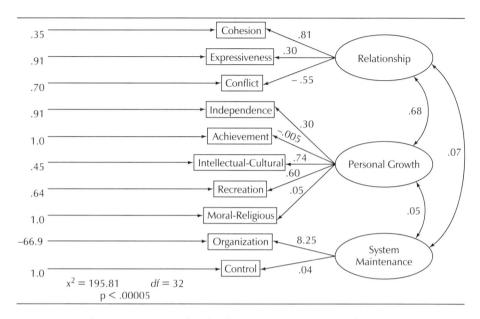

FIGURE 1. Confirmatory Factor Analysis for the Family Environment Scale

used as a guide in determining the number of factors to extract. Eigenvalues greater than 1 were 2.27, 1.94, and 1.39 for mothers and 2.63, 1.75, and 1.27 for children. The top three eigenvalues for fathers were 6.95, 1.02, and 0.68. Thus, the extraction of three factors for mothers and children was supported. Although eigenvalues for fathers supported retaining only two factors, extraction of three factors was performed for all groups to maintain consistency.

Variables were considered to load cleanly on a particular factor if the factor loading was greater than .40 (Nunnally, 1978) and its loading for that factor was .20 higher than its loading on other factors. Variables that loaded on each factor are different for each group and do not correspond to the conceptual groupings proposed by Moos (1979).

Several variables did not load cleanly on one factor (see Table 2) for mothers and for fathers. All variables loaded strongly and cleanly on one and only one factor for children. There is some consistency across groups for placement of several subscales, such as grouping Independence, Intellectual-Cultural, and Active-Recreation together on one factor and grouping Achievement, Moral-Religious, and Control together on another factor.

When a two-factor solution was requested for each group in an attempt to replicate findings reported in the literature, the resulting factors somewhat resembled those of Boake and Salmon (1983) and Fowler (1981) (see Table 3). Several variables did not load cleanly on only one factor. For fathers, Moral-Religious and Achievement loaded on both factors; for mothers and children, Organization loaded on both factors; and for mothers, Achievement did not load on either of the two factors.

TABLE 2
Family Environment Scale Subscale Factor Placements: Three-Factor Solution

	Mothers	*Fathers*	*Children*
Factor 1			
	Cohesion	Cohesion	
		Expressive	Expressive
	Independence[1]	Independence	Independence
	Intellectual-Cultural	Intellectual-Cultural	Intellectual-Cultural
	Recreation	Recreation	Recreation
		Organization	
Factor 2			
	Independence[1]		
	(Achievement)	Achievement	Achievement
	Moral-Religious	Moral-Religious	Moral-Religious
		Organization	
	Control	Control	Control
Factor 3			
	Expressive		Cohesion
	Conflict	Conflict	Conflict
	Organization		Organization

[1]Loaded on more than one factor.

Inspection of the correlation matrices for each group of respondents in the current study showed that the ranges in absolute values for each group are quite different. The mothers' matrix and the children's matrix were similar with correlations ranging from .004 to .50 and from .01 to .54 in absolute value, respectively. Negative correlations were obtained where expected conceptually. For example, Conflict and Cohesion were negatively correlated. Fathers' correlations ranged from .225 to .903, with only 3 out of 45 correlations below .50. There were no negative correlations in the fathers' matrix.

DISCUSSION

Overall, Moos' (1979) Family Environment Scale did not perform as well psychometrically in this sample as would have been anticipated from data published by Moos and Moos (1986). Internal consistency reliabilities were generally below levels considered acceptable. Confirmatory factor analysis using *LISREL VI* did not substantiate the three conceptual areas that Moos expected. Although sampling factors may have contributed to these results, it is also likely that different groups of respondents perceived the items differently.

Because of the unexpectedly poor results for this well used instrument, the use of the FES in published studies was reviewed. Of 34 articles 6 were methodologic and 28

TABLE 3
Family Environment Scale Subscale Factor Placements: Two-Factor Solution

	Mothers	*Fathers*	*Children*
Factor 1			
	Cohesion	Cohesion	Cohesion
		Expressive	Expressive
		Independence	Independence
	Intellectual-Cultural	Intellectual-Cultural	Intellectual-Cultural
	Recreation	Recreation	Recreation
	Organization[1]	Organization	Organization[1]
	Conflict		Conflict
		Moral-Religious[1]	
		Achievement	
Factor 2			
	Independence		
	Moral-Religious	Moral-Religious[1]	Moral-Religious
	Organization[1]		Organization[1]
	Control	Control	Control
	Expressive		
		Achievement[1]	
		Conflict	

[1]Loaded on both factors.
NOTE: Achievement did not load for mothers.

were substantive. None of the substantive and only one of the methodologic articles (Bloom, 1985) provided internal consistency reliabilities estimated for the reported study's sample. Thirteen studies cited Moos' original internal consistency estimates; the remainder made no mention of reliability.

The six methodologic articles reported results of factor analyses. Bloom (1985) and Robertson and Hyde (1982) investigated the structure of the individual items; the other studies (Bloom, 1985; Boake & Salmon, 1983; Fowler, 1981, 1982a, 1982b) used subscale scores in attempts to replicate the three dimensions Moos proposed. None of these reports supported Moos' conceptualization of the factor structure of the scale. Boake and Salmon and Fowler reported similar two-factor solutions. The two-factor solution for the current study resembled but did not replicate findings reported by Boake and Salmon and Fowler.

Many of the findings reported support the hypothesis that mothers, fathers, and children interpreted items differently. Children's scores were significantly different from both their parents' scores. The difference between children and parents was probably due to the type of family on which each is reporting. For children, the family of reference is the family of origin; for parents, it is the family of procreation. Position in the family may dramatically influence one's perspective. For example, parents may feel that they allow children considerable independence, but children may experience their parents' rules as restrictive. A related explanation by Moos and Moos (1986) attributes parent–child differences to different levels of authority and responsibility inherent in parent and child roles.

The finding that both the sign and the magnitude of the subscale correlations differed between mothers and fathers suggests that individual roles in the family may also influence the perspective of the family. For example, mothers reported more often than fathers that the family argued frequently. If the parents discussed their responses after the interview, mothers usually cited arguments between the children as the basis for their responses, but fathers referred to the lack of marital discord.

The results of this study and the review of the literature suggest several recommendations for the use of Moos' Family Environment Scale. First, because respondents in this study had difficulty with the dichotomous format, using a Likert response format may allow subjects to answer more consistently, thereby improving internal consistency estimates. In the only study reviewed that reported newly calculated alphas, Bloom (1985) reported acceptable internal consistencies for 8 of the 10 scales, ranging from .65 to .85 using a 4-point Likert response format. The Independence subscale had an alpha of .48 and Achievement Orientation had an alpha of .55.

Second, investigators are cautioned about three of the subscales. The Expressiveness, Independence, and Achievement Orientation subscales had alphas lower than .70 in the current study as well as in the studies by Bloom (1985) and Moos and Moos (1986). They also had the lowest KR20s in this study. A fourth subscale, Control, also had low reliability for Moos with a KR20 of .67 and for the current study at .55.

Third, it may be wise to redefine the subscales by changing the clustering of items and deleting items that do not load strongly and cleanly on one factor. Robertson and Hyde (1982) reported results of a factor analysis using items as the variables to be analyzed. The factor structure they obtained for the individual items did not support 10 separate factors, indicating that Moos's subscale definition may not be appropriate.

Research is needed with a larger, more representative sample to further investigate the factor structure of the items that make up the subscales. Unless the psychometric properties of the FES are documented as better than those suggested by this study and other published evidence, this instrument should be used and interpreted cautiously.

The study was conducted at the School of Nursing, The University of Michigan. The original project from which the data for this study were taken was supported by a grant from Sigma Theta Tau International to the first author for her doctoral dissertation completed at the College of Nursing, Wayne State University. The second author was supported in part by a National Research Service award, predoctoral fellowship from the National Center for Nursing Research, number f31-NR6152.

REFERENCES

Bloom, B. L. (1985). A factor analysis of self-report measures of family functioning. *Family Process, 24*(2), 225–239.

Boake, C., & Salmon, P. G. (1983). Demographic correlates and factor structure of the Family Environment Scale. *Journal of Clinical Psychology, 39,* 95–100.

Carmines, E. G., & Zeller, R. A. (1979).*Reliability and validity.* Newbury Park, CA: Sage Publications, Inc.

Enos, D., & Handal, P. (1985). Relation of sex and age to old and new family environment scale standard scores of white adolescent: Preliminary norms. *Psychological Reports, 57,* 327–330.

Fowler, P. C. (1981). Maximum likelihood factor structure of the Family Environment Scale. *Journal of Clinical Psychology, 37*(1), 160–164.

Fowler, P. C. (1982a). Factor structure of the Family Environment Scale: Effects of social desirability. *Journal of Clinical Psychology, 38,* 285–292.

Fowler, P. C. (1982b). Relationship of family environment and personality characteristics: Canonical analyses of self-attributions. *Journal of Clinical Psychology, 38,* 804–810.

Green, L. W. (1970). Manual for scoring socioeconomic status for research on health behavior. *Public Health Reports, 85*(9), 815–827.

Joreskog, K. G., & Sorbom, D. (1986). *LISREL VI.* Chicago: National Educational Resources.

Kim, J., & Mueller, C. W. (1978). *Factor analysis: Statistical methods and practical issues.* Newbury Park, CA: Sage Publications, Inc.

Long, J. S. (1983). *Confirmatory factor analysis.* Beverly Hills: Sage Publications, Inc.

Moos, R. H., Insel, P. M., & Humphrey, B. (1974). *Preliminary manual for family environment scale, work environment scale, group environment scale.* Palo Alto, CA: Consulting Psychologists Press.

Moos, R. H. (1979). Evaluating family and work settings. In P. I. Ahmed & G. V. Coelho (Eds.), *Toward a new definition of health: Psychosocial dimensions.* New York: Plenum Publishing.

Moos, R. H., & Moos, B. S. (1986). *Family environment scale manual* (2nd ed.). Palo Alto, CA: Consulting Psychologists Press.

Nunnally, J. C. (1978). *Psychometric theory.* New York: McGraw-Hill Book Co.

Robertson, D. U., & Hyde, J. S. (1982). The factorial validity of the family environment scale. *Educational and Psychological Measurement, 42,* 1233–1241.

CHAPTER 17

Family Coping: A Comparison of Stepfamilies and Traditional Nuclear Families During Pregnancy

Mildred A. Dietz-Omar

The experience of pregnancy brings about change affecting the total family. The anticipated addition of an infant alters coping processes operating within the family. Family coping includes the decisions that help family members move from a state of dependence to one of independence and interdependence within the family system. Klein (1983) described the use of effective family coping strategies benefiting family problem solving and the resolution of specific family problems. Differences in specific strategies used by family members are related to their particular stage of the family life cycle and learned patterns of behavior (King, 1983; Olson et al., 1983; Patterson, McCubbin, & Needle, 1983). LaRossa (1977) noted that the addition of a new family member may be associated with unity of the couple, but disunity may also occur due to the decreased involvement with the spouse. Miller and Myers-Walls (1983) addressed the need to study coping strategies in pregnancy and parenthood, yet there is a paucity of available, empirically based knowledge regarding family coping in expectant couples. In addition, marriages and families are also changing. The first-time married, traditional nuclear family is no longer the typical American family structure. Stepfamilies are emerging as a major family structure, with many of these remarried couples having mutual children of their own. Visher and Visher (1983) noted that stepfamilies used different coping strategies in dealing with some of the stresses of everyday living. Morris (1985) identified that the ability of stepfamilies to deal with difficulties arising within

Reprinted from *Applied Nursing Research, Vol. 4* (No. 1), February 1991, pp. 31–33. Used with permission of W. B. Saunders Company and the author.

their families is of great importance, often more so than the difficulties themselves. However, there is no documentation in the literature that addresses expectant stepfamily couples and their coping during pregnancy. The purpose of this study was to describe and compare coping strategies used by stepfamilies and traditional nuclear families during pregnancy.

This study was based on a descriptive, two-group comparison design of 40 stepfamily couples and 40 traditional nuclear family couples; all couples had wives in the third trimester of pregnancy and at least one child under the age of 18 living in the home. Stepfamily couples were experiencing a mutual birth for the first time, and traditional nuclear family couples were experiencing an other than first-time birth. Data were collected from paper and pencil questionnaires completed by both husbands and wives during in-home visits and included information on family coping strategies. A personal information form was used to obtain data on demographic characteristics and anticipated problems with the arrival of the baby.

The Family Crisis Oriented Personal Evaluation Scales (F-COPES), developed by McCubbin, Olson, and Larson (1981), were used to assess family coping, both internal (attitudinal) and external (behavioral) strategies used by families responding to problems or difficulties associated with life changes or difficult life events. This 30-item paper and pencil self-report instrument enabled husbands and wives to describe their family's level and type of coping strategies in dealing with the changes during pregnancy. Internal family coping strategies were defined as "the way[s] individual family members handle difficulties by using resources residing within the nuclear system" (McCubbin, Olson, & Larson, 1987, p. 196), such as knowing that we have the strength within our family to solve our problems. External family coping strategies were defined as "the active behaviors the family employs to acquire resources outside the nuclear system" (McCubbin et al., 1987, p. 196), such as sharing concerns with close friends.

The sample consisted of stepfamily couples who were married an average of 1.2 years and traditional nuclear family couples who were married an average of 7.3 years. The number of families with one child in the home was the same in each group; that is, 58% ($n = 23$) of the stepfamilies and 58% ($n = 23$) of the traditional nuclear families had one child. Thirty percent ($n = 12$) of the stepfamilies and 37% ($n = 15$) of the traditional nuclear families had two children, and 12% ($n = 5$) of the stepfamilies and 5% ($n = 2$) of the traditional nuclear families had three or more children. Children ranged in age from 1 to 19 years.

Interestingly, it was the traditional nuclear family wives (67%, $n = 27$) who anticipated the most family problems when the new baby arrived, as compared with 37% ($n = 15$) of the traditional nuclear family husbands and 47% ($n = 19$) of the stepfamily husbands and wives together. The traditional nuclear family wives expressed a primary concern about their ability to "make room" for and "love" this child as much as their first. Traditional nuclear family husbands, on the other hand, felt more confident about their ability to deal with this pregnancy and the new baby. Stepfamily husbands and wives together viewed this mutual baby as a means to connect or cement their family together.

Significant differences were found in the coping strategies used, both between and within groups. Stepfamily wives used significantly more internal family coping strategies than did traditional nuclear family wives, suggesting that stepfamily wives were coping with many new issues: a new marriage, a pregnancy as a new couple, and a new stepfamily. Interestingly, both traditional nuclear family husbands and stepfamily wives used significantly more external family coping strategies than did stepfamily husbands. This suggests that both traditional nuclear family husbands and stepfamily wives may have had established outside sources of support and viewed them as more useful than did stepfamily husbands.

Family coping strategies are important discussion topics during pregnancy. Internal family coping strategies may be of particular importance to newly formed stepfamilies as they seek to establish themselves as a family, share in the pregnancy experience as a couple and family for the first time, incorporate the new "mutual child/half sibling" into their existing family structure, and deal with the inherent difficulties of stepchildren in the home. Traditional nuclear family husbands and wives may have developed and established satisfactory coping strategies from managing prior family life experiences. They may only need to reinforce what family coping strategies they find useful as a couple in dealing with this pregnancy experience.

An understanding by health care professionals of family coping during pregnancy within various family structures can facilitate optimal family functioning in childbearing families. A primary function of the nurse caring for expectant couples is to support the family unit. Informing husbands and wives of the changes and concerns occurring both externally and from within the family helps expectant couples gain greater problem-solving ability and self-confidence. Husbands and wives who have a positive attitude about themselves and their families build solid foundations for meaningful relationships within their family structures and are better able to cope satisfactorily with a new addition to the family unit. Helping expectant couples who face the many demands and changes associated with pregnancy and parenthood to become proactive in terms of their own healthy functioning is a major direction for clinical practice.

Further research is needed on expectant stepfamily and traditional nuclear family husbands' and wives' experience of pregnancy and the degree to which the pregnancy is perceived as a stressor. Additional inquiry is needed on the effectiveness of different coping strategies during pregnancy for various family structures, including the single parent and extended kinship family structures.

REFERENCES

King, I. M. (1983). King's theory of nursing. In I. W. Clements & F. B. Roberts (Eds.), *Family health: A theoretical approach to nursing care* (pp. 177–188). New York: Wiley.

Klein, D. (1983). Family problem-solving and family stress. In H. I. McCubbin, M. B. Sussman, & J. M. Patterson (Eds.), *Social stress and the family: Advances and developments in family stress theory and research. Marriage and Family Review.* New York: Haworth.

LaRossa, R. (1977). *Conflict and power in marriage: Expecting the first child.* Beverly Hills, CA: Sage.

McCubbin, H. I., Olson, D. H., & Larson, A. (1981). F-COPES: Family Crisis Oriented Personal Evaluation Scales. In H. I. McCubbin & A. Thompson (Eds.), *Family assessment for research and practice.* (pp. 195–207). Madison, WI: University of Wisconsin, Madison.

McCubbin, H. I., Olson, D., & Larson, A. (1987). F-COPES: Family Crisis Oriented Personal Evaluation Scales. In H. I. McCubbin & A. Thompson (Eds.), *Family assessment for research and practice* (pp. 195–207). Madison, WI: University of Wisconsin, Madison.

Miller, B. C., & Myers-Walls, J. A. (1983). Parenthood: Stresses and coping strategies. In H. I. McCubbin & C. Figley (Eds.), *Stress and the family: Coping with normative transitions* (Vol. 1). (pp. 54–73). New York: Brunner/Mazel.

Morris, L. J. (1985). *A comparison of marital satisfaction and stepfamily integration in stepmother and stepfather remarriages.* Unpublished doctoral dissertation. United States University, San Diego.

Olson, D. H., McCubbin, H. I., Barnes, H., Larson, A., Muxen, M., & Wilson, W. (1983). *Families: What makes them work.* Beverly Hills, CA: Sage.

Patterson, J. M., McCubbin, H. I., & Needle, R. H. (1983). *A-COPE Adolescent Orientation for Problem Experiences* (Research Instrument). Madison, WI: University of Wisconsin, Madison.

Visher, E., & Visher, J. S. (1983). Stepparenting: Blending families. In H. McCubbin & C. Figley (Eds.), *Stress and the family, Vol. 1 Coping with marital transitions.* New York: Brunner/Mazel.

CHAPTER 18

Spouses' Experiences During Pregnancy and the Postpartum: A Program of Research and Theory Development

Jacqueline Fawcett

A program of nursing research was established to test a theory proposing that wives and husbands have similar pregnancy-related experiences. The research was guided by a conceptual framework of the family as a living open system. Findings were conflicting from three studies that investigated the relationship between spouses' strength of identification and similarities in changes in various body image components during and after pregnancy; taken together the findings suggested that spouses do not have similar patterns of change in their body images during pregnancy and the postpartum. Two other studies investigated the relationship between spouses' strength of identification and similarities in their reports of physical and psychological symptoms during pregnancy and the postpartum. In these studies the spouses reported similar physical and psychological symptoms during pregnancy and the postpartum. There was no evidence, however, in any of the studies of a relationship between spouses' strength of identification and similarities in their pregnancy-related experiences. The validity of the theory of similar pregnancy-related experiences and the credibility of the conceptual framework of the family as an open system are questioned.

A long-standing assumption underlying family-centered maternity nursing practice is that pregnancy is a family experience; that is, all family members are involved in a pregnancy. The validity of this assumption was never publicly challenged; nor was it

Reprinted from *IMAGE: Journal of Nursing Scholarship, Vol. 21* (No. 3), Fall 1989, pp. 149–152. Used with permission of the publisher.

tested empirically. The purpose of this paper is to outline the development of a conceptual-theoretical framework that characterizes spouses' pregnancy-related experiences as similar and to summarize the results of a program of research designed to test the theory.

CONCEPTUAL-THEORETICAL FRAMEWORK

The conceptual framework of the family as a living, open system guided theory development and testing (Fawcett, 1975). The conceptual framework is an extension and interpretation of Martha Rogers' (1970) Life Process Model. Rogers described the human being as a four dimensional energy field, an open system characterized by wholeness, pattern and organization, sentience and thought. The human energy field, according to Rogers, is coextensive with the four dimensional environmental energy field. Rogers claimed that human and environmental energy fields are engaged in mutual and simultaneous interaction.

Fawcett's (1975) conceptual framework of the family was based on the assumptions that one environmental field in which human beings are embedded is the family, and that the family is an open-system energy field. It was reasoned that if the family were an open-system energy field, the characteristics attributed by Rogers (1970) to the human open-system energy field could be attributed to the family. This line of reasoning is consistent with Rogers' (1983) own conceptualization of the family.

Briefly, the conceptual framework of the family describes the family as a living open system, an integral, unified whole characterized by a unique and ever-changing pattern and organization. Alterations in pattern and organization are described as being continuous; they reflect the mutual and simultaneous interaction between the family system and the environment.

The theory of similarities in spouses' pregnancy-related experiences was derived from the following conceptual framework concepts: open family system, pattern and organization, and mutual and simultaneous interaction. Pregnant and postpartal women and their husbands represent the open family system, pregnancy-related experiences represent pattern and organization, and strength of identification represents mutual and simultaneous interaction.

The following two conceptual framework postulates guided the development of theoretical propositions: (a) change in the pattern and organization of one family member is associated with a similar change in pattern and organization of other family members; and (b) mutual and simultaneous interaction is related positively to similarity of change in pattern and organization. These postulates represent an interpretation, or modification, of Rogers' (1970) statements about human beings, in that the postulates specify similarity of change in pattern and organization and a directional relationship between mutual and simultaneous interaction and change in pattern and organization. The theory therefore proposes that (a) wives and husbands have similar pregnancy-related experiences during pregnancy and the postpartum, and (b) the similarities in spouses' pregnancy-related experiences are positively related to the strength of their identification.

REVIEW OF THE LITERATURE

A review of the literature was undertaken in an attempt to identify specific pregnancy-related experiences of both pregnant women and their husbands. The literature revealed that women typically experience a number of physical symptoms including heartburn, nausea and vomiting, constipation or diarrhea, hemorrhoids, food cravings, changes in appetite, increased urination, backache, dyspnea, sensitivity to odors, skin irritations and fatigue. Some physical symptoms, especially fatigue, continue into the postpartum (Pritchard, MacDonald, & Gant, 1985; Reeder, Mastroianni, & Martin, 1983). Pregnant and postpartal women also experience some psychological symptoms such as mood swings, anxiety and depression (Cox, Conner, & Kendall, 1982; Glazer, 1980).

The literature also revealed that the profound and obvious change in the form and appearance of the woman's body during pregnancy and the postpartum is associated with considerable change in her body image. Studies have documented changes in attitude toward and perception of the body (Fisher, 1973; McConnell & Daston, 1961), which are the two main dimensions of body image (Schilder, 1950).

Investigators also have reported the occurrence of various physical and psychological symptoms in the husbands of pregnant women including gastrointestinal disorders, abdominal bloating, appetite changes, backache, toothache, lassitude, skin rashes, syncope, weight gain, leg cramps, anxiety, depression, tension, insomnia, irritability, nervousness and mood swings (Clinton, 1986, 1987; Lipkin & Lamb, 1982; Munroe, Munroe, & Nerlove, 1973; Strickland, 1987; Trethowan & Conlon, 1965). Investigators have reported that husbands of pregnant women express concerns about body intactness and dream about changes in their bodies (Colman & Colman, 1971; Liebenberg, 1969), suggesting that men experience body image changes during the childbearing period.

Male pregnancy-related experiences are referred to as the couvade syndrome (Trethowan & Conlon, 1965). Couvade phenomena are thought to be an expression of a man's involvement in pregnancy and his identification with his wife. It has been proposed that the more a husband identifies with his wife, the more likely he is to experience physical and psychological symptoms and body image changes during pregnancy and the postpartum (Colman & Colman, 1971; Trethowan & Conlon).

Most research related to the couvade syndrome has focused solely on the male partner, rather than comparing men's symptoms with those of their wives. One study compared spouses' symptoms and indicated that 10 couples experienced similar physiological and psychological changes during the pregnancy but did not specify what the changes were (Deutscher, 1969).

THEORY TESTING

The review of the literature led to the design of five studies that have tested the theory of similarities in spouses' pregnancy-related experiences. Three studies tested the theory as particularized for body image changes, and two studies tested the theory as particularized for physical and psychological symptoms. Inasmuch as all five studies have already been reported in detail, a summary of each is given below.

The three studies that focused on body image investigated the relationship between wives' and husbands' strength of identification and similarities in changes in various components of body image during and after pregnancy. These studies tested the theoretical propositions that (a) wives' and husbands' body image changes are similar during pregnancy and the postpartum and (b) similarities in spouses' body image changes are positively related to the strength of their identification.

The first body image study (Fawcett, 1978) focused on perceptions of the body. Perceived body space was defined as the amount of space individuals think that their bodies occupy; it was measured by the Topographic Device. Articulation of body space was defined as the extent to which individuals perceive their bodies as being separate from the surrounding environment; it was measured by the Figure Drawing Test. Strength of identification was defined as the amount of semantic similarity between spouses for a set of concepts related to identification; this was measured by the Identification Scale. Complete longitudinal data were available for 40 couples. Data were collected during the eighth and ninth months of pregnancy and the first, second, and twelfth postpartal months (articulation of body space was not measured at the twelfth postpartal month).

The second body image study was designed as a replication and refinement of the first study (Fawcett, 1987; Fawcett, Bliss-Holtz, Haas, Leventhal, & Rubin, 1986). This study also focused on perceptions of the body, again using the variable, perceived body space; and on attitudes toward the body, using the variable, global body attitude. Global body attitude was defined as individuals' general attitudes about the outward form and appearance of their bodies; it was measured by the Body Attitude Scale. Strength of identification, again, was measured by the Identification Scale. Longitudinal data were available on 54 couples. Data were collected during the third, sixth, and ninth months of pregnancy and during the first and second postpartal months. The third body image study was a replication of the second study, using a sample of 20 couples (Drake, Verhulst, Fawcett & Barger, 1988).

Content validity and acceptable levels of reliability were established for the population of interest for all instruments used in the three body image studies. The links among conceptual framework concepts, concepts of the theory as particularized for body image and empirical indicators are shown in Tables 1 and 2.

The two studies that focused on spouses' symptoms investigated the relationship between wives' and husbands' strength of identification and similarities in their reports of physical and psychological symptoms during pregnancy and the postpartum (Drake, Verhulst, & Fawcett, 1988; Fawcett & York, 1986, 1987). These studies tested the theoretical propositions that (a) wives' and husbands' reports of physical and psychological symptoms are similar during pregnancy and the postpartum and (b) similarities in spouses' reports of physical and psychological symptoms are positively related to the strength of their identification.

Physical symptoms were defined as reports of pregnancy-related bodily symptoms (e.g., nausea, appetite changes, leg cramps) and were measured by 20 items on a Symptoms Checklist. Psychological symptoms were defined as reports of psychological changes associated with childbearing (e.g., anxiety, depression) and were measured by 3 items on the Symptoms Checklist. In the first study, psychological symptoms also were

TABLE 1

Conceptual-Theoretical-Empirical Structure for First Study of Spouses' Body Image Changes during Pregnancy and the Postpartum

Conceptual Model Concepts	Open Family System	Pattern and Organization		Mutual and Simultaneous Interaction
Concepts of the theory	Pregnant and postpartal couples	Perceived body space	Articulation of body concept	Strength of identification
Empirical indicators	Couples in 8th, 9th months of pregnancy; 1st, 2nd, 12th postpartal months	Topographic device	Figure drawing test	Identification scale

SOURCE: Fawcett, J. (1978). Body image and the pregnant couple. *American Journal of Maternal Child Nursing, 3,* 227–233.

TABLE 2

Conceptual-Theoretical-Empirical Structure for Second and Third Studies of Spouses' Body Image Changes during Pregnancy and the Postpartum

Conceptual Model Concepts	Open Family System	Pattern and Organization		Mutual and Simultaneous Interaction
Concepts of the theory	Pregnant and postpartal couples	Perceived body space	Global body attitude	Strength of identification
Empirical indicators	Couples in 3rd, 6th, 9th months of pregnancy; 1st, 2nd postpartal months	Topographic device	Body attitude scale	Identification scale

SOURCES: Fawcett, J., Bliss-Holtz, V. J., Haas, M. B., Leventhal, M., & Rubin, M. (1986). Spouses' body image changes during and after pregnancy: A replication and extension. *Nursing Research, 35,* 220–223; Drake, M. L., Verhulst, D., Fawcett, J., & Barger, D. F. (1988). Spouses' body image changes during and after pregnancy: A replication in Canada. *IMAGE: Journal of Nursing Scholarship, 20,* 88–92.

measured by the Beck Depression Inventory. Strength of identification was again measured by the Identification Scale. The first study included data from 70 couples including 23 couples in an early pregnancy group, 24 in a late pregnancy group, and 23 in a postpartum group. The second study included data from 20 couples. Data from these couples were collected during the third, sixth, and ninth months of pregnancy and the first and second postpartal months. Content validity and acceptable levels of reliability were established for the population of interest for the instruments used in the two symptoms studies. The conceptual-theoretical-empirical structures for these studies are illustrated in Tables 3 and 4.

The findings from the body image studies are conflicting. The results of the first study indicated that both spouses experienced changes in perceived body space and that these changes were similar. This finding was not replicated in the second and third studies, where the findings indicated that although wives experienced changes in perceived body space, husbands did not. Thus there was no evidence of similarities in spouses' perceived body space changes. Neither wives nor husbands demonstrated any changes in articulation of body concept in the first study, obviously resulting in no evidence of similarities for spouses in this variable. Wives in the second and third studies experienced statistically significant changes in global body attitude. Husbands in the second study experienced no changes in global body attitude and those in the third study exhibited a tendency toward changes in this variable. There was therefore no evidence of similarities in spouses' global body attitude changes in either study. Furthermore, there was no evidence in any of the studies of a relationship between spouses' strength of identification and similarities in their body image changes.

The findings from the two symptoms studies indicated that spouses report similar physical and psychological symptoms during pregnancy and the postpartum. However, there was no evidence in either study of a relationship between spouses' strength of identification and similarities in their reports of symptoms.

DISCUSSION

Taken together, the findings of the five studies provide minimal support for the theory of similarities in spouses' pregnancy-related experiences. It is unlikely that the

TABLE 3

Conceptual-Theoretical-Empirical Structure for First Study of Spouses' Physical and Psychological Symptoms during Pregnancy and the Postpartum

Conceptual Model Concepts	Open Family System	Pattern and Organization		Mutual and Simultaneous Interaction
Concepts of the theory	Pregnant and postpartal couples	Physical symptoms	Psychological symptoms	Strength of identification
Empirical indicators	Early and late pregnancy groups, postpartal group	Symptoms checklist	Symptoms checklist; Beck Depression Inventory	Identification scale

SOURCES: Fawcett, J., & York, R. (1986). Spouses' physical and psychological symptoms during pregnancy and the postpartum. *Nursing Research, 35,* 144–148; Fawcett, J., & York, R. (1987). Spouses' strength of identification and reports of symptoms during pregnancy and the postpartum. *Florida Nursing Review, 2*(2), 1–10.

TABLE 4
Conceptual-Theoretical-Empirical Structure for Second Study of Spouses' Physical and
Psychological Symptoms during Pregnancy and the Postpartum

Conceptual Model Concepts	Open Family System	Pattern and Organization		Mutual and Simultaneous Interaction
Concepts of the theory	Pregnant and postpartal couples	Physical symptoms	Psychological symptoms	Strength of identification
Empirical indicators	Couples in 3rd, 6th, 9th months of pregnancy; 1st, 2nd post-partal months	Symptoms checklist	Symptoms checklist	Identification scale

SOURCE: Drake, M. L., Verhulst, D., & Fawcett, J. (1988). Physical and psychological symptoms experienced by pregnant Canadian women and their husbands. *Journal of Advanced Nursing, 13,* 436–440.

conflicting findings were the result of methodological flaws, since the instruments used in the studies were valid and reliable measures of the theory level concepts, and the sample sizes were adequate. Initial findings for the theoretical proposition asserting similarities in spouses' patterns of change in perceived body space during pregnancy and the postpartum were not upheld in two replication studies. There was no evidence of change in articulation of body concept for either spouse, suggesting that this component of body image may be more stable than previously thought. Although the wives experienced global body attitude changes, their husbands did not. Thus there was no evidence of similarities in wives' and husbands' changes in this variable.

Given the results of the body image studies, the findings for similarities in spouses' reports of physical and psychological symptoms must be interpreted with caution. Further replication of this research is warranted.

The lack of evidence for the theoretical proposition asserting a positive relationship between spouses' strength of identification and similarities in their pregnancy-related experiences may be because of a disparity between the definition of identification, as measured by the Identification Scale, and that implied by investigators, who claimed that identification is responsible for similarities in spouses' pregnancy-related experiences (Colman & Colman, 1971; Trethowan & Conlon, 1965). It is recommended that other definitions of identification such as imitation (Schilder, 1950) be considered in future research.

The collective findings of the five studies raise questions about the credibility of the conceptual framework of the family as a living open system. The results of the research provide inconsistent support for the postulate that change in pattern and organization of one family member is associated with a similar change in another member. No support is provided for the postulate that mutual and simultaneous interaction is related positively to similarity of change in pattern and organization. This could be because of an inappropriate choice of theoretical representatives of conceptual framework concepts. The conceptual framework concept, pattern and organization, might be better represented theoretically by pregnancy-related experiences other than body image and symptoms. Furthermore, the conceptual framework concept, mutual and simultaneous interaction, might be better represented theoretically as the quality of the marital relationship, the couple's desire for a child, the man's involvement in the pregnancy, intimacy, or empathy.

The findings also could be the result of flaws in the conceptual framework. A major flaw seems to be in the postulate of *similar* changes in pattern and organization of family members. The inclusion of this postulate may be a faulty interpretation of Rogers' (1970) work or a faulty modification of traditional open systems formulations, which assert that change in one component of a system is associated with change in another component of that system (Bertalanffy, 1968).

A serious threat to the credibility of the conceptual framework and to traditional open systems formulations is the finding that husbands did not always demonstrate observable pregnancy-related experiences. Thus, even a revised conceptual framework postulate stating that a change in pattern and organization of one family member is associated with a nonsimilar change in pattern and organization of another family member would not have consistent empirical support.

Perhaps it is too early to question the credibility of the conceptual framework. However, conceptual frameworks must be open to constant criticism or they will become ideologies rather than starting points for scientific work.

This program of research, derived from one conceptual framework of the family, provides mixed evidence regarding the assumption that pregnancy is a family experience. It remains for other research programs derived from other conceptual frameworks to yield the much-needed empirical data that will support or refute the assumption of family involvement in pregnancy.

REFERENCES

Bertalanffy, L. (1968). *General system theory.* New York: George Braziller.

Clinton, J. F. (1986). Expectant fathers at risk for couvade. *Nursing Research, 35,* 290–295.

Clinton, J. F. (1987). Physical and emotional responses of expectant fathers throughout pregnancy and the early postpartum period. *International Journal of Nursing Studies, 24,* 59–68.

Colman, A. D., & Colman, L. L. (1971). *Pregnancy: The psychological experience.* New York: Herder and Herder.

Cox, J. L., Connor, Y., & Kendall, R. E. (1982). Prospective study of the psychiatric disorders of childbirth. *British Journal of Psychiatry, 140,* 11–17.

Deutscher, M. (1969). First pregnancy and the origins of family: A rehearsal theory. *American Journal of Orthopsychiatry, 39,* 319–320.

Drake, M. L., Verhulst, D., & Fawcett, J. (1988). Physical and psychological symptoms experienced by pregnant Canadian women and their husbands. *Journal of Advanced Nursing, 13,* 436–440.

Drake, M. L., Verhulst, D., Fawcett, J., & Barger, D. F. (1988). Spouses' body image changes during and after pregnancy: A replication in Canada. *IMAGE: Journal of Nursing Scholarship, 20,* 88–92.

Fawcett, J. (1975). The family as a living open system: An emerging conceptual framework for nursing. *International Nursing Review, 22,* 113–116.

Fawcett, J. (1978). Body image and the pregnant couple. *American Journal of Maternal Child Nursing, 3,* 227–233.

Fawcett, J. (1987). Re: Spouses' body image changes during and after pregnancy: A replication and extension (Letter to the editor). *Nursing Research, 36,* 220, 243.

Fawcett, J., Bliss-Holtz, V. J., Haas, M. B., Leventhal, M., & Rubin, M. (1986). Spouses' body image changes during and after pregnancy: A replication and extension. *Nursing Research, 35,* 220–223.

Fawcett, J., & York, R. (1986). Spouses' physical and psychological symptoms during pregnancy and postpartum. *Nursing Research, 35,* 144–148.

Fawcett, J., & York, R. (1987). Spouses' strength of identification and reports of symptoms during pregnancy and the postpartum. *Florida Nursing Review, 2*(2), 1–10.

Fisher, S. (1973). *Body consciousness: You are what you feel.* Englewood Cliffs, NJ: Prentice-Hall.

Glazer, G. (1980). Anxiety levels and concerns among pregnant women. *Research in Nursing and Health, 3,* 07–113.

Liebenberg, B. (1969). Expectant fathers. *Child and Family, 8,* 265–278.

Lipkin, M., & Lamb, G. S. (1982). The couvade syndrome: An epidemiologic study. *Annals of Internal Medicine, 96,* 509–511.

McConnell, O. L., & Daston, P. G. (1961). Body image changes in pregnancy. *Journal of Projective Techniques, 25,* 451–456.

Munroe, R. L., Munroe, R. H., & Nerlove, S. B. (1973). Male pregnancy symptoms and cross-sex identity: Two replications. *Journal of Social Psychology, 89,* 147–148.

Pritchard, J. A., MacDonald, P. C., & Gant, N. F. (1985). *Williams' obstetrics* (17th ed.). Norwalk, CT: Appleton-Century-Crofts.

Reeder, S. R., Mastroianni, L., & Martin, L. L. (1983). *Maternity nursing* (15th ed.). Philadelphia: Lippincott.

Rogers, M. E. (1970). *An introduction to the theoretical basis of nursing.* Philadelphia: F. A. Davis.

Rogers, M. E. (1983). Science of unitary human beings: A paradigm for nursing. In I. W. Clements & F. B. Roberts, *Family health. A theoretical approach to nursing care* (pp. 219–227). New York: Wiley.

Schilder, P. (1950). *The image and appearance of the human body.* New York: International Universities Press.

Strickland, O. L. (1987). The occurrence of symptoms in expectant fathers. *Nursing Research, 36,* 184–189.

Trethowan, W. H., & Conlon, W. F. (1965). The couvade syndrome. *British Journal of Psychiatry, 111,* 57–66.

CHAPTER 19

Family Caregiving for a Relative with Alzheimer's Dementia: Coping with Negative Choices

Holly Skodol Wilson

The constant comparative method was used to generate a grounded theory explicating the process of family caregiving for a relative with Alzheimer's dementia. Findings from 20 in-depth, face-to-face interviews conducted with a purposive sample of family caregivers in their homes revealed that much of the caregiving experience consists of coping with negative choices wherein all possible alternatives are undesirable. The three stages of *Surviving on the Brink,* (1) Taking it on, (2) Going through it, and (3) Turning it over, capture the variation in behavior. Continued validation of this process of coping and decision making offers promise for substantive theory development on which nursing intervention programs for easing caregiver burdens might be based.

The purpose of this study was to explore and describe the process of family caregiving for elderly relatives with Alzheimer's dementia (AD) as experienced from the perspective of the caregiver. The approach used the constant comparative method for discovering grounded theory.

The constant comparative method (also called discovering grounded theory) is a method of theory-generating research used to explain basic patterns common to social life. Chenitz and Swanson (1987) wrote, "Grounded theory allows an investigator to create a new perspective or viewpoint on familiar problems or to delineate information about a phenomenon that has been little studied" (p. 7). The method is used to examine the empirical social world in a direct, naturalistic way (Glaser & Strauss, 1967) and offers an alternative or supplementary means for exploring problems when data are not easily quantified (Corbin, 1987). An assumption underlying grounded theory is that the resulting analysis can provide illuminating interpretive explanations in areas where it is important to grasp the experienced reality of others.

The significance of problems associated with care of an elderly person with Alzheimer's dementia (AD) is underscored by the unique demands these people make on a family member who is responsible for taking care of them. Isolation by virtue of being homebound; the need for constant supervision with little or no practical help or backup; the disruption of normal personal, household, and work activities; conflicting multiple role demands; lack of information from health professionals, and the psychological impact of caring for someone whose disorder follows a downhill course with needs progressively rising as hope is undermined all put family caregivers at serious risk for developing health problems of their own (Northouse, 1980; Ory et al., 1985; Reifer & Wu, 1982). In addition, the risk of institutionalization of the AD patient is increased when the ability of the family member to provide care goes over the brink of tolerability. In the words of one informant, "It becomes a question of how far up to the edge of our energy we go."

The importance of a broader understanding of family caregiving for demented elders has been emphasized in the published work of nurses as well as gerontologists (Archbold, 1980; Zarit et al., 1986). Goldman (1982) called the well-being of burdened family caregivers "the major public health issue of the next decade." Most research, however, has been limited to the composition of the elders' informal caregiving network and caregiver responsibilities. Worchester and Quayhagen (1983) reported that when psychological and behavioral problems were added to physical care, the potential for admission to a nursing home was increased for elders. Phillips and Rempusheski's (1986) study provided a beginning conceptual explanation of the phenomenon of elder abuse. The study reported here offers an in-depth analytic explanation of the process of family caregiving for an elderly relative with the seriously debilitating and ultimately terminal condition of Alzheimer's disease.

METHOD

Sample: The sample consisted of 20 family caregivers of AD relatives recruited from community agencies who gave their permission to be contacted by the investigator. A family caregiver was defined as a member of the patient's informal support system (family/friend) who: (a) carried primary responsibility for providing a range of care to the patient at home, (b) was identified by a referral source as having ongoing responsibility for the patient's care, (c) was not financially reimbursed for caregiving activities, and (d) had been a caregiver for a *minimum* of 6 weeks not more than 3 months prior to the interview. (The actual number of years of caregiving among study sample members ranged from 4 to 14 with a mean of 6, thereby far exceeding minimum criteria.) The mean age of caregivers was 62 years ($SD = 14.4$). Six were male and 14 female of whom 18 were married and 2 widowed. Education ranged from 6 to 21 years ($M = 13.9, SD = 3.8$ years).

Data Collection: Face-to-face interviews of approximately 2 hours were conducted in home settings with subjects. Open-ended interview questions and probes were used to explore topics including: greatest difficulties encountered, advice they would give to others, resources for support and direct help that were or would be important to deal better with difficulties and strains of caregiving.

Data Analysis: Interviews were tape recorded, then entered on an IBM—XT computer using the program *Ethnograph* for analysis.

Analysis was initially directed toward discovering the basic social-psychological problem (BSPP) experienced by the study sample members. A BSPP is a problem that is "shared by study sample members and may or may not be expressly articulated" (Hutchinson, 1986). Analysis of the 250 single-spaced pages of transcribed interview data revealed that family caregivers of Alzheimer's patients are constantly confronted with the problem of coping with negative choices. Negative choices are dilemmas in which all options represent "different degrees of impossibility." The most extreme example of a negative choice is between turning over their caregiving role by institutionalizing their relative in a nursing home versus persevering in the caregiver role to a point beyond their own tolerance and coping capacity. Negative choices also permeate day-to-day decisions. Examples are:

> To get anyone who can help is darn near impossible, particularly in this county because of the costs . . . I worry about the day coming when I'll have to ship her to a nursing home. Frankly, I'd rather see her dead.

> I have a feeling that I'm going to get myself in a terrible spot where I can't think correctly because I haven't had the time. Then I'll make a mistake and it's all going to fall apart.

> I didn't want to tell him he couldn't drive anymore, but do I wait until he's killed someone? What's the right time to tell a grown man he can't drive?

Once the grounded study problem was identified in the data, analysis was directed toward discovering the basic social process (BSP) that explained how the problem (BSPP) was managed given study conditions. The BSP provided a central integrative conceptual schema that encompassed most of the variation in behavior contained in the data (Glaser, 1978; Wilson, 1985).

The data coding procedures followed steps identified by Hutchinson (1986). (a) *Open coding* in which in vivo words used by interviewees themselves were identified to capture the theme in each sentence or episode in the text. Examples of in vivo codes in this study were "unburdening," "taking charge," "going under." (b) *Coding for categories* began once no new in vivo codes were discovered in the open coding step. Level II codes are categories that result from clustering and condensing in vivo codes. These become the core concepts in the grounded theory. In this study they were comprised of the three stages of *Surviving on the Brink*—Taking it on, Going through it, and Turning it over. (c) *Theoretical coding* involved comparing anecdote with anecdote, code with code, and category with category searching for relationships such as conditions, strategies, and consequences. (d) *Identifying the core variable or integrative scheme* was accomplished by sorting memos about Level II categories and their theoretical relationships. According to Glaser (1978), a core variable (or BSP) must have at least two stages to account for change over time. *Theoretical saturation* occurred when additional data analysis failed to discover any new ideas about the integrative scheme (Glaser, 1978).

FINDINGS

Family caregivers attempted to cope with the problem of negative choices through a three-stage process labeled here as *Surviving on the Brink* (see Figure 1). The stages that emerged in the data were: (1) Taking it on, (2) Going through it, and (3) Turning it over. Each stage had characteristic properties, problems, and coping strategies; however, the overall process is a consciously examined, self-reflective, strategic, and difficult means of surviving on a day-to-day, if not moment-to-moment basis under conditions of initial uncertainty and unpredictability, pressing demands with a paucity of support, and a dreaded future.

Stage 1: Taking It On

Taking on the responsibility of caregiving for a demented loved one at home occurs as an imperative to take action in the absence of any perceived alternatives. The context is one of uncertainty and unpredictability about the consequences of the caregiver's decision, overpowered by a keen sense of moral duty.

> The principal problem is I don't know what to expect. No one is able to say what will happen. You're constantly on a tightrope. At some point you have to decide whether you're the person to handle it. But, at first, you do what you have to do without knowing what's in store.

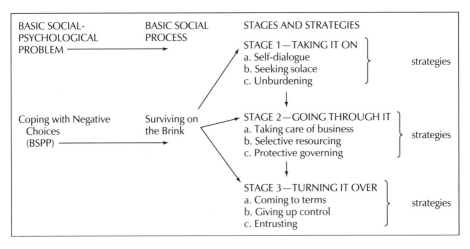

FIGURE 1. The Substantive Theory of Family Caregiving for a Relative with Alzheimer's Disease

Caregiving is taken on in addition to prior responsibilities, resulting in drastic life-style changes that leave caregivers feeling trapped.

> This situation has changed our life drastically. We used to do what we wanted—go to a movie or to lunch. Now we can't do any of that. It's a chore to even go grocery shopping. My social life is gone.

> I had to take over the entire household. It was a tremendous challenge to keep up all the rest—planning meals, paying bills, doing laundry. I had never done any of that.

Caregivers take on the responsibility of home care for their demented relative because they perceive themselves as the last and irreplaceable resort.

> Even if I had hired somebody, I don't think they could do what I am doing 24 hours a day. The only other option was my sister, and her situation at home is even more impossible than mine.

They make the decision despite a state of not "being in the know." They are not well informed about the disease and respite resources, and they lack information about what community services can offer. In short, taking on occurs in a context of the pervasive sense of not knowing.

> If only I'd have known a little ahead of time about how to cope with some of the problems, I might have been less stressed.

> I didn't know any resources to help me. I don't know where you'd get it unless you read it in the newspaper. Doctors and nurses should have lists.

Added to the conditions of uncertainty, unpredictability, lack of resources, and information which make up Stage 1, taking it on occurs in a context of financial strain because many of the costs associated with home-based, extended care are not reimbursable and those that are require "going through all that red tape." Yet, overriding the problematic conditions is a spectre of horror stories about nursing homes (called by some "melancholy institutions") and the caregivers' sense of moral duty.

> I'm afraid to involve anyone else. It's *my* mother; *my* responsibility. If it doesn't work, it's my fault, but I can live with that better than I could if someone else messes up.

Coping strategies in the first stage of caregiving included: (a) self-dialogue, (b) seeking solace, and (c) unburdening.

(a) Self-Dialogue

Almost all interviewees confided that they talked to themselves in an attempt to muster their own inner strength in the face of the decision to take on the caregiver role.

> I reminded myself that my life has been very rewarding to me—it makes the prospects easier to face.

> You must have to tell yourself that it's not a unique problem—it's not insurmountable, that you just have to keep at it.

> I tell myself to be patient. I can't keep thinking I should have done better. If I don't stop it, I will get angry and won't be able to do him any good.

(b) Seeking Spiritual Solace

Most caregivers turned to religious practices, rituals, and their belief in a higher power for motivation and strength given their decision to take on caregiving.

> My religion teaches us to serve and reminding myself of those teachings keeps me going . . . I don't see how a person without a belief in a higher power could possibly manage. My faith is the greatest help to me.

(c) Unburdening

The opportunity to talk about problems with others who are nonjudgmental and have been through it is identified as another major strategy used in this stage. A common response from caregivers was: "Just talking about it in the group, just letting all my worries out helped me to relax."

Yet, unburdening is used as a coping strategy very selectively. Caregivers separate potential sources of support into those who have and those who have not "been up this road themselves." They say, "the fact that others are going through the same thing you are lets you know you are not alone." Stage 1 becomes Stage 2 when caregivers experience what many call a "coming to terms," a realization of the reality of their decision and circumstances, which they described thus: "I think I finally accepted that life wasn't ever going to be the way it was nor can it ever again be more."

Gradually as time passes, the initial conditions of unpredictability and uncertainty characteristic of Stage 1 evolve into Stage 2, the process of going through it.

Stage 2. Going Through It

Once the decision to take on caregiving is made and the caregiver comes to terms with its implications, the mere passage of time unfolds as an ongoing sequence of problems. These problems, created by the demands of caregiving for a demented loved one, result in conflicting role demands that disrupt the rest of the family relations and routines. Most problems in this stage are solved on an emergent, trial-and-error basis, pushing caregivers to an awareness of their own physical erosion and emotional breaking points. Other family relationships are also seriously compromised and stressed by the demands of home-based caregiving by the primary caregiver.

> You become aware that the greatest difficulty is the wear and tear on your own emotions because you feel guilty about not doing what you should. If you don't look out, you get so wrapped up in the person that your own life will fall apart.

> My daughters insisted that I have someone come in and help with her bathing, something I've tried to do all on my own. They convinced me that otherwise I'll have a burnout.

Stage 2 is characterized by a long and formidable list of problems. Illness ambiguity, breakdown of shared meanings, maintaining activities of daily living, disrupted household patterns, family conflicts, and continuing financial strain represent only some of them.

In what seemed like a very short time, she resorted to her native language of Czech which, of course, I don't understand.

No one handles her communications very good. Sometimes I can read some of her signs but most of the time it's just gobbledygook and numbers and I just throw up my hands.

Lack of communication is the hardest part. I think it's because you are looking at the same person you communicated with and you're not getting through. It's like taking care of a dummy.

When your own wife doesn't know who you are, its extremely difficult. It's hard to come to grips with when you expect a response and it's never there again.

Active resistance, agitation, violence, the need for constant supervision, the depletion of the caregiver's energy due simply to the patient's progressive deterioration over time are other problems identified by caregivers that lead them to conclude, "It takes a saint to do this kind of work."

The consequence of Stage 2 is a prolonged state of fatigue, a sense of putting one's own life in suspension, physical and emotional exhaustion from continuous caring and responses from others that range from embarrassing praise to painful criticism. Yet family caregivers have evolved strategies that enable them to prolong their ability to sustain the caregiver role. These coping strategies for Stage 2 include: (a) taking care of business, (b) selective resourcing, and (c) protective governing.

Taking Care of Business

This strategy, particularly "putting one's legal house in order," occupies many caregivers in the early part of Stage 2. Although doing such pragmatic tasks is described as time-consuming and unfamiliar, they associate these accomplishments with a degree of satisfaction and achievement.

We had the nuptial agreement drawn up and shortly after that the durable power of attorney. Nowadays, you don't have to pauperize your entire estate if you get the right advice. But you have to search for that advice, which is so hard when every hour is busy.

Taking care of business also included accumulating some environmental interventions in the home to accommodate the circumstances of caregiving.

The waterbed has been very helpful—it must be something about the warmth. We've recommended it to others.

The smartest thing we did was get that prescription for Haldol. It made nighttime less of a disaster.

Selective Resourcing

Another strategy used in Stage 2 is influenced by several obstacles. Some caregivers are embarrassed and ashamed to tell anyone else what is happening, cutting themselves off from seeking help. Most caregivers report that an information gap separates them from getting help.

> We need an agency or some sort of program that works like a clearinghouse for information because when you start this (caregiving) you are in a fog.

Even when services are identified and accessed, they are perceived as generally inadequate.

> With day care help, she leaves here at 9:30 A.M. and gets back at 3:00 P.M. That about gives me enough time to do the paperwork, go shopping, and do something about our meal. But it doesn't make much of a dent in the 36-hour day.

> The day care center has given me a break but, then they don't have the professional staff to pick up on physical problems. She got into serious trouble because of the side effects from Haldol. It turned out to be more trouble than it was worth.

In contrast to the value attributed to unburdening in the early stage of taking on caregiving, instrumental help is cited as the most important resource as caregiving progresses.

> If somebody isn't here wiping the floor and taking him to the bathroom and changing his pants, they're really not much help. Being sympathetic doesn't do anything.

Protective Governing

Caregivers characterize themselves as "giving their all" before they seek help. But when they finally feel justified in so doing, they discover that numerous obstacles stand between them and resources that fit their needs. Based on individual tolerance levels, cutting points, and support resources available, caregivers reach the place where they become vividly aware that persevering in the caregiving role puts them at personal risk. This cutting point marks a shift to the strategy of protective governing, one that dominates later in Stage 2. Protective governing takes three forms that are used to sustain the energy and coping capacity of the caregiver: (a) situational positioning, (b) guarding personal time, and (c) recharging through personal diversions.

> I am a high energy person, but I have to admit that this just finally wore me down and it's going to get worse not better.

> I go to bed saying why am I doing this and how much longer can I go on?

> My burning out would add more social costs. We're supposed to have a safety net. Where's the safety net for AD caregivers?

> I think doctors and nurses should realize it isn't the AD patient you should ask about. It's more important to ask caregivers how they are doing.

Situational positioning is a strategy in which caregivers choose to eliminate situations that present problems and opt for those situations that are manageable.

> We only go to Chinese restaurants now because they respect their elders. They just carry her in and we don't get embarrassed. We stopped going to restaurants where other people get annoyed.

Protective governing also includes action taken to decrease the caregiver's vulnerability. For example, guarding private time occurs when caregivers place priority on activities judged as being likely to enhance their ability to go on. These choices must be made in face of other pressing demands on their time.

> The need to get educated about what to expect, the need for advice about caregiving, the need for support and affirmation in the caregiving role all take time.

> I don't go to many support group meetings now because after 6 years I know what it's like. I don't want to give up the time to sit there and listen to what others are going through. It's a couple of hours I could have for myself.

In the time caregivers designate for themselves they purposefully engage in diversions selected in order to recharge themselves.

> In the beginning, my own life was put into suspension. All my personal and social activities were cut off. Life became discouraging and repetitive and very difficult. I realized I was going to have to learn how to alter my life so the stress he put me under wouldn't make me sick. Now I take piano lessons and practice for an hour each day. It's like swimming. I can forget everything else while I do it.

Realizing what caregivers refer to as "my own breaking point" becomes a condition for using the strategies of protective governing. The sense that reaching that breaking point is imminent signals the third stage of Surviving on the Brink, Turning it over.

Stage 3. Turning It Over

The decision to turn over their caregiving role is a gradual, considered process of giving up control. It often requires that caregivers reverse their formerly held positions.

> In the beginning I couldn't think of putting her into a convalescent home even though it was a lot of trouble to have her here. I thought, how can a family dump their relative like a bag of garbage? Now I know I won't be able to keep it up.

No consistent patient problem marks the breaking point of caregiver tolerance. In some cases the decision to turn over caregiving occurs because the patient no longer recognizes anyone. In others, the patient develops serious physical problems such as incontinence or paralysis; in yet others, the patient cannot be left alone in the house. What is clear is that the ongoing sequence of problems with the concomitant time pressure and constant care demands force caregivers to question the consequences for their own lives.

> You can't help but eventually have difficulty reconciling the whole thing. You ask yourself, what's really going on here? What kind of person is it making me in the long run?

Deciding to give up control over the patient appears to precede the ultimate step of entrusting care to an institution.

> You begin to realize how pointless it is to try to make them do what you think they should do. She'd put her clothes on top of her night clothes. You end up thinking, what's the difference? She gets a bath everyday anyway. When other people ask about it, we tell them, "well, that's the way we do things."

Placing an AD relative in a nursing home is a dreaded eventuality and the decision poses the ultimate negative choice for caregivers.

I recognized that the time had come when I had to have her in a place where she could be taken care of. Yet it's the last thing I wanted to do because there aren't any proper places.

Caregivers readily speak of the paucity of acceptable alternatives once the emotional decision to turn over caregiving has been made.

I'm on the county medical health advisory committee and we've realized that there isn't an institution to care for them . . . The places where mental problems are handled are set up in such a fashion that they insist on people who are rehabilitative . . . that leaves the Alzheimer's patient out.

Despite lack of satisfaction with placement alternatives, the third stage culminates with the giving over of the active caregiving role and entrusting the family member to the care usually provided in an institutional facility such as a nursing home. Many family caregivers continue to engage in invisible caregiving by managing their relative's finances and legal matters and must cope with a range of social and psychological problems of visitation that, although important, go beyond this study's data.

DISCUSSION

The analysis of the process of caregiving clearly points to the inadequacy of health care services for both AD patients and their family caregivers, as well as to the need for changes in health care policy. Extended home care support services and survival strategies for family caregivers are neglected, yet sorely needed. Interviewees poignantly attested to the strain they experienced, and each stage in the caregiving process represented an opportunity to innovate and adapt psychoeducational approaches reported in the family burden literature to this growing population. Psychiatric nurses have traditionally valued support for families and health teaching. Nursing represents a logical discipline to generate and test intervention programs directed toward easing the burden for this population of underserved caregivers and their afflicted relatives.

Future research based on this study's findings should include attempts to identify and describe illness, caregiver, and contextual factors that influence the decision-making process of family caregivers. The notion that stage in the caregiving process (e.g., temporality or the caregiving trajectory) can be related to differential psychoeducation and support needs merits additional study as well. In this qualitative study common themes emerged across family caregiver data. A phenomenological interpretive study might portray specific exemplars that highlight the unique rather than the shared features of this experience. Expanding this research to family caregivers for relatives with other chronic and/or terminal conditions offers the promise of moving from substantive to formal theory.

This research was part of a UCSF Academic Senate supported study to develop a psychiatric specific measure of social support.

REFERENCES

Archbold, P. G. (1980). Impact of parent caring on middle-aged offspring. *Journal of Gerontologic Nursing, 6* (2), 79–85.

Chenitz, W. C., & Swanson, J. M. (1987). Qualitative research using grounded theory. In W. C. Chenitz and J. M. Swanson (Eds.), *From practice to grounded theory* (pp. 3–15). Menlo Park: Addison-Wesley.

Corbin, J. (1987). Qualitative data analyses for grounded theory. In W. C. Chenitz & J. M. Swanson (Eds.), *From practice to grounded theory* (pp. 91–101). Menlo Park, CA: Addison-Wesley.

Glaser, B. G., (1978). *Theoretical sensitivity: Advances in the methodology of grounded theory.* Mill Valley, CA: Sociology Press.

Glaser, B. G., & Strauss, A. L. (1967). The purpose and credibility of qualitative research. *Nursing Research, 15*, 56–61.

Goldman, H. H. (1982). Mental illness and family burden: A public health perspective. *Health and Community Practice, 34*(2), 129–134.

Hutchinson, S. (1986). Grounded theory: The method. In P. L. Munhall & C. J. Oiler (Eds.), *Nursing research: A qualitative perspective* (pp. 111–130). Norwalk, CT: Appleton-Century-Crofts.

Northouse, L. L. (1980). Who supports the support system? *Journal of Psychiatric Nursing and Mental Health Services, 18*(5), 11–15.

Ory, M. G., Williams, T. F., Emr, M., Lebowitz, B., Rabins, P., Salloway, J., Sluss-Radbaugh, T., Wolff, E., Zarit, S. (1985). Families, informal supports and Alzheimer's disease: Current research and future agendas. *Research on Aging, 7*, 623–644.

Phillips, L. R., & Rempusheski, V. F. (1986). Caring for the frail elderly at home: Toward a theoretical explanation of the dynamics of poor quality family caregiving. *Advances in Nursing Science, 8*(4), 62–84.

Reifer, B. V., & Wu, S. (1982). Managing families of demented elderly. *Journal of Family Practice, 14*, 1051–1056.

Wilson, H. S. (1985). *Research in nursing.* Menlo Park, CA: Addison-Wesley.

Worchester, M. I., & Quayhagen, M. P. (1983). Correlates of caregiving satisfaction: Prerequisites to elder home care. *Research in Nursing & Health, 6*, 61–67.

Zarit, S. H., Todd, R. A., & Zarit, J. M. (1986). Subjective burden of husbands and wives as caregivers: A longitudinal study. *The Gerontologist, 26*(3), 260–266.

CHAPTER 20

Family Involvement with Communication-Impaired Residents in Long-Term Care Settings

Kathleen C. Buckwalter, Donelle Cusack, Thomas Kruckeberg, Amy Shoemaker

This article describes the outcomes of a study involving family members of communication-impaired long-term care residents in a collaborative nursing/speech language pathology intervention designed to increase the residents' communication ability. Family members provided memorabilia and artifacts or produced audio or video tapes, for use in conjunction with a speech therapy enhancement program (STEP). Findings revealed that, despite a minimal improvement in speech ability, there was a dramatic increase in family members' satisfaction.

One important role of the family with a member in a long-term health care setting is to facilitate linkages that assist residents' interactions with the nursing staff and their environment (Buckwalter & Hall, 1987). However, this role is rarely actualized. Families may relinquish their dependent adults to staff care facilities (Clifford, 1985) or may become so overly involved in the activities of their loved ones as to be regarded as nuisances by nursing staffs. Whatever pattern is followed, the end result may be that families and staffs develop competitive or even adversarial relationships in their efforts to protect and care for long-term care residents.

Successful resident adaptation requires collaboration between the family system and facility personnel. This goal is fostered through creative use of the family, a neglected resource in many long-term care facilities (Buckwalter & Hall, 1987). Families can

Reprinted from *Applied Nursing Research, Vol. 4* (No. 2), May 1991, pp. 77–84. Used with permission of W. B. Saunders Company and the author.

aid resident adaptation to the facility through family-centered interventions and rehabilitative strategies. This article describes the creative use of families in a collaborative nursing/speech language pathology/family intervention to increase communication ability in primarily elderly, institutionalized residents with aphasia and/or dysarthria.

This study was centered on the nursing home care units (NHCUs) of a Veterans' Administration Medical Center (VAMC). Family members of aphasic and/or dysarthric residents had expressed interest in the residents' expressive disabilities and a desire to make constructive use of time spent visiting at the care facility. Many family members requested specialized information on communication deficits and indicated to the nursing staff that they would welcome the opportunity to participate in a program of consistent, coordinated activities focused on a goal of decreasing communication deficits.

LITERATURE REVIEW

The positive effects of family education and involvement in the rehabilitative process have been well documented (Anderson, Anderson, & Kottke, 1977; Shulman & Mandel, 1988). Aten et al. (1984) demonstrated that closely supervised, family members, well-trained in language treatment for aphasia, were able to effect positive changes in the communicative status of aphasic adults.

The acquisition of language in childhood develops spontaneously through purposeful, meaningful, repetitive practice based on memorable experiences. Similarly, the redevelopment of language skills may occur through the recreation of memorable events, verbally and pictorially. This knowledge provided the rationale underlying this project. Family members and nursing staff incorporated memorable pictures, photographs, and in-person or taped reminiscences into the speech therapy enhancement program (STEP), described in detail in Buckwalter, Cusack, Sidles, Wadle, and Beaver (1989) and reviewed briefly in the following section.

Nurses have used reminiscence as an intervention for the elderly for many years and with mixed results (Kovack, 1990). Reminiscence therapy has been shown to be effective in (a) resolving conflicts and coping with stress (Lewis, 1971); (b) maintaining ego integrity, a sense of identity, and self-worth (Baker, 1985; Bourestom, 1981); (c) promoting growth and development of personality (McMahon & Rhudick, 1967; Weinberg, 1974); (d) enhancing movement toward self-actualization and maintaining a sense of equilibrium and security (Butler, 1975); (e) facilitating communication (Liton & Olstein, 1969); (f) increasing socialization and decreasing isolation (Butler, 1974); and (g) improving cognitive function (Hughston & Merriam, 1982). All of these positive outcomes are relevant to the communication-impaired resident who may suffer frustration, embarrassment, irritation, depression (Topics in Geriatrics, 1986a), agitation, and aggression as a result of his or her inability to express and receive messages concerning needs, preferences, opinions, and emotions (Crickmay, 1977; Peterson & Olsen, 1965; Topics in Geriatrics, 1986b). Effective communication is regarded as an essential component of the rehabilitative process (Walton & MacLeod Clark, 1986) and is inextricably intertwined with quality of life issues (Shulman & Mandel, 1988). Not only is the ability to communicate closely tied to the long-term care resident's ability to perform activities of daily living, but it is also central to their maintenance of mental health and positive self-esteem. Thus, an intervention that would increase communication ability in this population would seem to be of benefit not only to the affected residents but to their family members and the nursing staff who care for them.

METHOD
Inclusion Criteria

Brain-damaged residents with diagnoses of aphasia, dysarthria, or both were included in this study. Residents with apraxia, speech problems secondary to psychiatric disorders, and late stage dementing disorders such as Alzheimer's disease were excluded. All subjects had a family member who consented to provide memorabilia and evaluative data for the project. Figure 1 is a copy of the informational summary sent to prospective family subjects to solicit their participation.

Design

Subjects with family members who agreed to participate in the study were non-randomly assigned to either the experimental (receiving the family-centered STEP intervention) or control (therapy as usual) condition. Pilot testing of the intervention had determined that random assignment of subjects to treatment condition was not feasible because of contamination issues in the clinical setting (e.g., more than one subject in a room). Rather, subjects were matched on the basis of speech ability according to a baseline battery of standardized speech assessment tests, including the Boston Diagnostic Aphasic Examination (BDAE; Goodglass & Kaplan, 1972), the Language Ability Screening Test (LAST), and the Assessment of Intelligibility of Dysarthric Speech (AIDS; 1981). Previous research on this population by Buckwalter et al. (1989) demonstrated that age, speech disorders, medical diagnoses, and time since brain injury did not influence speech results using this intervention. Analysis of variance on baseline speech scores confirmed no significant differences in speech ability between groups at the start of the study. Thus, the groups were considered to be equivalent, despite lack of randomization. In addition, subjects who received the STEP intervention using video cassette recordings were analyzed separately as a subgroup of the experimental condition.

Family-Centered Intervention

A quasi-experimental repeated measures design was used to test the effectiveness of family involvement in an individualized speech therapy enhancement program (STEP) over a 15-month period. This design enabled the investigators to study differences in non-randomized groups over time. Family involvement included the provision of memorable pictures and photographs accompanied by in-person (when the family was able to visit) or taped (either audio or video) reminiscences. Thus, a family who could only visit infrequently because of lack of proximity to the NHCU might record a

INFORMATION SHEET

TO THE FAMILY OF _____

NAME _____ RELATIONSHIP_____

ADDRESS _____

Dear Knoxville VAMC Family Member:

_____ has been participating in a study at the Knoxville
(Patient's Name)

VAMC funded by a grant from the Robert Wood Johnson Foundation to the University of
Iowa. A Speech/Language Pathologist has devised an individualized therapy program for
your veteran and administered it, conducted tests, etc. In addition, the nursing staff were
taught to conduct the practice exercises during the time they ordinarily spent with the
patient every day. There are no known risks associated with participation in this study. The
patients are making progress in regaining their ability to communicate.

If you would like _____ to continue in this
(Patient's Name)

project, please sign here: _____

We are entering the second phase of the study, which involves family members. Each
veteran's individual therapy program will be developed from memorable events in his past
life. We hope the memory of pleasurable events will help him advance further in regaining
his speech skills. We are seeking your involvement in any one of the following ways: (Please
mark with an X all you are willing to do.)

____ Provide photographs, snapshots, or other items of meaningful events in the patient's
     life.

____ Make 6 audio (voice) tapes reminiscing about meaningful past events. Tapes should
     run 3 to 5 minutes. All materials will be provided.

____ Make a brief (15 to 30 minute) video tape of you and/or any interested family
     members reminiscing about meaningful past events in the patient's life. The videos
     will be filmed at the Knoxville VAMC at the convenience of family members. We feel
     these videotapes will be an effective mechanism for stimulating speech therapy,
     particularly for patients whose family members are unable to visit frequently.

The tapes and memorabilia will be shown only to your veteran and will be returned to you
at the end of the study. Your confidentiality will be respected and maintained throughout.
You will be asked to fill out and return (by mail) a brief questionnaire once a month.

Please indicate when you might be available to make the tapes or bring in the pictures and
other items. _____ (date) We hope to start this phase of the project by
early summer.

FIGURE 1. Information sheet.

60-minute video segment featuring spouse, children, and grandchildren relating meaningful past and current events. The speech language pathologist working with the project would then divide the tape into six 10-minute sessions and devise the individual speech tasks related to the content presented by the family on the tape. Speech tasks were individualized both in the sense that they highlighted communication deficits unique to each subject (e.g., naming of objects) and incorporated reminiscences unique to each subject's experience (e.g., the name of the family dog is "Sparky"). In this way, family members reinforced both verbally and visually content used in the STEP program. This content was meaningful and memorable to the resident, as opposed to the often boring, repetitive exercises associated with more traditional speech therapies (Draizar, 1981). Figure 2 is an example of a traditional speech therapy exercise.

For experimental subjects, the STEP intervention devised by the speech therapist and based on family reminiscences was implemented by nursing personnel for 10 minutes daily on both the day and evening shifts and the night shift when feasible (i.e., without awakening the resident). The speech intervention was administered during

---

Communication Checklist

Patient: _____ I.D.# _____
Date: _____, 198___
Shift: _____ Night _____ Day _____ Evening
Initials: _____

	+/−	The Patient will accurately—	+/−
1. chest	_____	1. I sleep on a _____. (bed)	_____
2. ankle	_____	2. When I'm cold, I cover up with a _____. (blanket)	_____
3. neck	_____	3. You hit a baseball with a _____. (bat)	_____
4. middle finger	_____	4. You wear a ring on your _____. (finger)	_____
5. thigh	_____	5. We fly up in the air in a _____. (plane)	_____
6. lips	_____	6. You write checks to pay _____. (bills)	_____
7. eyebrow	_____	7. You cut meat with a _____. (knife)	_____
8. left cheek	_____	8. I like to watch my _____. (TV)	_____
9. right index finger	_____	9. You cut paper with a _____. (scissors)	_____
10. right wrist	_____	10. We see with our _____. (eyes)	_____
		11. Ronald Reagan used to act in _____. (movies)	_____
		12. I hear with my _____. (ears)	_____
		13. I mop the floor with a _____. (mop)	_____
		14. You drink beer from a _____. (bottle, can)	_____
		15. We can look out the _____. (window, door)	_____
		16. They mow the grass with a _____. (mower)	_____
		17. At noon, we eat _____. (lunch, dinner)	_____
		18. They use a lawn-mower to cut _____. (grass)	_____
		19. During the war, I served in the _____. (Navy, Army)	_____
		20. We ride to Des Moines in a _____. (car, van)	_____
Total	_____	Total	_____

FIGURE 2. Example of a traditional speech therapy task.

the course of routine nursing activities (e.g., while making the bed or dressing or feeding the resident). For those residents whose families had developed audio or video tapes, the tape would be played in the resident's room. Pictures and photographs supplied by families were laminated for preservation purposes, enlarged if the resident was visually impaired, and left in a drawer in the resident's room.

Control subjects received the usual biweekly speech therapy treatment from speech language pathologists. Control subjects and their family members were administered the same evaluative measures at the same intervals as subjects and family members in the experimental group.

Instruments

Data were collected weekly on the STEP speech tasks and every 3 months on the standardized speech measures (BDAE, LAST, AIDS) as described in Buckwalter et al. (1989). In addition, every 3 months family members in both groups provided mailed evaluations of their satisfaction with the treatment program using a Family Perception Scale (FPS) developed expressly for this purpose. Using a 5-point Likert scale (1 = *strongly agree* to 5 = *strongly disagree*), the FPS assessed family attitudes in seven major areas: (a) satisfaction with care the resident was receiving, (b) concern of the nursing staff, (c) resident progress, (d) family involvement in care, (e) family willingness to work with resident in the institution, (f) interest in working with the resident after discharge, and (g) interest in caring for their family member after discharge. Ample space was also provided on the instrument for families to provide information about the frequency of their visits and anecdotal information about the content and quality of the visit, as well as to express any concerns they might have. For the FPS, lower scores are indicative of higher levels of family satisfaction. Pilot testing had established the utility and psychometric properties of the scale (test-retest reliability of r = .92). Interestingly, return rates for the family data over the 25-month course of the study differed significantly by group: 90% for those in the experimental group and 65% for those in the control group, suggesting differential degrees of family investment in the project according to group.

HYPOTHESES

Two sets of hypotheses were tested in this study. With regard to family-centered outcomes, it was hypothesized that family members who were involved in implementing the STEP program under the guidance of nursing personnel would: (a) demonstrate higher levels of satisfaction with the care of their family member; (b) have a more positive attitude toward participating in other rehabilitative programs associated with post brain injury recovery; and (c) demonstrate a greater willingness to accept the resident into the home setting after discharge from the care facility, which has been shown to increase survival rates in this population. In summary, it was hypothesized that family members involved in the rehabilitative process would experience greater satisfaction than those not involved. With regard to speech outcomes, it was hypothesized that residents in the experimental group would demonstrate more improved speech performance on the STEP tasks and the standardized speech measures (BDAE, LAST, and AIDS) than residents in the control group.

FINDINGS

Subjects

Thirty-seven resident subjects were entered into the study: 19 in the experimental group and 18 in the control group. Over the 15-month study period, there were five deaths (three in the experimental group and two in the control group) and two discharges to acute care facilities for treatment of illness (one in each group). This attrition rate is consistent with the frail and dependent nature of the population under study. Residents ranged in age from 30 to 86 years, with an average age of 61. Because of the setting (a rural VAMC), all subjects were male. They had been aphasic ($n = 22$), dysarthric ($n = 10$), or both ($n = 5$) for an average of 12.5 years, ranging from 4 to 24 years post brain injury. Subjects had resided on the NHCU where the study took place and had been without active speech therapy for an average of 10 years. Their primary medical diagnoses included cerebrovascular accident ($n = 18$), organic brain syndromes ($n = 11$), head trauma ($n = 6$), and progressive degeneration ($n = 2$). A summary profile reflects a primarily elderly, aphasic resident sample, institutionalized for many years on the NHCU of a rural VAMC. Most had been without active speech therapy or family involvement in their care for a long period of time. The majority were also seriously physically ill and geographically removed from family members, who visited an average of once per month.

The mean age of experimental family member subjects was 63.4 years and 61.1 years for family members in the control group. Table 1 illustrates the relationship of family members to resident subjects.

TABLE 1
Relationship of Family Members to Resident Subjects

Relationship	Experimental Group (n = 19)	Control Group (n = 18)
Spouse	11	10
Adult child	5	4
Sibling	2	3
Parent	1	1
Total	19	18

Speech Tasks

Using a two-way (time by group) repeated measures analysis of variance (RM-ANOVA), there were no significant differences in speech task scores between the experimental and the control groups ($p = .32$) over time, and no interaction effects between time and group. Thus, residents in the experimental group did not improve more than control subjects on this measure of speech ability. However, the factor of time itself was significant for both groups ($p = .03$); that is, both experimental and control subjects improved their scores on speech tasks as the study period progressed. This unexpected finding can perhaps best be explained by the fact by the fact that task data were collected weekly on control group members, and the act of data collection and the inherent attention to communication may have served as a speech intervention. There were also no significant differences between video and nonvideo (e.g., pictures or audio recordings) interventions within the experimental group, although qualitative analysis of staff and subject comments revealed that they *liked* the video intervention better.

Standardized Speech Tests

Using similar two-way (time-by-group), RM-ANOVA format, subjects in the experimental and control groups were compared on the three standardized speech tests: BDAE, LAST, and AIDS. For the BDAE, experimental subjects performed significantly better than controls on only 4 of 43 dimensions: reciting ($p = .04$), articulation ($p = .02$), phrase length ($p = .008$), and melodic line ($p = .01$). A fifth dimension, verbal agility, showed significant ($p = .01$) improvement over time for both groups, with no interaction (time by group) effects ($p = .36$).

In the LAST data, overall there were no significant differences between experimental and control groups ($p = .18$) and no time by group interaction effects ($p = .21$), but time itself was a significant factor ($p = .02$). That is, subjects in both groups improved on their LAST scores over the 15-month study period. Analysis by components of this test (completeness, promptness, accuracy) confirmed significant interactions only over time. For the AIDS test, which consists of two components—sentences and words—there were no significant differences between experimental and control groups.

Family Satisfaction Data

Again, using a two-way RM-ANOVA, family members who participated in the experimental protocol were significantly ($p = .016$) more satisfied with the care their family member received than family members in the control group. Families of experimental subjects also reported they would be more willing ($p = .0006$) to care for their family member in the home if that family member were to be discharged. Family members of experimental subjects also differed significantly from control family members in their positive perception of nursing staff concern ($p = .006$), believed they were more involved in their loved one's care ($p = .0003$), and believed the speech therapy intervention would be effective both while their family member was hospitalized ($p = .002$)

and after discharge (p = .0001). The only variable for which no statistical difference was evident between control and experimental families was "family member doing as well as can be expected" (p = .07), which approached significance. This latter finding is not surprising given the level of frailty of resident subjects and sample attrition due to morbidity and mortality. Table 2 compares mean scores for family members of the two groups on the FPS at 3, 6, 9, 12, and 15 months.

DISCUSSION

The speech-related hypotheses were not supported, as findings on standardized speech tests suggest that the STEP intervention does not globally improve speech. Those dimensions on the BDAE that were shown to differ between experimental and control groups (reciting, articulation, phrase length, and melodic line) were also the factors most often rehearsed in the speech (STEP) tasks. The finding that in many areas both experimental and control subjects improved suggests that increased staff/resident interaction, even from testing encounters, may improve selected aspects of communication. Examination of means at systematic intervals of analysis over the study period (baseline, 3, 6, 9, 12, and 15 months) consistently showed peaks in scoring at the 3-month interval (although the RM-ANOVAs were not statistically significant). This may be attributed to either a Hawthorne-like effect of newness of the study and subject response to the increased attention this entailed in the study period or to the fact that over time the physical condition of many subjects deteriorated (see prior discussion of subject attrition by death/disability). Preliminary analysis to determine the influence of the factor "change in health status" suggests that controlling for health status markedly affects differences in performance between experimental and control subjects on speech data.

The family-related hypotheses, on the other hand, were strongly supported. Inclusion of family members in the speech therapy program, by audiotaped or videotaped reminiscences and/or by providing significant family memorabilia such as photographs and artifacts, significantly increased their satisfaction with many aspects of the residents' care. It also increased their sense of positive involvement, suggesting they would be more likely to accept the resident post-discharge.

TABLE 2
Comparison of Experimental and Control Group Family Member Total Scores on the PS over the Study Period

Study Period (months)	Experimental Group (n = 19)	Control Group (n = 18)
3	11.70	13.62
6	12.22	14.00
9	15.00	16.83
12	13.00	15.20
15	13.00	15.50

Lower score indicates higher satisfaction.

The findings of this study are in keeping with recent research by Shulman and Mandel (1988), who evaluated a series of workshops called CONNECT (Communication Need Not Ever Cease Totally) for families of communication-impaired residents. The CONNECT workshops resulted in increased understanding, increased satisfaction with visits, and increased skill in communication between family and residents. Similarly, the response from families in the experimental group of this study was overwhelmingly positive. A serendipitous finding from those families who videotaped their reminiscences was an almost cathartic psychological therapy for them to resolve some issues they may have avoided confronting. In the open-ended section of the FPS, many reported feeling better about themselves and the institutionalization of their family member, feeling less frightened by their loved one, and enjoying their visits to the VAMC more. It is notable that, over the study period, experimental family members increased the number of their visits by 23% whereas visits by family members of control subjects increased only 6%. This anecdotal finding deserves further systematic investigation using videotapes of family members as a potential nursing intervention to help families adapt to institutionalization and prevent a sense of abandonment.

IMPLICATIONS FOR NURSING

In this study family members brought photographs or made video/audio cassettes of memorable family occasions. The rationale for family involvement in this manner was twofold. First, if the speech subject is personally meaningful it will be more motivating; that is, residents may be more eager to discuss a photograph of their wedding or a grandchild than a flashcard of a cup and saucer from traditional speech therapy activities. Second, the reminiscence therapy of recalling happy days before institutionalization may evoke spontaneous expressions.

Data analysis revealed that, although speech improved minimally (not surprising in this highly debilitated population), satisfaction of family members involved in the speech therapy enhancement program (STEP) increased dramatically. Family members involved in this study were significantly more satisfied with all aspects of care, which generalized to their reported desire to become more involved in the institutional setting as well as after discharge. The collaborative speech/nursing/family intervention developed and tested in this study needs to be replicated with a larger, more heterogeneous sample to validate these initial findings and to test the feasibility of this strategy in a variety of settings. A major limitation of this study was lack of randomization, and future research should include random assignment to condition. The notion of this approach as an effective *family-centered communication* intervention rather than a *patient-centered speech therapy* intervention deserves further study, with attention to family responses and outcomes. As cogently expressed by Shulman and Mandel (1988):

> The role of the family must be recognized as vital to enhancing the quality of life for older people in institutions. Coping strategies and interventions which enable families to maintain relationships with the impaired relatives must be developed. Techniques which can enhance their communication skills must be made known to them in a

supportive environment. In this way, families will be helped to remain connected to their older relatives in institutional settings and to play a continuing role in their lives. (p. 798)

ACKNOWLEDGMENTS

We thank the Veterans Administration Medical Center, Knoxville, IA, speech language pathologists Elise Sidles, Darrel Wheeler, and Elizabeth Sayers; Administrative Assistant Margaret Beaver; and Nursing Research Coordinator Karen Wadle for their assistance with the work described herein. Appreciation is also expressed to Robert Oppliger, PhD, for assistance with data analysis and to Nancy Goldsmith for manuscript preparation.

Supported by Grant No. 9062 to K.C.B. from The Robert Wood Johnson Foundation, Princeton, NJ.

REFERENCES

Anderson, E., Anderson, T. P., & Kottke, F. J. (1977). Stroke rehabilitation: Maintenance of achieved gains. *Archives of Physical Medicine and Rehabilitation, 58,* 352–354.

Assessment of intelligibility of dysarthric speech. (1981). Tigard, OR: C. C. Publishing Company, Inc.

Aten, J. L., Wertz, R. T., Weiss, D., Brookshire, R. H., Garcia-Bunnel, L., Holland, A. L., LaPointe, L. L., Kurtzke, J. F., Milianti, F. J., Brannigan, R., Greenbaum, H., Marshall, R. C., Vogel, D., Carter, J., Barnes, N. S., & Goodman, R. (1984). Veterans administration cooperative study on aphasia: A comparison of clinical, home and deferred treatment. *Archives of Physical Medicine and Rehabilitation, 65,* 666.

Baker, N. (1985). Reminiscing in group therapy for self-worth. *Journal of Gerontological Nursing, 11*(7), 21–24.

Buckwalter, K. C., & Hall, G. R. (1987). Families of the institutionalized older adult: A neglected resource. In T. H. Brubaker (Ed.), *Aging, health and family: Long term care* (pp. 176–196). Newbury Park, CA: Sage.

Buckwalter, K. C., Cusack, D., Sidles, E., Wadle, K., & Beaver, M. (1989). Increasing communication ability in aphasic/dysarthric patients. *Western Journal of Nursing Research, 11,* 736–747.

Bourestom, N. (1981). *The role of reminiscence in therapy with the aged.* Grant No. 470–26–1540, U.S. Veterans Administration, Department of Medicine and Surgery.

Butler, R. (1974). Successful aging and the role of the life review. *Journal of American Geriatrics Society, 12,* 529–535.

Butler, R. (1975). *Why survive? Being old in America.* New York, NY: Harper and Row.

Clifford, A. (1985). Your mother is ours now. *Journal of Gerontological Nursing, 10*(9), 44.

Crickmay, M. C. (1977). *Help the stroke patient to talk.* Springfield, IL: Charles C. Thomas.

Draizar, A. (1981). *Rapid linguistic change in recovery from aphasia.* Bethesda, MD: National Institute of Education, Department of Health, Education and Welfare.

Goodglass, H., & Kaplan, E. (1972). *Boston diagnostic aphasia examination.* Philadelphia, PA: Lea & Febiger.

Hughston, G., & Merriam, S. (1982). Reminiscence: A non-formal technique for improving cognitive functioning in the aged. *International Journal of Aging and Human Development, 15,* 132–141.

Kovack, C. R. (1990). Promise and problems in reminiscence research. *Journal of Gerontological Nursing, 16*(4), 10–14.

Language ability screening test. [Unpublished test developed at the Veterans Administration Medical Center, Knoxville, IA.]

Lewis, C. N. (1971). Reminiscing and self-concept in old age. *Journal of Gerontology, 26*, 240–243.

Liton, L., & Olstein, S. C. (1969). Therapeutic aspects of reminiscence. *Social Casework, 50*, 263–269.

McMahon, A. W., & Rhudick, P. J. (1967). Reminiscing in the aged. In S. Levin & R. J. Kohana (Eds.), *Psychodynamic studies on aging: Creativity, reminiscing, and dying.* New York, NY: International Universities Press.

Peterson, J. C., & Olsen, A. P. (1965). *Language problems after a stroke.* Minneapolis, MN: American Rehabilitation Foundation.

Shulman, M. D., & Mandel, E. (1988). Communication training of relatives and friends of institutionalized elderly persons. *The Gerontologist, 28*, 797–799.

Topics in Geriatrics. (1986a). Treatment of poststroke depression with ECT. *Massachusetts General Hospital Newsletter, 5*(1), 1–3.

Topics in Geriatrics. (1986b). Management and pseudobulbar emotional symptoms. *Massachusetts General Hospital Newsletter, 5*(4), 13–16.

Walton, L., & MacLeod Clark, J. (1986, August 13). Making contact. *Nuring Times,* pp. 28–32.

Weinberg, J. (1974). What do I say to my mothers when I have nothing to say? *Geriatrics, 29*(11), 155–159.

CHAPTER 21

Living with
a Wife Undergoing
Chemotherapy

Sharon Wilson, Janice M. Morse

This study explicates the experience of living with a woman undergoing chemotherapy from the perspective of her husband. Data include 48 unstructured, open-ended face-to-face or telephone interviews with 14 informants and the diary of one informant. A substantive theory depicts the process through which husbands experience their wives' chemotherapy treatment for cancer. A three-stage model was developed, consisting of identifying the threat, engaging in the fight and becoming a veteran. Buffering was identified as the basic social process that explained the behaviors of husbands throughout this experience. It is proposed that when the disease reoccurs and chemotherapy is recommended, the process begins again.

Cancer is feared as a life-threatening disease that conveys a threat of intractable pain, hopelessness and wasting away before death occurs (Klagsbrum, 1983). Although advanced and successful forms of cancer treatment such as chemotherapy are available many adverse and unrelenting side-effects must be endured. Precious little is known about the coping strategies of those undergoing chemotherapy; still less is known about the experiences of the husband supporting his wife undergoing such treatment. Understanding these experiences would provide health professionals with valuable insights into ways families cope, thus enhancing their quality of life. The purpose of this quality of life study was to explore the experiences of the husband supporting his wife undergoing chemotherapy for cancer.

From *IMAGE: Journal of Nursing Scholarship, Vol. 23* (No. 2), Summer 1991, pp. 78–84. Reprinted by permission of the publisher.

In the literature, the patient's response to chemotherapy is described primarily from the health professional's perspective. Studies on spousal response are often reported collectively without identifying the unique reactions of being either the well husband or the well wife. Most do not address inherent changes as the disease progresses. Although cancer is a disease of multiple stages, frequently data collection is based on one interview at a particular stage rather than many interviews done over time and during various stages of treatment. The one-shot approach ignores the changing nature of the disease progression as well as the spousal response to these changes. Thus, there is a scarcity of longitudinal information regarding day-to-day management of chemotherapy for both the patient and spouse.

Very little is known about the experiences of a husband responding to his wife's reaction to a diagnosis of cancer. Husbands describe a deterioration of their own health as well as disturbed thought processes during their wives' terminal illness (Howell, 1986). Husbands who are involved in the decision-making process leading to mastectomy are able to adjust more readily during their wives' postoperative recovery (Wellisch, Jamison, & Pasnau, 1978). Husbands report an increased desire for physical closeness with a decreased sexual desire when wives undergo chemotherapy for advanced disease (Leiber, Plumb, Gerstenzang, & Holland, 1976). During chemotherapy, husbands deny their own feelings (Sabo, Brown & Smith, 1986). Other studies report husbands have a need to be constantly cheerful and hopeful while experiencing ambivalent feelings of anger and guilt (Oberst & James, 1985), hostility and rejection (Gates, 1980) during chemotherapy. These studies indicate a negative reaction, with the possibility of a potentially harmful outcome, for the husband whose wife receives chemotherapy. This study addresses the research question: How does the husband describe his day-to-day experience of living with a wife undergoing chemotherapy for cancer?

METHOD

The methods of grounded theory (Chenitz & Swanson, 1986; Glaser, 1978; Glaser & Strauss, 1967) were used to identify the husbands' experience over time and to develop an explanatory model.

Sample and Data Collection

The interviews began using a purposeful, nonprobability sample of husbands whose wives were currently undergoing chemotherapy treatment. Later, theoretical sampling facilitated "densifying" the categories (Chenitz & Swanson, 1986, p. 96), and increased the richness and thickness of the data. Concurrent data collection and analysis permitted the delimitation and refinement of categories, and guided sampling strategies as possible questions included: Does the husband's experience differ depending on the presence or absence of chemotherapy treatment? Does length of time or length of chemotherapy affect the husband's experience either during or after conclusion of chemotherapy? Does the wife's longevity affect the husband's experience? In response to these questions, the sample was expanded to explore comparative data and included husbands whose wives were newly diagnosed, undecided about undergoing chemotherapy, had completed chemotherapy and were either living or had died after conclusion of chemotherapy.

Demographic characteristics of husbands in this study are shown in Table 1. The mean age of husbands was 47 years, the mean length of marriage was 17 years, and the mean length of time living with a wife receiving chemotherapy was 17 months.

Fourteen informants volunteered to participate. The 15th informant kept a diary throughout his wife's illness, and gave permission to include this information as research data. Forty-eight interactive tape-recorded interviews were conducted face-to-face or by telephone. These were later transcribed verbatim and were sufficient to obtain an appropriate and adequate amount of data to saturate all emergent categories (Morse, 1986).

Interview questions were descriptive and initially were used to allow informants to tell their stories. Husbands were asked to relate their experiences from the time "it all began" and most chose to begin from the moment when the first symptoms were observed. Attempts to focus questions came out of comparative analysis and expanded upon expressed thoughts or behavioral patterns described by husbands. The search for commonalities and differences among husbands and within categories was of constant concern. For example, anger was a dominant theme in all of the evolving categories. It

TABLE 1
Biographical Characteristics of Husbands

			Characteristics			
Informant	Age in Years	Years of Marriage	Type of Cancer	Months of Chemo-therapy	Under-going Chemo-therapy	Total Number of Interviews
1	46	20	Breast	90	Currently	8
2	32	12	Lymphoma	15	Currently	4
3	46	12	Breast	3	Currently	1
4	44	12	Breast	3	Currently	4
5	46	20	Breast	3	Currently	4
6	32	1	Breast	3	Currently	2
7	60	4	Lymphoma	16	Completed	5
8	65	37	Lymphoma	14	Completed	5
9	54	37	Breast	24	Completed	3
10	48	14	Breast	11	Completed	2
11	50	26	Breast	4	Completed	2
12	43	22	Breast	10	Completed	3
13	49	25	Breast	26	Completed	3
14	46	10	Breast	9	Completed	3
15	nk[1]	9	Leukemia	11	Completed	Diary

[1]*Not known.*

became important to focus on questions such as: What contributed to feelings of anger? How did husbands reduce their angry feelings? How did husbands resolve their angry feelings? How did anger influence the ability to cope with experiencing the wife's response to chemotherapy?

Reliability and Validity

Reliability was enhanced by the process of theoretical sampling, by deliberately selecting appropriate informants according to the theoretical needs or by probing and clarifying ambiguity. The assumption that all informants are not equally able to share information relevant to the purpose of the study enabled the choice of husbands who were motivated, interested, knowledgeable and willing to be interviewed over time. Interviews over time were used to corroborate recurrent or changing data, and categories were saturated, thus ensuring adequacy (Morse, 1986).

Data Analysis

Using methods described by Glaser (1978) and Glaser and Strauss (1967), systematic analysis of interview transcripts proceeded with the assistance of the *Ethnograph* program (Seidel, Kjolseth, & Clark, 1985). *Ethnograph* was used to manage, cut and paste the field notes. Data codes were entered to code and recode all interviews, memos and voluminous amount of data. The coding process involved several levels of increasing complexity and abstractness. Initial level 1 coding represented action verbs used by informants such as nurturing, listening, touching, humoring or assisting. After interpretation of these behaviors, the codes were grouped to form a more complex code called "cherishing." In turn, cherishing was grouped with other similarly complex codes such as "being there," "normalizing," "taking charge" or "being positive" to form the more abstract code of "softening the blow." As the coding became greater in scope, it became clear that softening the blow was one strategy used by husbands to endure their wives' response to chemotherapy. Similarly, other strategies of "resisting disruption" and "preserving self" were formulated. Eventually, "strategies of enduring" were grouped with other experiences husbands described. Three distinct categories, identifying the threat, engaging in the fight and becoming a veteran were identified. The process of concurrent data collection and analysis led to the discovery of the core variable, buffering, which explained the experiences of husbands who respond to their wives' reactions to chemotherapy. In addition, throughout data collection and analysis, two activities which served to formulate abstract ideas and generate creative thinking were memos and field notes. The emphasis on the generation of new relationships between datum and evolving categories helped to clarify and define the grounded theory and eventually led to the basic social process. Variation was accounted for by comparing cases with the presence or absence of concepts and developing 2 × 2 typologies to illustrate each scenario (Glaser, 1978).

BASIC SOCIAL PROCESS

The basic social psychological problem for the husband was coping with his wife's reaction to chemotherapy. The basic social process, buffering, is illustrated in Figure 1.

"Buffering" was a process by which husbands filtered and reduced the stresses of day-to-day living to protect their wives. It required a delicate balance of patience, persistence, understanding and compassion within a caring relationship. Husbands constantly evaluated the effectiveness of their buffering strategies, revising and/or developing new ones. The buffering process involved two active components: constant vigilance and cognitive action. Constant vigilance consisted of watching his wife's response to chemotherapy and her interactions with others. Cognitive action involved the interpretation of his perceptions, judging whether his wife was in a harmful situation and then planning an action designed to buffer.

Buffering was manifested in the form of behavioral strategies designed to reduce or eliminate a potential threat to the wife's well-being, to alter her perception of the threat or to enhance her coping abilities. Buffering strategies were designed to "soften the blow," "resist disruption" and "preserve self."

"Softening the blow" included behaviors that were supporting (by "being there") and endearing (by "cherishing"). This made day-to-day life easier for their wives. "Being there" was being supportive but knowing enough not to hover. "Cherishing," the

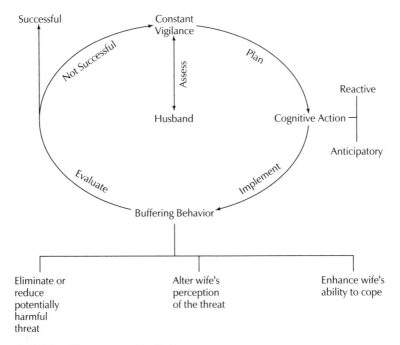

FIGURE 1. The process of buffering.

most obvious form of endearment, consisted of nurturing, listening, touching, humoring and assisting. An example of assisting would be bathing the wife or helping her in the bathroom. Husbands became more attentive, compassionate and considerate. They no longer took their wives for granted. Although sexual relations decreased, husbands continued to experience intense emotions of affection, gratitude and love for their wives.

"Resisting disruption" included disguising one's feelings. One husband said: "I tried to do a good job of hiding my feelings from her. I never wanted to show weakness in front of her." They avoided talking to their wives about their own excessive drinking, smoking, outside friendships or dismay at their wives' appearance. They maintained self-control at all times so that disruption to the household would be minimal despite their wives' mood swings, physical illness and mental apathy.

"Preserving self" consisted of maintaining their own self-control, health and energy. Conserving energy, for example, might include "power naps" before leaving the office at the end of the day. Work provided an escape from the feeling of helplessness they experienced in the home and, therefore, became a strategy to promote self-control and energy restoration. Exercise became an important way of releasing stress and providing time for private thought. In order to maintain self-control, husbands focused on the present, getting through each day. Long-term goals were non-existent.

As shown in Figure 2, the ability to plan and implement buffering behavior depended on whether the husband was able to dissipate his anger. If the husband could dissipate his anger, maintain a positive attitude and develop effective buffering strategies, he was able to effectively assist his wife during chemotherapy (cell a). If the husband was able to dissipate his anger but was unable to identify effective buffering strategies, he felt useless or powerless and his attitude became apathetic (cell b). Husbands in this group tended to project a lack of concern for others and often became emotionally and physically ill. If the husband suppressed his anger, but was able to develop effective buffering strategies, he became domineering (cell c). Husbands in this group were stressed and spent more time at work. If the husband suppressed his anger and was unable to identify effective buffering strategies, he became cynical (cell d). Husbands in this group felt like failures, withdrew from the marital relationship, never spoke to anyone about the cancer experience and were the most likely ones to leave the relationship.

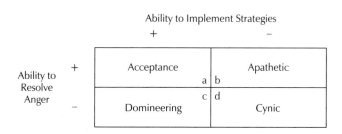

FIGURE 2. Typology illustrating the relationship between the husband's ability to resolve anger and the ability to assist his wife endure chemotherapy.

As a husband's strategies of buffering were consciously planned and carried out, he described an ongoing attempt to evaluate their effectiveness. Evaluation took two forms. First, the husband was vigilant of his wife's response, i.e., he watched to determine if his buffering action reduced his wife's stress. The husband perceived this as a valid means of evaluation because he was so familiar with his wife. The husband believed that he could determine his wife's level of stress by the way she behaved or acted throughout the day. Secondly, the husband evaluated the manner which his wife communicated, verbally and nonverbally. The ultimate success of buffering occurred when she verbalized feeling more comfortable because of her husband's actions. Then the husband felt secure in knowing that his buffering actions reduced the stress of daily living for his wife. When the buffering strategy was evaluated and found to be ineffective in protecting, filtering or reducing the stress for his wife, then the husband persistently began to re-enact the buffering process by reassessing the situation causing stress.

A model depicting the husband's experience was developed. Husbands exemplify buffering behavior throughout the three-stage process, and the model provides a structure which can be used to assess the specific stage of the husband's experience. Clearly, buffering is the underlying behavioral response of husbands in all stages of their experience as they react to their wives' response to chemotherapy. Figure 3 illustrates this three-stage process juxtaposed with the medical course of illness.

For the husband whose wife undergoes chemotherapy, the three-stage process differed from that associated with the medical model of illness. The stages, categorized as identifying the threat, engaging the fight and becoming a veteran, are independent. Each stage has specific boundaries and characteristics of responses. Categories were linked to describe the dynamic process through which a husband progresses as he reacts to his wife's response to chemotherapy.

Stage 1: Identifying the Threat

The first stage, "the threat," began when cancer was suspected, but not confirmed. Husbands developed a suspicion of cancer when their wives discovered an abnormality or consulted a physician. This stage ended following diagnosis.

Suspecting: Husbands became apprehensive that something was "not right" and worried about the well-being of their wives. They were doubtful when their wives discovered a lump. They were fearful after the physician noted "it does not look good" and ordered a biopsy. Feelings of sadness, apprehension, worry and doubt increased as husbands waited for verification of cancer. Self-control was expressed in the form of guarded optimism, a state of disciplining the mind to think positively so as to counter the fear associated with the "worst scenario." The "worst scenario" was the confirmation of cancer and with it, the dreaded expectation of a painfully prolonged death for their wives.

Finding out: A rapid flow of events took place from the uncertainty of "suspecting" to the beginning of treatment, once the diagnosis of cancer was verified. Husbands, who were already overwhelmed by the shock of the diagnosis, now grappled with the speed of events, such as surgery. Consequently, regaining control was important for

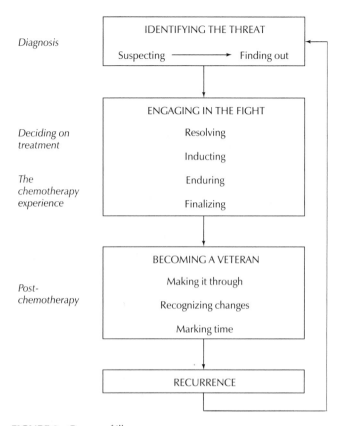

FIGURE 3. Course of illness.

husbands to take charge and spare their wives the stress of informing others of the diagnosis. Waiting and wondering produced fear, uncertainty and anxiety, and spouses mirrored each other's emotional responses. Although he mentally prepared for the "worst thing that could happen" and was emotionally drained, he projected an optimistic outlook about the prognosis to his wife and others.

The presence of cancer forced husbands to acknowledge their own terror, despair and sadness while continuing to "cover up" their own response of horror to the situation. The wife's hospitalization further reinforced the reality of a life-threatening situation. It was during quiet times, such as driving to and from the hospital, that husbands expressed their grief by crying privately. They also described feelings of powerlessness: "There was nothing you could do about it," and a sense of feeling lost and unbalanced which resulted in a lack of direction.

As husbands experienced painful feelings, they also experienced an increased closeness in the marital relationship and the ability to express compassion toward their wives. They asked questions such as "What do I know of cancer?" "Why my wife? Why not me?" and "What do I do now?" They became angry at inanimate "things" such as the disease per se (but not their wives) or the treatment institution (but not their physicians). It is important to note that the target of the anger was never their wives nor anything that jeopardized their treatment.

Stage 2: Engaging in the Fight

This stage began when husbands resolved to participate in "fighting" the disease with their wives and ended with completion of the current chemotherapy program. Fighting behaviors included accompanying their wives to chemotherapy, waiting, acting as an advocate or intermediary and assuming some of the household tasks.

Resolving: Deciding to fight the cancer provided husbands with an immediate sense of control. While fearful of becoming too hopeful for a cure, they compensated by becoming immersed in the struggle of helping their wives endure chemotherapy. This active participation in their wives' treatment compensated for the paralyzing effects of fear. In addition, it motivated them to get information about their wives' condition. Husbands noted that their ability to cope with their wives' condition was dependent upon the kind of information obtained. Receiving a poor diagnosis was preferable to "being [left] in the dark" and fearing the worst.

Inducting: Inducting was the period leading up to and experiencing the initial chemotherapy treatment. Husbands described financial difficulties (with their wives no longer working), and household difficulties (particularly with the added role of child care), which drained energy. An additional stressor for the couple was the lack of sexual relations because husbands feared causing their wives psychological or physical pain.

The first chemotherapy treatment was the time to "learn under fire," even though husbands had been given information and explanations about the drugs used. Experiential learning had the greater impact on reducing their anxiety about the unknown:

> It doesn't compute until you start seeing it happen. You know, it just doesn't register. After seeing the first session and seeing everything happen, the [following] ones were a lot easier to cope with because you knew what was going to happen.

Enduring: The struggle of watching their wives suffer ensued as the encounter with chemotherapy progressed and was the most prolonged aspect of the "fight:"

> It hits you when the person that's beside you gets sick, has never been sick, and goes through chemo and comes home and vomits, and holds her teeth in her hand. You start seeing a person so differently. You know, you have to help them to the washroom because they're dizzy. Then you really get to love somebody beyond their physical being.

"Struggling" involved apprehending, waiting and committing. The struggle was assessed by observing their wives' response and evaluating the efficacy of treatment by assessing side effects, such as hair loss, fatigue, weight loss or temperament. The struggle permeated their lives and husbands became obsessed:

> It was hell on wheels, watching her go downhill. Hardly being able to talk and eat. Just wasting away in front of your eyes, and in really, really terrible pain. There didn't seem to be much they could do about it.

Husbands were proud of their wives' determination, fortitude and strength, and developed a deep respect for their wives' resilience to pain and suffering. They felt increasing admiration for their wives' acceptance of the "poison," and reported: "I never figured that she would take as much abuse as she was able to." There was a mutual conspiracy of silence around such topics as dying and "facing the future." Husbands were dismayed when they observed their wives broke this agreement by reading the obituaries in newspapers or quietly planning their own funerals.

As chemotherapy progressed, a change in physical appearance became obvious and was a constant reminder of the impact of the illness. Husbands did not perceive hair loss due to chemotherapy to be as frightening as it was to their wives, even if hair loss occurred over the entire body. Some used humor to comfort and counteract their wives' humiliation and fear of feeling "neutered." As their wives became increasingly drawn and fatigued, social events were curtailed. Watching and listening to nausea and vomiting made husbands feel "impotent:"

> It's a terrible thing, when you start getting out of the liquid vomit into the dry heaves. It's even worse, you just sit there and what can you do? It's just a helpless feeling—it's just a terrible helpless feeling.

Husbands felt guilty when they met their own basic needs. For example, while preparing a meal, husbands kept kitchen doors closed so that cooking odors would not cause nausea for their wives.

The level of intensity of "being ill" was dependent on the drug type and dosage. One of the most distressing effects for husbands was their response to the dramatic and rapid change in their wives' temperament. Behaviors such as screaming one moment and being compassionate the next were described as the "chemo crazies," or "Jekyll and Hyde." A lack of understanding for these behaviors induced anger and frustration in husbands. They tried to tolerate and rationalize these temperamental behaviors. Husbands learned to assume a passive role, not arguing or saying anything, but rather "accepting" the mood swings as they were "not her fault."

The paradoxical gap between the husband's overt and optimistic support for his wife and his covert and internalized fear of an eventual death continued. Self-control was maintained by hiding sadness and fear. Husbands felt that crying in front of their wives was a mistake. For many, crying represented weakness, pain, sorrow or lack of control. Crying was a constant pain "in their heart," a pain they could not express because they had to be strong.

Although overworked, husbands helped children continue their day-to-day activities. Husbands acquired a submissive doer role, which meant they dealt with the effects of chemotherapy even though they were not the recipient of the drugs. For example, husbands were awake for long periods during the night to listen to their wives when the effects of the chemotherapy interrupted sleep patterns. This participation helped to dissipate the guilt that husbands felt from being the well spouse.

Fear and sadness were constantly in evidence: "You're always scared, I was always afraid. Deep in your mind, you knew she wasn't going to get well and you were so afraid of that." Husbands had difficulty witnessing their wives' reaction to pain and the sight of needles or injections was upsetting. Their difficulty was often not so much with the present "real pain," but with the idea of future pain they feared their wives would have. In order to retain sufficient energy to fight, they took care not to be overwhelmed with sadness or to be depressed.

Couples became calendar-watchers. This enabled them to normalize their life by "keeping track of what was going on." Because the acute stage of illness was associated with receiving chemotherapy, calendar-watching was a way to see how many days the sickness would last following treatment. It was important to plan ahead:

> You just knew that you were going to be home all weekend. Your wife was going to be awfully sick. There's not a heck of a lot you can do about it . . . just hang in there.

The waiting was timeless, and fluctuated with the "ebb and flow of the disease:"

> The whole thing was a waiting game for me—waiting for results, waiting to see if there was any improvement, waiting to see if she was getting worse, waiting for the end of chemotherapy. It went on and on and on.

Husbands waited for their wives to get ready, for a parking place at the treatment facility, for the physician, for the results of blood work, for prescriptions to be filled, and for an end to the treatment. Waiting was incessant, prolonged, boring, extremely irritating, anxiety provoking and predictable.

Husbands rarely were given information by health care professionals; the men hoped to hear something positive. Anger at the system, at the lack of compassion of health care providers and at having to wait for test results, strained their ability to cope. For example, being forced to wait up to five days for test results was common. It was demeaning when scans were not shown to the couple, particularly when wives who used visualization to understand their disease, needed to see the scans. Requesting information or phoning the physician was often unsuccessful.

Finalizing: Relief was expressed when chemotherapy was finished and the couple realized they were still alive and together. The experience of "fighting" was described "as a bit of an omen," and husbands gained a new appreciation of life as "a gift" to be treasured.

Stage 3: Becoming a Veteran

Husbands shared their doubt and fear about the progress of the disease. They were relieved and happy when chemotherapy was over. Buffering decreased as wives resumed their independence. For example, without the doer role to keep them physically active, many felt lost and helpless. This disturbing and puzzling change led to role re-evaluation for husbands. This was the time to accept their wives' cancer and to begin to attribute meaning to the experience. Some considered this a time of personal and change growth in the way they perceived the world around them. As "veterans" or survivors, they now considered themselves experts and wanted to help others experiencing a similar situation.

Making It Through: This stage was labeled "the veteran" because the experience was devastating: "an unforgettable memory." Husbands emerged from the last chemotherapy session with a sense of fulfillment regarding the fight and making it through.

They expressed admiration for their wives: "I think that is just incredible to go through that horrendous experience and still come out with a sense of humor."

Recognizing Changes: Husbands were relieved when their wives' moods stabilized and their hair came back: Their perception was that their wives became "more like [they] used to be."

Marking Time: Nevertheless, husbands remained vigilant. Again, they were acutely aware of waiting: Waiting for the "magical five-year point" or waiting for test results that would show progress. They did not consider recurrence of the disease and noted, "We will have to deal with that particular crisis at that time."

Recurrence

With a recurrence of the disease, the cycle of experiencing "the threat," "the fight" and "the veteran" resumed. Although now feeling "better equipped" about what to expect, nevertheless, the feelings of devastation and loss of control persisted. Metastases was feared because it meant "game over." Death was a topic which was never discussed between spouses. Therefore, recurrence of cancer represented an extremely stressful time for husbands as they tried desperately to continue to think positively and second-guess their wives' responses. Frantic worry was evident, but not shared. Waiting began again. Test results became the pivotal milestones upon which decisions were made for further chemotherapy.

DISCUSSION

Even though the attention of health care providers is "patient-focused" and they recognize the significance of the family support system for home care of the sporadically ill, little is known about the actual experience and the contribution the primary support person makes caring for the ill after chemotherapy. Although support groups to assist couples are becoming more common, these may be of little help to those who do not express fears. Therefore, there remains a need to assist the healthy spouse, "the primary supporter." Health care professionals can help them maintain their critical role within the family while dealing with the wife's reaction to chemotherapy.

The Canadian Cancer Society widely publicizes the slogan, "Cancer can be Beaten." This implies that cancer is a disease that can be fought. This analogy of battling or fighting is an activity one must participate in if one is to win. Thus, fighting is a prerequisite to winning. A further implication in the slogan is: if one fights, then one can be hopeful of beating or curing the cancer. Thus, the fighting process provides hope. Finally, the slogan also places the onus on the "person" to do battle and win rather than on the caregivers or the therapy. The demand that one must fight in order to succeed assumes that if one fights hard enough then one will succeed. If one does not win the fight, then blame is not placed on the caregiver or the chemotherapy because neither the caregiver nor the treatment are fighting the battle. The only ones left to blame are the patient and spouse. Husbands feel responsible to seek ways of winning so they can help their wives beat cancer. When they do not appear to be winning, husbands feel an overwhelming sense of guilt.

This attitude was so pervasive that the response of husbands could be sorted into phases according to the analogy of warfare. Although deliberately chosen so that the patient is not a passive participant in the therapy, this analogy also implies hope that an associated psychosomatic response may trigger the immunological system to facilitate its own "cure." The negative consequence is placing the burden of cure on the patient and the patient's support system.

Literature on victim-blaming further supports the use of this metaphor (Allison, 1982; Labonte & Penfold, 1981; Wikler, 1987; Wortman, 1983). Several elements serve to intensify a husband's obligation to do anything to ease his wife's suffering. These elements include the guilt associated with being the well spouse, the pain of watching a wife suffer and marital commitment. By encouraging his wife to choose treatment, he also assumes responsibility for the consequences of his wife's suffering. Husbands feel obligated to be loyal, protective and supportive, to assume responsibility for commitment to the household and to assist their wives in fighting the disease. The commitment made at the onset of treatment tends to deny the option to leave the relationship during the current program of chemotherapy. Husbands who left the relationship usually did so after the disease was in remission.

In this study, the husband remained focused on his wife and on his own needs. Apart from coping with day-to-day household tasks, the emotional needs of children were tangentially noted and rarely of concern to the father. It was apparent that the severity of the crisis was so preoccupying that he did not have enough energy left to give to other members of the family. This aspect of the husband's buffering role should be carefully assessed by health professionals.

The process of "buffering" has not been described in the literature. From the perspective of role theory, buffering has two major components. First is the "doer role" where the husband waits upon his wife by meeting her physical needs, following her instructions for completion of household chores, and taking care of children. The other component is the protector and advocacy role where the husband acts as an intermediary among his sick wife, their friends and relatives. Although the husband does not interfere with the relationship between his wife with her physician, he hovers in a protective fashion, i.e., waiting in the hallway or driving her to appointments, as well as being vigilant in monitoring her condition. Each of these components is essential and complements the other for the purpose of preventing burnout. The doer role is clearly asymmetrical, with little reciprocity from the wife, and emotionally draining for the husband. Through providing for the necessary input from those outside the family to renew the vigor needed by the husband to function with day-to-day living, the protector role balances the lack of marital reciprocity. Husbands countered the loss of self-esteem in a subordinate role by the management roles and by the admiration (albeit, sometimes silent) from those outside the family for the way he was coping. Thus, the spousal system did not become imbalanced (Minuchin, 1974; Wright & Leahey, 1984); rather, it developed a different structure as roles changed.

CONCLUSIONS

This three-stage model can be used by health care professionals to understand the experiences of husbands as they progress through three distinct phases of responding to their wives' reaction to chemotherapy. Including the model in the form of an assessment tool to be used by health care professionals would help determine how to support husbands. Further research is needed to address the following questions: How do other family members cope with the wife's chemotherapy experience? How do their experiences differ from the husband's? Are there specific interventions, and at distinct stages, that would facilitate the buffering abilities of husbands?

In summary, this study illustrates the importance of inductive inquiry into the experience of the husband who tries to reduce the stress of day-to-day living for his wife as she receives chemotherapy. This study explicates the reality of the husband's buffering behaviors during a three-stage process previously overlooked by health professionals. The findings describe a model which may be used by nursing practitioners to develop supportive interventions designed to assist the husband's need to engage in buffering behavior.

REFERENCES

Allison, K. (1982). Health education: Self-responsibility vs. blaming the victim. *Health Education, 20*(3), 11–13, 21.

Chenitz, W. C., & Swanson, J. M. (1986). *From practice to grounded theory.* Menlo Park, CA: Addison-Wesley.

Gates, C. C. (1980). Husbands of mastectomy patients. *Counselling and Health Education, 1,* 38–41.

Glaser, B. G. (1978). *Theoretical sensitivity: Advances in the methodology of grounded theory.* Mill Valley: The Sociology Press.

Glaser, B. G., & Strauss, A. L. (1967). *The discovery of grounded theory, strategies for qualitative research.* Chicago: Aldine.

Howell, D. (1986). The impact of terminal illness on the spouse. *Journal of Palliative Care, 2,* 22–30.

Klagsbrum, S. (1983). The making of a cancer psychotherapist. *Journal of Psychosocial Oncology, 1*(4), 55–60.

Labonte, R., & Penfold, S. (1981). Canadian perspectives in health promotion: A critique. *Health Education, 19* (3–4), 4–9.

Lieber, L., Plumb, M. M., Gerstenzang, M. L., & Holland, J. (1976). The communication of affection between cancer patients and their spouses. *Psychosomatic Medicine, 38,* 379–388.

Minuchin, S. (1974). *Families and family therapy.* Cambridge, MA: Harvard University Press.

Morse, J. M. (1986). Quantitative and qualitative research: Issues in sampling. In P. Chinn (Ed.), *Nursing research methodology: Issues in nursing, 8* (4), 46–57.

Oberst, M. T., & James, R. H. (1985). Going home: Patient and spouse adjustment following cancer surgery. *Topics in Clinical Nursing, 7* (4), 16–57.

Sabo, D., Brown, J., & Smith, C. (1986). The male role and mastectomy: Support groups and men's adjustment. *Journal of Psychosocial Oncology, 4*(1/2), 19–31.

Seidel, J. V., Kjolseth, R., & Clark, J. A. (1985). *The ethnograph, A users guide.* Littleton, CO: Qualis Research Associates.

Wellisch, D. K., Jamison, K. R., & Pasnau, R. O. (1978). Psychosocial aspects of mastectomy: II. The man's perspective. *American Journal of Psychiatry, 135,* 543–546.

Wikler, D. (1987). Who should be blamed for being sick? *Health Education Quarterly, 14* (1), 11–25.

Wortman, C. B. (1983). Coping with Victimization: Conclusions and implications for future research. *Journal of Social Issues, 39,* 195–221.

Wright, L. M., & Leahey, M. (1984). *Nurses and families.* Philadelphia: F. A. Davis.

CHAPTER 22

Psychosocial Predictors of Maternal Depressive Symptoms, Parenting Attitudes, and Child Behavior in Single-Parent Families

Lynne A. Hall, Diana N. Gurley,
Barbara Sachs, Richard J. Kryscio

The purposes of the study were to identify psychosocial predictors of depressive symptoms among low-income, single mothers and to investigate the effects of maternal psychosocial factors, depressive symptoms, and parenting attitudes on children's behavior. In-home interviews were conducted with 225 mothers to obtain data on their everyday stressors, coping strategies, social resources, depressive symptoms, and parenting attitudes, as well as reports of their children's behavior. High depressive symptoms occurred among 59.6% of the women. Higher depressive symptoms were associated with greater everyday stressors, fewer social resources, and greater use of avoidance coping. Neither social resources nor coping strategies buffered the relationship between everyday stressors and depressive symptoms. Maternal depressive symptoms predicted parenting attitudes. Parenting attitudes, in turn, predicted child behavior. These findings suggest that depressive symptoms are indirectly associated with mothers' reports of child behavior through their influence on parenting attitudes.

Low-income, single mothers and their children constitute a rapidly growing population at high risk for adverse health outcomes. The mental health of these women is particularly at risk. In turn, there is evidence that parental psychological disturbance places children at increased risk for negative outcomes and may lead to abusive parenting behavior.

In this report, the findings from the first wave of a three-wave panel study of predictors of health outcomes among low-income, single mothers and their children are presented. The purposes of the study were: (a) to determine the prevalence of depressive symptoms among a sample of low-income, single mothers with children between 1 and 4 years of age; (b) to identify psychosocial predictors of depressive symptoms and parenting attitudes of the women; and (c) to examine the effects of maternal psychosocial factors, depressive symptoms, and parenting attitudes on children's behavior. The interrelationships of maternal depressive symptoms, parenting attitudes, and child behavior, and the effects of chronic stressors, social resources, and coping on these variables were investigated. The question of main or modifying effects of both social resources and coping on these variables was investigated. The question of main or modifying effects of both social resources and coping was examined, as well as the question of direct or indirect effects of maternal depressive symptoms on child behavior.

RELATED LITERATURE

In studies of mothers with young children, prevalence estimates of high depressive symptoms vary from 35% (Orr & James, 1984) to 57% (Hall & Farel, 1988). The highest rates are among women, young adults, those with young children, the unmarried, those with low income, the poorly educated, and the unemployed (Brown, Bhrolchain, & Harris, 1975; Comstock & Helsing, 1976; Eaton & Kessler, 1981). The high prevalence of depressive symptoms among mothers with young children, coupled with the fact that depressive symptoms tend to persist over time (Richman, Stevenson, & Graham, 1982), is of particular concern because of the potential ramifications for both mothers and their children.

Adverse health outcomes for the child may be consequences of maternal depression. Parental psychological disturbance and a stressful family environment have been associated with child morbidity (Beautrais, Fergusson, & Shannon, 1982) and with problems in children's social, emotional, and behavioral functioning (Orvaschel, Weissman, & Kidd, 1980). The family environment of depressed mothers has been characterized by conflict and decreased expressiveness, cohesion, and organization (Billings & Moos, 1983); hostility toward the child (Weissman & Paykel, 1974); and diminished maternal involvement, affection, and communication (Weissman, Paykel, & Klerman, 1972). Maternal depression may affect attitudes about child-rearing that are critical to the perception, assessment, and interpretation of child behaviors (Elster, McArnaney, & Lamb, 1983). It is unclear from previous research whether a mother's depressive symptoms directly influence child outcomes or whether their effects occur through their impact on parenting attitudes and behavior (Hall & Farel, 1988).

In comparison to acute stressors, chronic stressors have a greater etiologic role in the development of depressive symptoms (Kanner, Coyne, Schaefer, & Lazarus, 1981; Kaplan, Roberts, Camacho, & Coyne, 1987). Among low-income mothers of young children, chronic stressors such as inadequate income, unemployment, inadequate housing, parenting worries, and problematic interpersonal relationships were associated with high depressive symptoms (Belle, 1982; Hall, 1990; Hall, Williams, & Greenberg, 1985). The effects of chronic stressors on both maternal depressive symptoms and child behavior have not been investigated simultaneously.

In comparison to married mothers, single mothers have been found to be more socially isolated, receive less emotional and parental support, and have more unstable social networks (Weinraub & Wolfe, 1983). Single mothers also were less successful in gaining behavioral compliance from preschool children, were more authoritarian, and were less affectionate (Hetherington, Cox, & Cox, 1978). They also had more restrictive child-rearing attitudes and behaviors and reacted inconsistently toward their children (King & Fullard, 1982). Among single mothers of preschool children, parenting problems were associated with the absence of a close friend, the absence of close family relationships, and a lack of assistance (Norbeck & Sheiner, 1982). In contrast, mothers with support had more appropriating parenting behaviors (Coletta & Gregg, 1981), were less punitive (Field, Widmayer, Stringer, & Ignatoff, 1980), and provided a more organized, stimulating environment (Elster et al., 1983).

There is considerable debate in the literature concerning the relationships of social support to mental and physical well-being. While interaction effects supporting the buffering hypothesis were reported by some investigators (e.g., Boyce, 1981), others reported only main effects (e.g., Schaefer, Coyne, & Lazarus, 1981). Some researchers, not investigating stress, found significant positive relationships between social support and health outcomes (e.g., Hall, Schaefer, & Greenberg, 1987). Evidence for the beneficial effects of social support on mental health is stronger when social support is measured in terms of the quality as opposed to the quantity of social ties (Hall et al., 1987). Family support (Holahan & Moos, 1985) and a close relationship with an intimate or confidant (Brown et al., 1975) are important to the mental health of women. There is no consensus on whether coping is directly related to mental health or whether it modifies the relationship between stressors and mental health (Aldwin & Revenson, 1987; Folkman & Lazarus, 1988). Problem-focused coping strategies moderated the negative effects of stressful life events on psychological functioning (Billings & Moos, 1981). In contrast, avoidance strategies were positively correlated with psychological distress (Billings & Moos, 1981) and a lack of family support (Cronkite & Moos, 1984). Similarly, the use of emotional release was associated with greater depression and was a more frequently used coping strategy among women (Billings & Moos, 1984).

METHOD

Sample

Mothers were recruited in clinics of a county health department. Inclusion criteria were: (a) at least 18 years of age; (b) never married, widowed, divorced, or separated at least 6 months; (c) family income at or below 185% of poverty level; and (d) at least one child between one and four years of age. Of the women approached, 89% agreed to participate. The final sample consisted of 225 mothers. At the time of recruitment, one child for each mother was identified as the index child.

The mean age of the mothers was 25.8 years ($SD = 4.9$), with a range of 18 to 48 years. More than 90% of the sample reported an annual household income under $10,000. The majority had never married (63.6%) and were unemployed (66.7%). The mothers had a mean of 11.4 years of education (SD = 2.0), but more than half (54.6%) had at least a high school education. The mothers had a mean of 2.4 children (SD = 1.2, range = 1–7). The majority of the index children were females (57%).

Measures

Depressive Symptoms

The 20-item Center for Epidemiological Studies–Depression Scale (CES-D; Radloff, 1977) was used by mothers to rate how frequently each symptom was experienced during the past week on a scale ranging from *rarely or none of the time* (0) to *most or all of the time* (3). The positive items were reversed and added to the negative items, forming a summary score ranging from 0–60 (Radloff, 1977). A score greater than 15 indicates a high level of depressive symptoms and it corresponds to the 80th percentile of scores in community samples (Comstock & Helsing, 1976). The CES-D has good internal consistency and test-retest reliability (Comstock & Helsing, 1976; Hall et al., 1985; Radloff, 1977). Cronbach's alpha in this sample was .86. Substantial correlations of the CES-D with other self-report measures of depressive symptoms and with clinical ratings of depression support the scale's validity (Berkman et al., 1986).

Parenting Attitudes

Parenting attitudes were measured by 20 items of the Index of Parental Attitudes (Hudson, 1982). The mother indicated the degree to which each statement described her attitude toward the index child on a scale of *rarely or none of the time* (0) to *most or all of the time* (4). The 10 negative items were reversed and summed with scores on the 10 positive items to form a cumulative score, with a range of 0 to 80. Higher scores indicate more favorable parenting attitudes. Internal consistency and construct validity were supported (Hudson, 1982). Cronbach's alpha in this study was .86.

Child Behavior

The 30-item Preschool Behavior Questionnaire (PBQ; Behar & Stringfield, 1974) was used to measure mothers' perceptions of the index child's behavior. Each item was rated on a scale of *does not apply* (0), *sometimes applies* (1), or *frequently applies* (2). The score was obtained by summing responses to all items. The PBQ distinguished preschoolers with and without emotional disturbance (Behar & Stringfield, 1974). Good internal consistency, interrater, and test-retest reliability were reported (Bee, Hammond, Eyres, Barnard, & Snyder, 1986; Behar & Stringfield, 1974). Cronbach's alpha in this sample was .84.

Chronic Stressors

The 20-item Everyday Stressors Index (ESI; Hall, 1983) measures chronic daily stressors faced by mothers with young children. Mothers rated how much each problem worried, upset, or bothered them from day to day on a 4-point scale ranging from *not at all bothered* (0) to *bothered a great deal* (3). Item values were summed for a total score ranging from 0 to 60. Construct validity of the index was supported by discrimination of everyday stressors from maternal depressive and psychosomatic symptoms (Hall, 1983; Hall, 1987). Cronbach's alpha in this sample was .82, comparing favorably to previous alphas of .80 to .85 (Hall et al., 1985; Hall, 1987).

Coping Strategies

Mothers' coping strategies were measured with indices developed by Billings and Moos (1981) that assess active-behavioral, active-cognitive, and avoidance-oriented strategies. Respondents indicated how often they used each of 32 strategies to deal with stressful situations or problems on a scale ranging from *not at all* (0) to *fairly often* (3). Scores were derived for each of the three strategies by summing the responses to their respective items. The measures distinguished depressed patients, depressives in remission, and community controls (Billings & Moos, 1985). Holahan and Moos (1987) reported Cronbach's alphas of .62 for active-cognitive, .74 for active-behavioral, and .60 for avoidance. Cronbach's alphas in this sample were .66 for active-behavioral, .66 for active-cognitive, and .39 for avoidance.

Social Resources

Four dimensions of social resources were measured: functional support, the quality of family relationships, tangible support, and the quality of primary intimate relationships.

Functional social support was assessed with the 8-item Duke-UNC Functional Social Support Questionnaire (FSSQ; Broadhead, Gehlbach, de Gruy, & Kaplan, 1988, 1989). The mothers indicated for each item their perception of the amount of support they received on a scale of *much less than I would like* (0) to *as much as I would like* (4). A cumulative score was derived. Estimates of internal consistency of the scale were not reported by Broadhead et al. (1988, 1989), but evidence for validity was demonstrated by correlations with other measures of social support (Broadhead et al., 1988) and by the ability of the scale to distinguish high and low users of medical care (Broadhead et al., 1989). Cronbach's alpha in this sample was .78.

The quality of family relationships was measured with the 31-item Family Function Questionnaire (FFQ; Zyzanski, Reeb, Graham, & Kitson, 1987). It assesses four dimensions: satisfaction with family functioning, family cohesion, family adaptability, and quality of family life. For each item, the mothers identified the response that best described the people they thought of as close family on a scale of *almost never* (1) to *almost always* (5). A composite family function score was derived by summing the four mean subscale scores. The reliability and validity of each instrument from which the FFQ was derived have been strongly supported (Hudson, 1982; Olson, Russell, & Sprenkle, 1983; Smilkstein, 1978). The FFQ predicted intrapartum complications and low birth weight (Reeb, Graham, Zyzanski, & Kitson, 1987). Lower family function scores were associated with higher rates of physician visits for respiratory illness and otitis media in infants during the first 15 months of life (Foulke, Reeb, Graham, & Zyzanski, 1988). Cronbach's alpha in the present study was .96.

Tangible social support was measured using the tangible aid subscale of the Interpersonal Support Evaluation List (ISEL; Cohen & Hoberman, 1983). Respondents indicated whether each of 10 statements was *true* (1) or *false* (0) about themselves. Responses were summed to form a cumulative score; higher scores indicate greater tangible support. This measure has been used extensively and has demonstrated good internal consistency and test-retest reliability as well as support for construct validity (Cohen & Hoberman, 1983; Cohen, Sherrod, & Clark, 1986). Cronbach's alpha in this study was .83.

The primary intimate was defined as the person to whom the respondent felt closest (excluding her children). The *quality of the intimate relationship* was measured with the Autonomy and Relatedness Inventory (ARI; Schaefer & Edgerton, 1982). Respondents rated 32 descriptors of the intimate's behavior toward them on a scale of *not at all like* (0) to *very much like* (4) the intimate. Negative items were reversed and ratings summed to form a cumulative score ranging from 0 to 128; higher scores denote more positive ratings of the relationship. Support for the construct validity and internal consistency of the ARI have been reported (Hall & Kiernan, 1991; Hall et al., 1987). Cronbach's alpha in this sample was .94.

Social desirability. The M-C (20) (Strahan & Gerbasi, 1972), a 20-item version of the Marlowe-Crowne Social Desirability Scale (Crowne & Marlowe, 1960), was used to measure socially desirable response set. Respondents rated each item as either *true* or *false*. Reliability coefficients ranged from .73 to .83 in four samples (Strahan & Gerbasi, 1972). In this sample, the reliability coefficient (Kuder-Richardson 20) was .74.

Procedure

Women were approached in clinic waiting areas of a county health department. The purpose of the study was explained, and women meeting the inclusion criteria were invited to participate. Those interested were given further information about the nature of participation, and written informed consent was obtained. Trained interviewers, using a structured questionnaire, conducted in-home interviews lasting approximately one hour and 15 minutes. Each mother was paid $15 for participating in this interview.

RESULTS

Descriptive Analyses

The mean CES-D score of the mothers was 19.2 ($SD = 10.3$; range 0–52); 59.6% of the mothers scored in the high range (CES-D $\geq$ 16). Employed mothers reported lower CES-D scores than unemployed mothers (16.1 versus 20.7; $t_{223} = 3.23, p = .001$). There were no significant differences in depressive symptoms by race. Mean scores on the CES-D were higher for separated mothers than for divorced mothers (20.8 versus 14.6; $p = .04$). There were no differences among other marital status categories.

The mean score for parenting attitudes was 66.2 ($SD = 8.8$; range 34–80). Employed mothers reported more positive parenting attitudes than unemployed mothers ($t223 = -2.51, p = .01$). There were no differences in parenting attitudes by mothers' race or marital status, or by gender of the index child.

The mean PBQ score was 19.5 (SD = 8.1; range 3–42). PBQ scores did not differ by the mothers' employment status, race, or marital status, nor did they differ by gender of the index child.

The four measures of social resources were significantly correlated with one another, with correlations ranging from .23–.54. The fewer the social resources, the higher the level of chronic stressors reported, a relationship that held for all measures of social resources. Women reporting higher everyday stressors also reported greater use of avoidance coping. Greater use of active-behavioral coping and less use of avoidance coping were associated with higher social resources.

T-tests for differences in the means of study variables by depressive symptom status are shown in Table 1. In comparison to mothers with CES-D scores less than 16, mothers with high depressive symptoms (CES-D ≥ 16) reported more everyday stressors, less use of active-behavioral coping strategies, and greater use of avoidance coping strategies. They also reported fewer social resources, less favorable parenting attitudes, and more child behavior problems.

Regression Analyses

The results of backward stepwise elimination to identify the best predictive models for depressive symptoms, parenting attitudes, and child behavior are shown in Table 2. The psychosocial variables included in each initial model were the four measures of social resources, the three coping strategies, and everyday stressors. These variables were allowed to eliminate at p > .05. Inspection of the correlations among these variables indicated no multicollinearity. Although income, employment status, race, and

TABLE 1

T-Tests for Differences in Means of Study Variables by Depressive Symptom Status (N = 225)

	CES-D Score				
	< 16 (LOW) (n = 91)		≥ 16 (HIGH) (n = 134)		
Variable					t_{223}
	M	(SD)	M	(SD)	
Everyday Stressors	18.7	(8.7)	26.1	(10.1)	5.7***
Active-Cognitive Coping	22.9	(4.5)	21.8	(4.1)	−1.9
Active-Behavioral Coping	22.6	(5.6)	20.5	(4.5)	−3.0*
Avoidance Coping	6.2	(2.7)	8.7	(3.0)	6.5***
Quality of Primary Intimate Relationship	105.2	(19.2)	94.3	(22.1)	−3.8**
Quality of Family Relationships	11.7	(3.2)	9.0	(3.7)	−5.7***
Functional Social Support	22.9	(7.0)	17.0	(7.4)	−5.9***
Tangible Social Support	8.6	(2.2)	7.4	(2.7)	−3.6**
Parenting Attitudes	70.0	(6.6)	63.6	(9.2)	−6.1***
Child Behavior	16.3	(6.9)	21.7	(8.2)	5.2***

*p < .01; **p < .001; *** p ≤ .0001.

TABLE 2
Multiple Regression Estimates for the Best Predictive Models of Depressive Symptoms, Parenting Attitudes, and Child Behavior ($N = 225$)

Outcome	Variables in Model	Regression Coefficient	Standardized Estimates (β)
Depres-sive Symptoms	Income	− 0.9820	−.11
	Employment Status	− 1.8845	−.09
	Race	− 1.7614	−.08
	Social Desirability	− 0.1183	−.04
	Quality of Family Relationships	− 0.3445	−.12*
	Tangible Support	− 0.5670	−.14*
	Everyday Stressors	0.1706	.17*
	Avoidance Coping	1.2002	.37***
	Model $R^2 = .42$; ($F_{8,216} = 19.46$)***		
Parenting Attitudes	Income	0.0831	.01
	Employment Status	1.5339	.08
	Race	− 0.1298	−.01
	Social Desirability	0.4713	.20**
	Depressive Symptoms	− 0.2042	−.24**
	Quality of Primary Intimate Relationship	0.1035	.25***
	Model $R^2 = .24$; ($F_{6,218} = 11.61$)***		
Child Behavior	Income	− 0.7886	−.11
	Employment Status	0.5252	.03
	Race	0.5313	.03
	Social Desirability	− 0.1128	−.05
	Everyday Stressors	0.1369	.17**
	Active-Cognitive Coping	0.3707	.20**
	Parenting Attitudes	− 0.5178	−.56***
	Model $R^2 = .45$; ($F_{7,217} = 25.29$)***		

*$p \le .05$; ** $p \le .001$; *** $p \le .0001$.

social desirability were retained in each regression model as controls, only social desir-ability was associated with any study variable, that being parenting attitudes.

Predictors of Depressive Symptoms

Poorer family functioning, less tangible support, higher everyday stressors, and greater use of avoidance coping predicted higher depressive symptoms. The standard-ized regression coefficients indicated that everyday stressors and avoidance coping were the strongest predictors. The strength of the association of avoidance coping with depressive symptoms ($\beta = .37$) was twice that of everyday stressors ($\beta = .17$) and three times greater than that of the quality of family relationships ($\beta = -.12$). Together these four variables plus the four control variables accounted for 42% of the variance in depressive symptoms.

The potential buffering effects of social resources and coping strategies on the relationship of everyday stressors with depressive symptoms were tested for each social resource and coping strategy measure using the approach recommended by Baron and Kenny (1986) for assessing moderating effects. After entering the control variables and main effects, individual interaction terms (everyday stressors × social resources and everyday stressors × coping strategies) were entered into separate regression models, each using one of the four measures of social resources or one of the three measures of coping strategies. None of the interaction terms was significant, providing no support for the buffering hypothesis.

Predictors of Parenting Attitudes

A similar backward stepwise elimination procedure was conducted to determine the best predictors of parenting attitudes, but with depressive symptoms as an additional predictor in the initial model. The only variables that added significantly to the prediction of parenting attitudes were social desirability, depressive symptoms, and one measure of social resources—the quality of the primary intimate relationship. The standardized regression weights indicated modest partial correlations of parenting attitudes with depressive symptoms ($\beta = .24$) and the quality of the primary intimate relationship ($\beta = .25$). The higher the depressive symptoms and the poorer the quality of the primary intimate relationship, the less favorable the parenting attitudes. The model accounted for 24% of the variance in parenting attitudes.

Predictors of Child Behavior

Child behavior was predicted using the same initial model, but incorporating both depressive symptoms and parenting attitudes on the first step. Higher everyday stressors, greater use of active-cognitive coping, and less favorable parenting attitudes were related to more child behavior problems. Parenting attitudes displayed the strongest effect ($\beta = -.56$). This variable was approximately three times more strongly associated with child behavior problems than were everyday stressors ($\beta = .17$) and active-cognitive coping ($\beta = .20$). The model accounted for 45% of the variance in child behavior problems.

DISCUSSION

The findings document the high-risk status of low-income, single mothers for depressive symptoms. The prevalence of high depressive symptoms (59.6%) in this sample is greater than that reported in other studies using the CES-D with similar samples (Orr & James, 1984; Hall & Farel, 1988). The mean CES-D score of 19.2 is also high in comparison to the mean of 8.7 found in the general population (Sayetta & Johnson, 1980). The substantial prevalence of depressive symptoms among this high-risk group has serious implications not only for their mental health but also for the well-being of their children.

All four measures of social resources were inversely related to avoidance coping and positively correlated with active-behavioral coping. While active-cognitive coping was moderately correlated with active-behavioral coping, it was significantly correlated with only two of the measures of social resources—functional social support and the quality of family relationships. These findings are similar to those of Dunkel-Schetter, Folkman, and Lazarus (1987) who found different coping strategies associated with different types of social support. The findings also correspond to those of Billings and Moos (1981) who reported fewer social resources to be associated with greater use of avoidance coping. There was no evidence that any of the dimensions of social resources or coping strategies buffered the relationship between everyday stressors and depressive symptoms. As in previous research, everyday stressors were directly associated with maternal depressive symptoms (Belle, 1982; Hall, 1990; Hall et al., 1985). Only main effects for everyday stressors, avoidance coping, the quality of family relationships, and perceived tangible support were observed. Mothers who lack support from family and friends may be more likely to use avoidance as a strategy to deal with chronic stressors. This approach may result in greater depression, since direct attempts to reduce stressors are not made. Billings and Moos (1981), using the same measure of avoidance coping, found a direct correlation with psychological distress as was found in this study. In contrast, they reported that problem-focused coping buffered the relationship between stressful life events and psychological functioning, although they measured acute rather than chronic stressors.

The finding that various indicators of social resources predicted different outcomes underscores the importance of a multidimensional approach to the assessment of social resources. This finding is consistent with previous theoretical formulations of social support as a multidimensional construct (House, 1981; Kahn, 1979). In contrast, Brown (1986) did not find emotional, material, informational, and appraisal support were separate dimensions; instead, support was a unidimensional construct. Further investigation of the dimensionality of social resources is needed to advance our knowledge of this construct. Also, greater attention to the source of support is warranted in future studies, as this may be a key to addressing the question of dimensionality.

Only depressive symptoms and the quality of the primary intimate relationship predicted parenting attitudes. These two factors plus controls explained relatively little of the variance in parenting attitudes. Other explanatory variables, untapped by the measures used in this study, apparently were operating. Panaccione and Wahler (1986) emphasized the importance of the contextual influence of maternal depression and adult social relationships on parenting behavior. This contention is supported by the study findings. Further exploration of the predictors of parenting attitudes is warranted.

The quality of the mothers' primary intimate relationship was negatively associated with their parenting attitudes, but was not associated with the mothers' reports of child behavior. Snyder and his colleagues (Snyder, Klein, Gdowski, Faulstich, & La-Combe, 1988) found that parents' reports of emotional or behavioral difficulties of their children were positively associated with dissatisfaction with the parent-child relationship, but were not correlated with the quality of the marital relationship. While the sample of Snyder and his colleagues consisted of married couples, their findings are similar.

The findings of this study and others (Dumas, Gibson, & Albin, 1989; Goodman & Brumley, 1990; Sachs & Hall, in press) suggest that parenting attitudes mediate the relationship between maternal depressive symptoms and child behavior. This indirect relationship between maternal depressive symptoms and child behavior is in contrast to the findings of Fendrich, Warner, and Weissman (1990). They reported both parental depression and family discord predicted conduct disorder in children. Similarly, Hammen, Adrian, Gordon, Burge, and Jaenicke (1987) found that both maternal depression and chronic stress predicted psychopathology in children. In other studies, depressed mothers reported their children had more behavior problems than nondepressed mothers (Brody & Forehand, 1986; Webster-Stratton & Hammond, 1988). However, the effects of parenting attitudes were not examined or controlled in these studies. Depressed mothers may have lower confidence in their parenting skills than nondepressed mothers (Cutrona & Troutman, 1986), which may be expressed negatively in their parenting attitudes. Children, in turn, may react to this negativity with more behavior problems.

The cross-sectional nature of these data permits several alternative explanations. Depressed mothers may have a distorted perception of the support available to them and their behavior may alienate social network members or erode existing support from family and friends. Aversive child behaviors may negatively influence parenting attitudes which, in turn, may lead to greater depressive symptoms because of guilt or feelings of parental incompetence.

Both low-income single mothers and their children may be affected by the social and psychological environment in the family when there are fewer social resources, increased chronic stressors, and greater use of avoidance coping strategies. Greater attention should be paid by health professionals to the potential negative consequences of these factors on single mothers and their young children. Assessment of mothers' social resources, chronic stressors, coping strategies, depressive symptoms, and parenting attitudes may lead to identification of areas for intervention to enhance the well-being of low-income, single-mother families.

Data for this study were collected under grant #1 R01 NR01960–01 awarded to Drs. Hall and Sachs by the National Center for Nursing Research, National Institutes of Health.

The authors wish to express appreciation to Dr. Margaret R. Grier, Dr. Elizabeth R. Lenz, Ms. Melanie Lutenbacher-Webne, and Ms. Betsy Neale for constructive suggestions on the manuscript and to Ms. Linda Mitchell and Ms. Elizabeth Janecek for manuscript preparation.

An earlier version of this manuscript was presented at the 117th Annual Convention of the American Public Health Association, Chicago, IL, October 1989.

REFERENCES

Aldwin, C., & Revenson, T. (1987). Does coping help? A re-examination of the relation between coping and mental health. *Journal of Personality and Social Psychology, 53,* 337–348.

Baron, R. M., & Kenny, D. A. (1986). The moderator-mediator variable distinction in social psychological research: Conceptual, strategic, and statistical considerations. *Journal of Personality and Social Psychology, 51,* 1173–1182.

Beautrais, A. L., Fergusson, D. M., & Shannon, F. T. (1982). Life events and childhood morbidity: A prospective study. *Pediatrics, 70,* 935–940.

Bee, H., Hammond, M., Eyres, S., Barnard, K., & Snyder, C. (1986). The impact of parental life change on the early development of children. *Research in Nursing & Health, 9,* 65–74.

Behar, L., & Stringfield, S. (1974). A behavior rating scale for the preschool child. *Developmental Psychology, 10,* 601–610.

Belle, D. (Ed). (1982). *Lives in stress.* Beverly Hills: Sage.

Berkman, L. F., Berkman, C. S., Kasl, S., Freeman, D. H., Leo, L., Ostfeld, A. M., Coroni-Huntley, J., & Brody, J. A. (1986). Depressive symptoms in relation to physical health and functioning in the elderly. *American Journal of Epidemiology, 124,* 372–388.

Billings, A. G., & Moos, R. H. (1981). The role of coping response and social resources in attenuating the stress of life events. *Journal of Behavioral Medicine, 4,* 139–157.

Billings, A. G., & Moos, R. H. (1983). Comparisons of children of depressed and nondepressed parents. *Journal of Abnormal Child Psychology, 11,* 463–486.

Billings, A. G., & Moos, R. H. (1984). Coping, stress, and social resources among adults with unipolar depression. *Journal of Personality and Social Psychology, 46,* 877–891.

Billings, A. G., & Moos, R. H. (1985). Psychosocial processes of remission in unipolar depression. *Journal of Consulting and Clinical Psychology, 53,* 314–325.

Boyce, W. T. (1981). Interaction between social variables in stress research. *Journal of Health and Social Behavior, 22,* 194–195.

Broadhead, W. E., Gehlbach, S. H., De Gruy, F. V., & Kaplan, B. H. (1988). The Duke-UNC Functional Social Support Questionnaire. Measurement of social support in family medicine patients. *Medical Care, 26,* 709–723.

Broadhead, W. E., Gehlbach, S. H., De Gruy, F. V., & Kaplan, B. H. (1989). Functional versus structural social support and health care utilization in a family medicine outpatient practice. *Medical Care, 27,* 221–233.

Brody, G. H., & Forehand, R. (1986). Maternal perceptions of child maladjustment as a function of the combined influence of child behavior and maternal depression. *Journal of Consulting and Clinical Psychology, 54,* 237–240.

Brown, G. W., Bhrolchain, M. N., & Harris, T. (1975). Social class and psychiatric disturbance among women in an urban population. *Sociology, 9,* 225–254.

Brown, M. A. (1986). Social support during pregnancy: A unidimensional or multidimensional construct? *Nursing Research, 35,* 4–9.

Cohen, S., & Hoberman, H. (1983). Positive events and social supports as buffers of life change stress. *Journal of Applied Social Psychology, 13,* 99–125.

Cohen, S., Sherrod, D. R., & Clark, M. S. (1986). Social skills and the stress-protective role of social support. *Journal of Personality and Social Psychology, 50,* 963–973.

Coletta, N. D., & Gregg, C. (1981). Adolescent mothers' vulnerability to stress. *Journal of Nervous and Mental Disease, 169,* 50–54.

Comstock, G. W., & Helsing, K. J. (1976). Symptoms of depression in two communities. *Psychological Medicine, 6,* 551–563.

Cronkite, R., & Moos, R. H. (1984). The role of predisposing and moderating factors in the stress-illness relationship. *Journal of Health and Social Behavior, 25,* 372–393.

Crowne, D., & Marlowe, D. (1960). A new scale of social desirability independent of psychopathology. *Journal of Consulting Psychology, 24,* 349–354.

Cutrona, C. E., & Troutman, B. R. (1986). Social support, infant temperament, and parenting self-efficacy: A mediational model of post-partum depression. *Child Development, 57,* 1507–1518.

Dumas, J. E., Gibson, J. A., & Albin, J. B. (1989). Behavioral correlates of maternal depressive symptomatology in conduct-disordered children. *Journal of Consulting and Clinical Psychology, 57,* 516–521.

Dunkel-Schetter, C., Folkman, S., & Lazarus, R. S. (1987). Correlates of social support receipt. *Journal of Personality and Social Psychology, 53,* 71–80.

Eaton, W. W., & Kessler, L. G. (1981). Rates of symptoms of depression in a national sample. *American Journal of Epidemiology, 114,* 528–538.

Elster, A., McArnaney, E., & Lamb, M. E. (1983). Parental behavior of adolescent mothers. *Pediatrics, 71,* 494–503.

Fendrich, M., Warner, V., & Weissman, M. M. (1990). Family risk factors, parental depression, and psychopathology in offspring. *Developmental Psychology, 26,* 40–50.

Field, T., Widmayer, S., Stringer, S., & Ignatoff, E. (1980). Teenage, lower-class, black mothers and their preterm infants. *Child Development, 51,* 426–436.

Folkman, S., & Lazarus, R. S. (1988). The relationship between coping and emotion: Implications for theory and research. *Social Science and Medicine, 26,* 309–317.

Foulke, F. G., Reeb, K. G., Graham, A. V., & Zyzanski, S. J. (1988). Family function, respiratory illness, and otitis media in urban Black infants. *Family Medicine, 20,* 128–132.

Goodman, S. H., & Brumley, H. E. (1990). Schizophrenic and depressed mothers: Relational deficits in parenting. *Developmental Psychology, 26,* 31–39.

Hall, L. A. (1983). *Social supports, everyday stressors, and maternal mental health.* Unpublished doctoral dissertation, University of North Carolina, Chapel Hill.

Hall, L. A. (1987). *Psychometric evaluation of the Everyday Stressors Index (ESI).* Unpublished manuscript.

Hall, L. A. (1990). Prevalence and correlates of depressive symptoms in mothers of young children. *Public Health Nursing, 7*(2), 71–79.

Hall, L. A., & Farel, A. M. (1988). Maternal stresses and depressive symptoms: Correlates of behavior problems in young children. *Nursing Research, 37,* 156–161.

Hall, L. A., & Kiernan, B. S. (1991). *Psychometric assessment of a measure of the quality of primary intimate relationships: Preliminary findings.* Unpublished manuscript.

Hall, L. A., Schaeffer, E. S., & Greenberg, R. S. (1987). Quality and quantity of social support as correlates of psychosomatic symptoms in mothers with young children. *Research in Nursing & Health, 10,* 287–298.

Hall, L. A., Williams, C. A., & Greenberg, R. S. (1985). Supports, stressors, and depressive symptoms in low-income mothers of young children. *American Journal of Public Health, 75,* 518–522.

Hammen, C., Adrian, C., Gordon, D., Burge, D., & Jaenicke, C. (1987). Children of depressed mothers: Maternal strain and symptom predictors of dysfunction. *Journal of Abnormal Psychology, 96,* 190–198.

Hetherington, E., Cox, M., & Cox, R. (1978). The aftermath of divorce. In J. Stevens & M. Mathews (Eds.), *Mother/child father/child relationships* (pp. 149–176). Washington, DC: National Association for the Education of Young Children.

Holahan, C., & Moos, R. H. (1985). Life stress and health: Personality, coping, and family support in stress resistance. *Journal of Personality and Social Psychology, 49,* 739–747.

Holahan, C., & Moos, R. H. (1987). Personal and contextual determinants of coping strategies. *Journal of Personality and Social Psychology, 52,* 946–955.

House, J. (1981). *Work, stress, and social support.* Menlo Park, CA: Addison-Wesley.

Hudson, W. (1982). *The Clinical Measurement Package: A field manual.* Homewood, IL: Dorsey.

Kahn, R. L. (1979). Aging and social input. In M. W. Riley (Ed.), *Aging from birth to death* (pp. 77–91). New York: Westview Press.

Kanner, A. D., Coyne, J. C., Schaefer, C., & Lazarus, R. S. (1981). Comparison of two modes of stress measurement: Daily hassles and uplifts versus major life events. *Journal of Behavioral Medicine, 4,* 1–39.

Kaplan, G., Roberts, R., Camacho, T., & Coyne, J. (1987). Psychosocial predictors of depression. *American Journal of Epidemiology, 125,* 206–220.

King, T., & Fullard, W. (1982). Teenage mothers and their infants: New findings on home environment. *Journal of Adolescence, 5,* 333–346.

Norbeck, J., & Sheiner, M. (1982). Sources of social support related to single-parent functioning. *Research in Nursing & Health, 5,* 3–12.

Olson, D., Russell, C., & Sprenkle, D. (1983). Circumplex Model of marital and family systems: VI. Theoretical update. *Family Process, 22,* 69–83.

Orr, S., & James, S. (1984). Maternal depression in an urban pediatric practice: Implications for health care delivery. *American Journal of Public Health, 74,* 363–365.

Orvaschel, H., Weissman, M., & Kidd, K. (1980). The children of depressed parents; the childhood of depressed patients; depression in children. *Journal of Affective Disorders, 2,* 1–16.

Panaccione, V. F., & Wahler, R. G. (1986). Child behavior, maternal depression, and social coercion as factors in the quality of child care. *Journal of Abnormal Child Psychology, 14,* 263–278.

Radloff, L. S. (1977). The CES-D scale: A self-report depression scale for research in the general population. *Applied Psychological Measurement, 1,* 385–401.

Reeb, K. G., Graham, A. V., Zyzanski, S. J., & Kitson, G. C. (1987). Predicting low birthweight and complicated labor in urban black women: A biopsychosocial perspective. *Social Science and Medicine, 25,* 1321–1327.

Richman, N., Stevenson, J., & Graham, P. J. (1982). Preschool to school: A behavioral study. New York: Academic Press.

Sachs, B., & Hall, L. A. (in press). Maladaptive mother-child relationships: A pilot study. *Public Health Nursing.*

Sayetta, R. B., & Johnson, D. P. (1980). *Basic data on depressive symptomatology: United States, 1974–75* (National Center for Health Statistics, Vital and Health Statistics Series 11, No. 216). DHEW Publication No. (PHS) 80–166. Washington, DC: U.S. Government Printing Office.

Schaefer, C., Coyne, J. C., & Lazarus, R. S. (1981). The health-related functions of social support. *Journal of Behavioral Medicine, 4,* 381–406.

Schaefer, E. S., & Edgerton, M. (1982). *The Autonomy and Relatedness Inventory (ARI).* Unpublished manuscript, University of North Carolina, Chapel Hill, NC.

Smilkstein, G. (1978). The Family APGAR. *The Journal of Family Practice, 6,* 1231–1239.

Snyder, D. K., Klein, M. A., Gdowski, C. L., Faulstich, C., & LaCombe, J. (1988). Generalized dysfunction in clinic and nonclinic families: A comparative analysis. *Journal of Abnormal Child Psychology, 16,* 97–109.

Strahan, R., & Gerbasi, K. (1972). Short, homogeneous version of the Marlowe-Crowne Social Desirability Scale. *Journal of Clinical Psychology, 28,* 191–193.

Webster-Stratton, C., & Hammond, M. (1988). Maternal depression and its relationship to life stress, perceptions of child behavior problems, parenting behaviors, and child conduct problems. *Journal of Abnormal Child Psychology, 16,* 299–315.

Weinraub, M., & Wolf, B. (1983). Effects of stress and social supports on mother-child interactions in single- and two-parent families. *Child Development, 54,* 1297–1311.

Weissman, M. M., & Paykel, E. S. (1974). *The depressed woman: A study of social relationships.* Chicago: University of Chicago Press.

Weissman, M. M., Paykel, E. S., & Klerman, G. (1972). The depressed woman as a mother. *Social Psychiatry, 7,* 98–108.

Zyzanski, S. J., Reeb, K. G., Graham, A. V., & Kitson, G. C. (1987, May). *Performance of measures of family function in a population of pregnant urban black women.* Paper presented at the North American Primary Care Research Group Annual Meeting, Minneapolis, MN.

CHAPTER 23

Adolescent Reactions to Sibling Death: Perceptions of Mothers, Fathers, and Teenagers

Nancy S. Hogan, David E. Balk

Fourteen families in which a child had died participated in this study; the mother, father, and one teenager from each family were interviewed. All participants completed a sibling bereavement inventory consisting of 109 scaled items that measured self-concept perceptions and grief reactions. The teenagers completed the inventory in terms of their own reactions; the mothers and fathers were instructed to complete the inventory as they anticipated their teenager would answer it. Mothers held significantly different views of their teenagers' self-concept and grief than did the fathers or the teenagers. Fathers' responses resembled those of their teenagers. In addition to accenting the need to study more fully the family dynamics involved when a child dies, the results call into serious question commonly held views regarding the accuracy and reliability of mothers' perceptions of bereaved children. The results suggest that more credence be given to fathers' observations about the phenomena of bereavement engaging their teenage children.

A child's death produces intrapersonal and interpersonal changes for each surviving family member as parents and siblings strive to cope and adapt to lives that are changed forever (Bank & Kahn, 1982; Bowlby-West, 1983; Brent, 1983; Osterweis, Solomon, & Green, 1984). Clinicians and researchers have documented an increase in the incidence of psychological dysfunction for children following a sibling's death (Cain, Fast, & Erickson, 1964; Cobb, 1956; Hilgard, 1969; Krell & Rabkin, 1979). Both applied clinical researchers and developmental psychologists have found that adolescent bereavement can produce both short-term and long-term debilitating effects (Gray, 1987).

While there is ample evidence of the negative outcomes that can occur following sibling death, an emerging body of research suggests that many children attain an increased sense of maturity, resiliency, and psychological growth following sibling bereavement that include perceptions of being more mature than friends, belief in ability to cope better with distress, increased empathy and compassion toward parents, and an increased sense of creativity (Balk, 1981, 1983; Hogan, 1987, 1988a; Pollock, 1978, 1986). After an extensive study of sibling relationships and the effects of sibling death, Bank and Kahn (1982) concluded that "the dead sibling's legacy can be a force for sickness and stagnation or, under beneficent circumstances, can serve as an inspiration for maturation and creativity" (p. 287). Offer (1969) was impressed not only with the resiliency of his teenage subjects in the face of severe family tragedies, but noted that for most of the teenagers these crises served as catalysts that spurred personal growth and impelled the youth more quickly into adulthood than their peers.

Sibling bereavement during adolescence occurs within the context of a grieving family. During such a life crisis, social transactions between family members give children information about their self-worth and about the degree to which social support is available to facilitate coping with crisis and change (Cobb, 1976). During sibling bereavement, surviving children struggle to redefine their sense of self within their traumatically altered family constellation. In addition, bereaved teenagers must cope with normal developmental tasks within a family that has lost its equilibrium (Bowlby-West, 1983; Krell & Rabkin, 1979; Leon, 1986).

It has been commonly believed that there is a negative shift in self-concept following parental and sibling bereavement (Kliman, 1980; Rochlin, 1965). Recent research has not supported these earlier findings. For instance, Martinson, Davies and McClowry (1987) examined the long-term effects of sibling death on children's self-concept. Using the Piers-Harris Self-Concept Scale with 29 children whose siblings had died within the previous seven to nine years, Martinson and colleagues found that the bereaved children had statistically higher self-concept scores than Piers-Harris norm groups. In addition, using content analysis of interview data, they identified factors that appeared to contribute to high and low levels of self-concept in the bereaved children. Balk (1981, 1983) studied 33 bereaved adolescent siblings and found that the respondent scores on the Offer Self-Image Questionnaire (OSIQ) were similar to Offer norm groups on all scales except for the Morals Scale; on the Morals Scale, the bereaved teenagers had scores significantly higher than the norm groups. Balk concluded that the OSIQ results—in tandem with interview data about lessons learned from the death, perceptions of personal maturity, attitudes toward religion, and the serious demeanor of the bereaved teenagers during the interviews—supported the inference that the development of values in research participants had been influenced positively following sibling death. These findings were confirmed by Hogan (1988b) in a sibling bereavement study using the OSIQ with 144 adolescents. Data revealed that the teenagers were comparable to the normed group on all 12 scales, with the Morals subscale the highest score.

A child's sex plays an important interactive role with family dynamics to influence personality development in areas such as sense of warmth and closeness toward siblings (Furman & Buhrmester, 1985), sibling rivalry and friendship bonding (Dunn & Kendrick, 1982), identity formation, sexual identification and role entitlement (Bank

& Kahn, 1982), reactions to a family member's death (Balk, 1981; Gray, 1987; Hilgard, Newman, & Fisk, 1960; Hogan, 1987), and self-esteem (Demo, Small & Savin-Williams, 1987). Fathers appear to have a stronger influence on adolescent self-esteem than mothers (Gecas & Schwalbe, 1986); mothers are disclosed to more by their children than are fathers (Jourard, 1971); and there is greater congruence between mothers' and adolescents' reports than between fathers' and adolescents' reports (Demo, et al., 1987).

Demi and Gilbert (1987) focused on the congruence of parents' and children's reactions to grieving, coping, and adaptation following sibling death. Using the Impact of Events Scale, these researchers studied 22 child-parent pairs from 9 bereaved families and determined that parents' intrusion scores were correlated with children's avoidance scores. The findings suggest that whereas parents became highly distressed with intrusive thoughts about their deceased child, surviving siblings avoided thinking about the dead child as a means to keep from being overwhelmed by intrusive thoughts.

Members of The Society of Compassionate Friends, a national self-help support group for bereaved parents, have described the complex differences between the grieving reactions of fathers and mothers (Rosenthal, 1987; Schatz, 1984; Schiff, 1977). Clinicians and researchers also have reported gender differences in parental responses following the death of a child (Gyulay, 1975; Hogan, 1987, 1988a; Pollock, 1986; Soricelli & Utech, 1985). Block (1957) used semantic differential techniques to identify gender differences in perceptions of grief. On emotions such as love, anger and guilt the scores of males and females had a high correlation of .84 to .98; for the emotion of grief, however, the correlation dropped to .66. Balk (1981, 1983) reported that as time passed adolescent females expressed significantly more confusion than males about a sibling's death. Hogan (1987) indicated that, among her bereaved teenage subjects, females scored significantly higher than males on items related to difficulty sleeping at night, feeling closer to their father, believing that they should have died rather than their sibling, and sensing the incompleteness of the family.

Family bereavement researchers typically have grouped mothers and fathers under the common heading of "parents." However, the congruence of the perceptions of mothers and fathers with the perceptions of their sons and daughters regarding the teenagers' grief reactions and self-concept following sibling death have not been examined. Thus, the purpose of the present study was to investigate the perceptions of bereaved mothers and fathers regarding self-concept and grief reactions of their teenagers following a child's death and the congruence of those perceptions with those of the bereaved teenagers.

METHOD

Sample

Fourteen bereaved families participated in this study. Mothers, fathers, and one teenager were interviewed in each family. Informed consent was obtained from all participants. In addition, parents consented to the involvement of their teenagers in the investigation. Care was taken to ensure that the rights and dignity of each participant were protected. All the participants had been contacted through the Society of Compassionate Friends, a mutual support group for families bereaved over the death of a child. The teenage participants were part of a larger sample of bereaved adolescents studied by Hogan (1987). The parents were identified by randomly selecting the names of 20 adolescents in this larger sample and then contacting their parents to take part in the new study. In three cases the adolescents no longer lived with both parents, and in three cases fathers declined to participate. This left 14 families that completed data sets for the investigation. No more than two months elapsed between the adolescents' and parents' completion of the instrument.

The 42 participants were white (76.2%), Hispanic (11.9%), and other racial/ethnic identity (11.9%). There were 14 fathers, 14 mothers, 7 teenage girls, and 7 teenage boys. The teenage subjects ranged in age from 13 to 18, with a mean age of 14.7 and a modal age of 13.

The deaths of siblings had been caused by accidents (42.9%), illness (42.9%), and other causes (14.2%). At the time of their deaths, the ages for the children ranged from one day to 19 years, with a mean age of 10.7 years and a standard deviation of 5.5 years. The children who had died were divided evenly between males and females. No family had endured multiple deaths of children. Time elapsed since the death ranged from 7 to 36 months, with a mean of 22.7 months and a standard deviation of 9.4 months.

Instrument

The Hogan Sibling Inventory of Bereavement (HSIB) (Hogan, 1987, 1990) was used to collect data for this investigation. The HSIB consists of 109 items, each prefaced with the words: "Since my brother/sister died I feel that. . . . " Each item is answered on a 5-point scale ranging from 1 *almost always true* to 5 *hardly ever true*. The phrasing on several items was varied to prevent respondents from focusing on only one end of the scale; during data analysis responses to several items were recorded to adjust for this scaling technique.

The 109 items in the HSIB were written after an extensive review of theory and literature and consultation with experts in the field of adolescent bereavement. The instrument gathers data on such distinct categories as perceptions of peer relations, bereavement of family members, relationship with mother, relationship with father, self-concept perceptions, grief reactions, and school-related issues. Analyses have consistently demonstrated that responses to specific categories are independent (Hogan, 1989).

Internal consistency of the complete instrument has been calculated using Cronbach alpha. In two earlier studies the Cronbach alpha coefficients were .88 (Hogan, 1987) and .95 (Hogan, 1988b). Responses of all the subjects in this present study to the complete instrument had a Cronbach alpha of .73. When the internal consistency of responses of each group to the total instrument in this study was calculated, Cronbach alphas were .93 for the mothers, .85 for the fathers, and .88 for the adolescents. Research categories of interest for this study were perceptions of self-concept and grief reactions following the death of a sibling, two of the dimensions measured by the HSIB.

Self-concept perceptions include items such as "I am a better person," "I am stronger because of the grief I have had to deal with," and "I must lead two lives, my own and my dead brother's/sister's." Eight items comprised the self-concept scale. Possible scores on the self-concept scale range from 8 to 40, with scores closer to 8 indicative of better self-concept. In this sample, the average score for the self-concept scale was 23.2, with a standard deviation of 4.4, a minimum score of 12, and a maximum score of 30. The mode was 21 (5 persons). Internal consistency of the self-concept scale, using Cronbach's alpha, was found to be .62.

The grief reaction items include statements such as "I am uncomfortable about having fun," "I am guilty that I lived and my brother/sister died," and "I am depressed when I think about him/her." Seventeen items were included in the grief reactions scale. Possible scores on the grief reactions scale range from 17 to 85, with scores closer to 17 indicative of less-enduring grief reactions. In this sample, the average score for the grief reactions scale was 32, with a standard deviation of 7.5, a minimum score of 21, and a maximum score of 50. The mode was 26 (5 persons). Internal consistency of the grief reactions scale was analyzed using Cronbach's alpha and was .77. Canonical correlation analysis indicated that response to the self-concept scale and the responses to the grief scale were independent.

The adolescents completed the inventory in the presence of one of the investigators (Hogan, 1987). Eighty-two percent completed the inventory in their homes, and the others completed it at a church where parents' bereavement meetings were held. Identical copies of the inventory were mailed to parents, who were instructed to complete the inventory on their own and not to discuss the responses with each other.

The teenagers answered the inventory in terms of their own reactions since their siblings' deaths. The teenagers' mothers and fathers were instructed to answer the inventory as if they were their teenager, that is, to answer the inventory as they thought their teenager had answered it.

RESULTS

Means and standard deviations to the self-concept and grief reactions scales are given in Table 1. Scores are provided for mothers, fathers, all parents, and teenagers.

Mothers' and fathers' scores were averaged to form parents' scores, and then compared to the average scores of all teenagers. T-tests demonstrated no differences between the mean scores of parents ($M = 22.8$) and their teenagers ($M = 24.1$) on self-concept perceptions of adolescents following sibling deaths, $t(37) = -0.88, p = .382$. Similarly, t-tests demonstrated no differences in the mean score of parents ($M = 32.9$) and the mean score of teenagers ($M = 30.4$) on grief reactions of teenagers following sibling death, $t(37) = .98, p = .332$.

Mothers held a much more favorable view of their teenagers' self-concept following sibling death than the fathers ($M = 19.5$ and 26.3, respectively), $t(23) = -4.74, p <$

TABLE 1
Means and Standard Deviations of All Participants to the Self-Concept
and Grief Reactions Scales

| | Self-Concept | | Grief Reactions | |
	M	SD	M	SD
Mothers	19.5	4.2	36.6	7.3
Fathers	26.3	2.7	28.8	3.7
All parents	22.8	4.9	32.9	7.0
Teenagers	24.1	3.5	30.4	8.3

.001. Fathers' mean scores indicated that they considered their teenagers' grief reactions to be less enduring than the mothers ($M = 28.8$ and 35.6, respectively), $t(23) = 3.32$, $p = .003$.

The fathers and their teenagers shared self-concept perceptions ($M = 26.3$ and 24.1, respectively), very much unlike the mothers' perceptions ($M = 19.5$) of their teenagers' self-concept following sibling death, $F(2,37) = 11.90$, $p = .0001$. The mothers had a much more favorable opinion of their teenagers' self-concept than the fathers or the teenagers themselves. The mean scores of the mothers, fathers and teenagers regarding adolescent grief reactions also showed significant differences. The mean score of the mothers ($M = 36.6$) indicated they considered grief reactions to be more enduring for adolescents than did the fathers ($M = 28.8$) or the teenagers ($M = 30.4$), $F(2,37) = 4.27$, $p = .023$.

DISCUSSION

Some researchers have identified a greater congruence between the reports of mothers and adolescents than between the reports of fathers and adolescents (Demi, et al., 1987). The present findings do not corroborate those results. When compared to the responses of their teenagers, the responses of the mothers and fathers were expected to be more alike than dissimilar. Because teenagers mentioned that they primarily seek out mothers as confidants after a sibling's death (cf. Balk, 1981; Hogan, 1987), we assumed that, if there were going to be shared perceptions between children and a parent, they would exist between mothers and teenagers. The similarity between fathers' and teenagers' responses was thus surprising, especially since this similarity was in striking contrast to what the mothers reported about their perceptions of their teenagers.

As a first step in formulating a means to explain the greater reliability of the perceptions of the fathers in our study, it might be suggested that socialization processes lead males to become private, intellectual, and introspective when dealing with life crises ("detached observers") while females are socialized to become public, emotional, and extroverted when dealing with life crises ("involved participant observers"). Male coping processes may enable fathers to assess more accurately than mothers how their children are coping despite the fact that children disclose more in discussions with their mothers. We do not know, however, whether fathers are privy to these mother-child interactions and whether fathers process the information regarding the child more accurately than mothers.[1]

Mothers seem to believe their role is to actively assess and monitor the quality and quantity of their children's grief. Fathers seem to have a "quiet faith" in their children's ability to process the grief on their own while keeping a careful watch over the children with less intrusiveness than the mothers.

The marked contrasts between parental perceptions of adolescent self-concept and grief reactions led to a recheck of the data. We wondered why mothers' perceptions of adolescent self-concept were so favorable and yet mothers' perceptions of their adolescents' grief reactions were so filled with a sense of trouble. The mothers seemed to be saying their teenagers had stronger self-concepts since the death but at the same time were struggling with grief. Are mothers more sensitive instruments to the identity and emotional responses of their children than fathers? Or do fathers have a clearer, more reliable picture of teenagers' reactions? Because the fathers' and the teenagers' responses are alike, and differ significantly from the mothers' perceptions, the issue is not simply explained as a matter of women being more empathic or sensitive to interpersonal and intrapersonal issues than are men. It could be that mothers may be working from a faulty database; an adolescent may be telling his/her mother what they think she wants to hear.

An alternative explanation is suggested by considering what is at stake for a bereaved mother in her reflections about a surviving teenager. To the mother, the well-being of this teenager would be a clear indication of the quality of her nurturing the growth and development of her child. A prominent sign of quality mothering would be manifested by a youth with a healthy identity. The bereaved mothers in our study had already lost a child and needed some sense, if only by means of self-confirmation, that their surviving teenager had developed well and could handle the difficulties of mourning. These personal needs could have influenced mothers to overestimate a teenager's self-concept and, at the same time, exaggerate the grief reactions of the youth. Bereaved fathers also care about their surviving teenagers, but the socialization patterns of fathers may have enabled them to remain more detached in nurturing the development of their children and, perhaps, to gain more reliable estimates not only of their teenager's identity but also of their teenager's grief reactions.

The findings indicate that health professionals and others who work with teenagers bereaved over a sibling's death need to recognize the complex family dynamics related to the bereavement process. Grieving children and their parents need to be assessed for normative as well as nonnormative grieving. However, it is striking that without a clear picture of the trajectory of adolescent sibling bereavement gained by means of prospective studies, the notion of normative versus nonnormative grieving may be informed by misguided opinion rather than by reliable, valid data.

---

[1]The revised HSIB (Hogan, 1988a) includes two parallel items: "My grief is the same as my father's grief" and "My grief is the same as my mother's grief;" the teenagers' mean scores on the items (1.85 and 2.22) demonstrate much greater sense of identification with the father's grief.

The authors contributed equally in the preparation of this manuscript.

The authors gratefully acknowledge the assistance of Dr. Dallas Johnson, Department of Statistics, Kansas State University, who served as a statistical consultant, and Susan Boxer, a graduate student at Kansas State University, whose ideas helped generate alternative explanations to our findings.

REFERENCES

Balk, D. E. (1981). *Sibling death during adolescence: Self concept and bereavement reactions.* Unpublished doctoral dissertation, University of Illinois, Champaign-Urbana.

Balk, D. E. (1983). Adolescents' grief reactions and self-concept perceptions following sibling death: A study of 33 teenagers. *Journal of Youth and Adolescence, 12,* 137–161.

Bank, S. P., & Kahn, M. D. (1982). *The sibling bond.* New York: Basic Books.

Block, J. (1957). Studies in the phenomenology of emotions. *Journal of Abnormal and Social Psychology, 54,* 358–363.

Bowlby-West, L. (1983). The impact of death on the family system. *Journal of Family Therapy, 5,* 279–294.

Brent, D. (1983). A death in the family: The pediatrician's role. *Pediatrics, 72,* 645–651.

Cain, A., Fast, I., & Erickson, M. (1964). Children's disturbed reactions to the death of a sibling. *American Journal of Orthopsychiatry, 34,* 741–754.

Cobb, B. (1956). Psychological impact of long-term illness and death of a child on the family circle. *Journal of Pediatrics, 49,* 746–751.

Cobb, S. (1976). Social support as a moderator of life stress. *Psychosomatic Medicine, 38,* 300–314.

Demi, A., & Gilbert, C. (1987). Relationship of parental grief to sibling grief. *Archives of Psychiatric Nursing, 6,* 385–391.

Demo, D., Small, S., & Savin-Williams, R. (1987). Family relations in the self-esteem of adolescents and their parents. *Journal of Marriage and the family, 49,* 705–715.

Dunn, J., & Kendrick, C. (1982). *Siblings: Love, envy & understanding.* Cambridge: Harvard University Press.

Furman, W., & Buhrmester, D. (1985). Children's perceptions of the quality of sibling relationships. *Child Relationships, 56,* 448–461.

Gecas, V., & Schwalbe, M. (1986). Parental behavior and adolescent self-esteem. *Journal of Marriage and the Family, 48,* 37–46.

Gray, R. E. (1987). Adolescent reactions to the death of a parent. *Journal of Youth and Adolescence, 16,* 511–525.

Gyulay, J. (1975). The forgotten grievers. *The American Journal of Nursing, 75,* 1476–1479.

Hilgard, J. R. (1969). Depressive and psychotic states as anniversaries of a sibling death in childhood. *International Psychiatry Clinics, 6,* 197–211.

Hilgard, J. R., Newman, M. F., & Fisk, F. (1960). Strength of adult ego identity following childhood bereavement. *American Journal of Orthopsychiatry, 30,* 788–798.

Hogan, N. S. (1987). An investigation of the adolescent sibling bereavement process and adaptation (Doctoral dissertation, Loyola University of Chicago, 1987). *Dissertation Abstracts, International,* 4024A.

Hogan, N. S. (1988a). The effects of time on the adolescent sibling bereavement process. *Pediatric Nursing, 14,* 333–335.

Hogan, N. S. (1988b). [Sibling bereavement reactions and self concept of 144 adolescents]. Unpublished raw data.

Hogan, N. S. (1990). Hogan Sibling Inventory of Bereavement. In J. Touliatos, B. Perlmutter, & M. Straus (Eds.), *Handbook of family measurement techniques,* p. 524, Newbury Park, CA: Sage.

Jourard, S. M. (1971). *The transparent self.* New York: D. Van Nostrand Co.

Kliman, G. (1980). Death: Some implications in child development and child analysis. *Advances in Thanatology, 4,* 43–50.

Krell, R., & Rabkin, L. (1979). The effects of sibling death on the surviving child. *Family Process, 18,* 471–477.

Leon, I. G. (1986). Intrapsychic and family dynamics in perinatal sibling loss. *Infant Mental Health Journal, 7,* 200–213.

Martinson, I. M., Davies, E. B., & McClowry, S. G. (1987). The long-term effects of sibling death on self concept. *Journal of Pediatric Nursing, 24,* 227–235.

Offer, D. (1969). *The psychological world of the teenager.* New York: Basic Books.

Osterweis, M., Solomon, F., & Green, M. (Eds.). (1984). *Bereavement: Reactions, consequences, and care.* Washington, DC: National Academy Press.

Pollock, G. (1978). On siblings, childhood sibling loss and creativity. *The Annual of Psychoanalysis, 6,* 443–481.

Pollock, G. H. (1986). Childhood sibling loss: A family tragedy. *Pediatric Annals, 15,* 851–855.

Rochlin, G. (1965). *Grief and discontents.* Boston: Little, Brown.

Rosenthal, H. (1987, July 24). Men have more trouble handling grief than do women. *Chicago Tribune,* p. 5.

Schatz, W. H. (1984). *Healing a father's grief.* Redmond, WA: Medic Publishing Co.

Schiff, H. S. (1977). *The bereaved parent.* Boston: G. K. Hall & Co.

Soricelli, B. A., & Utech, C. L. (1985). Mourning the death of a child: The family and group process. *Social Work, Volume 30,* 429–433.

CHAPTER 24

Parental Stress Response to Sexual Abuse and Ritualistic Abuse of Children in Day-Care Centers

Susan J. Kelley

The purpose of this study was to examine the stress responses of parents to the sexual and ritualistic abuse of their children in day-care centers. Sixty-five mothers and 46 fathers of children sexually abused in day-care centers completed the Symptom Checklist-90-Revised (SCL-90-R), a measure of psychological distress. These scores were compared with a carefully matched comparison group of parents of 67 nonabused children. Parents of abused children also completed the Impact of Event Scale (IES), a measure which indexes symptoms that characterize posttraumatic stress disorder. Parents of sexually abused children reported significantly more psychological distress than parents of nonabused children, with parents of ritually abused children displaying the most severe psychological distress. Parents of abused children reported symptom profiles on the SCL-90-R and IES consistent with posttraumatic stress disorder.

The sexual abuse of a child constitutes a major crisis for the victims and their parents. While existing empirical evidence indicates that sexually abused children are negatively affected by the experience (Anderson, Bach, & Griffith, 1981; Conte & Schuerman, 1987; Friedrich, Urquiza, & Beilke, 1986; Gomes-Schwartz, Horowitz, & Sauzier, 1984; Tong, Oates, & McDowell, 1987), to date there has been no systematic examination of parental responses to sexual victimization. The literature, largely anecdotal, lacks standardized measures of parental reactions. The purpose of this study was to empirically validate parental stress responses to extrafamilial sexual and ritualistic abuse.

RELEVANT LITERATURE

Impact of Sexual Abuse on Parents: Sexual victimization and the resulting disclosure is a stressful event that alters the balance of the family and interferes with previously effective coping abilities (Sesan, Freeark, & Murphy, 1986). The few studies that have attempted to examine the reaction of parents to sexual abuse have primarily involved cases of intrafamilial sexual abuse (Anderson et al., 1981; de Young, 1982; Gomes-Schwartz et al., 1984; Herman, 1981). This poses a serious problem, as it is difficult to separate the effect of sexual abuse from membership in a dysfunctional incestuous family.

It is generally believed that sexually abused children incorporate their parents' reactions to the abuse (DeVine, 1980; Esquilin, 1987; MacFarlane & Waterman, 1986). Anderson et al. (1981) found increased behavioral symptomatology in children who had encountered negative reactions from their parents, such as blaming the child, compared with victims whose parents were responsive to their needs. Gomes-Schwartz et al. (1984) reported that when mothers reacted to disclosure of sexual abuse with anger and punishment, children manifested more behavioral disturbances. Friedrich and Reams (1987) suggested that the symptoms seen in sexually abused children reflect not only the trauma they have experienced directly, but also their family environment, the amount of support the child feels, and the level of disruption that follows the disclosure of abuse. Thus, based on the available data, it appears that the reactions of parents to their child's victimization critically influence the child's reaction.

Although the majority of sexual abuse is committed by relatives, there has been a sharp rise in the number of reported sexual abuse cases in day-care centers. In a national study of day-care centers, researchers (Finkelhor, Williams, & Burns, 1988) identified 270 day-care centers where sexual abuse occurred from 1983 to 1985, involving a total of 1,639 child victims. Thirteen percent of these cases involved ritualistic abuse.

Ritualistic abuse is a particularly disturbing type of child maltreatment that has recently come to the attention of law enforcement officials and mental health professionals (Gould, 1987; Hollingsworth, 1986; Kagy, 1986; Kaye & Klein, 1987). Ritualistic abuse refers to the systematic and repetitive sexual, physical, and psychological abuse of children by adults engaged in cult worship (Kelley, 1988). The purpose of ritualistic abuse is to induce a religious or mystical experience for the adult participants. Perpetrators of ritualistic abuse involve children in group religious practices and ceremonies that often include the ingestion of human excrement, semen, or blood; witnessing the mutilation of animals; threats with supernatural or magical powers; ingestion of drugs; and use of songs or chants. The child victims are threatened with supernatural powers and physical harm to prevent disclosure of the ritualistic activities. For example, children may be threatened that the devil or demons will harm them.

A major hypothesis of this study was that parents whose children were sexually abused in day care would demonstrate greater psychological distress than a comparison group of parents of nonabused children. Furthermore, because of the extreme nature of ritualistic abuse, it was hypothesized that parents whose children were ritually abused would demonstrate more psychological distress than parents of children sexually abused without rituals.

METHOD

Sample

The sample consisted of the parents of 134 children, 67 of whom were sexually abused in day-care centers, and a carefully matched comparison group of 67 nonabused children. The sexually abused children and their parents were divided into two groups based on whether the sexual abuse involved ritualistic abuse. Allegations of sexual abuse were substantiated by the child protective agency in the jurisdiction responsible for investigating charges of sexual abuse for all cases involved in this study. Types of abuse are based on statements made by the children to parents or their therapists.

Group I consisted of the parents of 32 children who were sexually abused (without ritualistic abuse). The parents in Group I included 32 mothers and 25 fathers. The mean age of the mothers was 33.5 years (range = 26 to 42) and for fathers 36 years (range = 30 to 45). The majority of families were of middle to high socioeconomic status, with 82% falling into social classes I and II on the Hollingshead Index of Social Status (Hollingshead, 1975). Forty-four percent were college graduates and 72% of the families earned more than $26,000 a year.

The age of the children at the time the abuse began ranged from 1 to 4 years ($M = 2.38$ yr.). There were equal numbers of males and females. The time elapsed since the abuse ended and data were collected ranged from 8 to 36 months ($M = 26$). The mean duration of the abuse was 13 months (range = 1 to 36). The types of abuse ranged from fondling of the genitals to vaginal and rectal intercourse. Fifty-nine percent were forced to perform oral-genital sexual activity, 15.6% of females were vaginally penetrated by a penis, and 28.1% had foreign objects placed in their vaginas. Twenty-eight percent of the children were rectally penetrated with a penis and 56.3% had a foreign object inserted into their rectum. The children experienced a mean of 4.81 different types of sexual acts (range = 1 to 10) by an average of 1.97 different offenders (range = 1 to 5). Three percent of the children were abused on only one occasion, 43.7% were abused between 5 to 20 times, and 53.1% were abused more than 20 different times.

Group II included the parents of 35 children who were ritually abused. The parents in this group included 33 mothers and 21 fathers, representing all 35 children. The mean age of the mothers was 34.6 years (range = 28 to 43); mean age of the fathers, 37 years (range = 26 to 55). The majority of the families were of middle to upper SES, with 75% scoring within social classes I and II of the Hollingshead Index of Social Status (Hollingshead, 1975). Fifty-nine percent were college graduates and 91.2% of the families earned over $26,000 per year.

The ages of the children at the onset of the abuse ranged from 1 to 7 years ($M = 3.2$ yrs.). Sixty percent were female and 40% male. The time elapsed since the abuse ended and the data were collected ranged from 6 to 47 months ($M = 29$).

The children in Group II were physically, sexually, and psychologically abused within the context of cult worship. Children in this group described forced participation in religious ceremonies as well as threats with supernatural powers. In addition to ritualistic abuse, children in Group II experienced more extensive sexual abuse than the children in Group I. The mean duration of the abuse was 16.57 months (range = 1 to 81). The types of abuse ranged from fondling the genitals to vaginal and rectal intercourse, with a mean of 8.34 different types of abuse (range = 1 to 11) per child. Eighty-eight percent were forced to perform oral-genital sexual activity, 42.9% of females were vaginally penetrated by a penis, and 40% had foreign objects placed in their vaginas. Sixty-three percent of the children were rectally penetrated with a penis, and 77.1% had a foreign object inserted into their rectums. Each child was abused by an average of 4.82 different offenders (range = 1 to 17). Twenty percent of the children were abused between 5 to 20 times, and 80% were abused more than 20 times.

Group III, the comparison group, was comprised of the parents of 67 nonabused children aged 4 to 11 years (M = 6.6). The subjects in the comparison group were matched to the children in Groups I and II on the following variables: age, gender, socioeconomic status, and length of attendance at a day-care center. Group III included 66 mothers and 53 fathers representing families of all 67 non-abused children. The Hollingshead Index of Social Status was employed to match abused subjects on SES. Sixty-three percent of the parents were college graduates and 90% of the families earned over $26,000 annually.

The parents in Groups I and II (abuse groups) were recruited nationally through three sources: a nonprofit organization for parents of sexually and ritually abused children, a district attorney's office, and a mental health center. A total of 81 parents whose children had been abused in day-care centers were contacted by the sources cited above to solicit their participation in the study. Each family contacted expressed a willingness to participate; therefore 81 sets of questionnaires were mailed. Sixty-seven of the 81 parents who were mailed questionnaires returned them to the researcher, resulting in a response rate of 83%. The subjects represented 16 different day-care centers in 12 states where abuse had occurred.

Subjects in Group III, the comparison group, were recruited through three day-care centers and two public school systems in the Northeast. Two-hundred-and-fifty questionnaires were mailed to potential subjects for the comparison group. Of these, 189 were returned, resulting in a response rate of 76%. The first 67 comparison subjects who matched individual subjects in Groups I and II on age, gender, SES, and history of having attended day-care, were selected for the comparison group.

Instruments

Symptom Checklist-90-R

The Symptom Checklist-90-R (SCL-90-R) (Derogatis, 1977), a 90-item multidimensional self-report symptom inventory, was used to measure symptomatic psychological distress in the parents. The SCL-90-R reflects psychopathology in terms of nine primary symptom dimensions (somatization, obsessive–compulsive, interpersonal sensitivity, depression, anxiety, hostility, phobic anxiety, paranoid ideation, and psychoticism) and three global indices of distress (General Severity Index [GSI], Positive Symptom Total, and Positive Symptom Distress Index). The GSI combines information on numbers of symptoms and intensity of distress, and is considered to be the best single indicator of distress in subjects. It was therefore chosen as the summary measure of psychological distress. Each item of the SCL-90-R represents distress in terms of a discrete 5-point scale ranging from *not at all* (0) to *extremely* (4). The SCL-90-R scores reported are normalized T scores for adult nonpatient normals ($M = 50$; $SD = 10$).

The SCL-90-R has shown high levels of both internal consistency and test-retest reliability. Derogatis (1977) reported coefficient alphas between .77 and .90 for the nine primary symptom dimensions, and test-retest coefficients between .78 and .90. Cronbach's alpha, computed on the responses of subjects in this sample, resulted in a reliability coefficient of .98.

Validity of the SCL-90-R has been well established. A very high convergent and discriminate validity between the SCL-90-R and the Minnesota Multiphasic Personality Inventory (MMPI) has been established. The SCL-90-R is highly sensitive to stress related changes.

Impact of Event Scale (IES)

The IES is a 15-item instrument which focuses on the quality of conscious experiences related to a specific stressful event. The stressful event of interest is written on the form as the referent for response to the list of experiences. For the purposes of this study the event is the sexual abuse of the subject's child in a day-care center.

The IES was developed through sequential refinement of items and studies or reliability and validity of the instrument (Horowitz, Wilner, Kaltreider, & Alvarez, 1980). Subscales of coherent items were found to be both logically and empirically consistent and yielded intrusion and avoidance subscales. The split half reliability of the total scale is .86. The internal consistency of these subscales, using Cronbach's alpha, was .78 and .82, respectively. The test-retest reliability was .87 for the total stress score, .80 for the intrusion subscale, and .79 for the avoidance subscale. Cronbach's alpha was computed for internal consistency of items on the IES. The reliability coefficient for mothers was .93; for fathers, .94.

The two subscales of avoidance and intrusion index symptoms on the two dimensions that characterize the DSM-III diagnosis of posttraumatic stress disorder. These are: intrusion into consciousness of unbidden ideas, feelings, and images; and consciously recognized denial or avoidance of stress-related themes and emotional responses (Horowitz, Wilner, & Alvarez, 1979).

Procedure

Data were collected through mailed questionnaires. Subjects in Groups I and II completed the two self-administered standardized instruments described above, the Child Behavior Checklist (Achenbach & Edelbrock, 1983), as well as a questionnaire developed by the researcher to collect information related to the sexual abuse, a brief inventory of 12 stressful life events, and demographic data. Comparison subjects completed the Child Behavior Checklist, the SCL-90-R, and the questionnaire on demographic data and stressful life events.

A letter for informed consent was included; anonymity and confidentiality of responses were assured.

RESULTS

Initial analyses were performed to examine potential sources of confounding by demographic, stressful life events, and abuse-related variables. There were no significant differences between the three groups on socioeconomic status, income, marital status, race, number of children in the family, length of time the child attended day care, or total number of stressful life events.

Results of analysis of variance (ANOVA) and planned comparisons of mean T scores of parents on the GSI and the nine subscales of the SCL-90-R are presented for mothers and fathers in Table 1 and Table 2. As hypothesized, parents of sexually abused children (Groups I and II) reported greater psychological distress than parents of nonabused children as indicated by their significantly higher mean T scores on the GSI (mothers, $t = -9.32, p < .0001$; fathers, $t = -8.86, p < .0001$). Fifty-two percent of parents of abused children had GSI T scores ≥ 63, which are at the 90th percentile and considered in the clinical range (Derogatis, 1977).

Parents of abused children (Groups I and II) scored significantly higher on each of the nine subscales of the SCL-90-R than parents of nonabused children. Mothers and fathers of abused children had the highest elevations in five primary dimensions: depression, interpersonal sensitivity, hostility, paranoia, and anxiety.

As predicted, parents of ritually abused children reported the most psychological distress, with significantly higher mean GSI T scores than parents of children abused without rituals (mothers, $t = 1.79, p < .05$; fathers, $t = 2.08, p < .05$). Sixty-five percent of parents whose children were abused with rituals scored in the clinical range compared with 40% of parents whose children were abused without rituals.

Next, paired t tests were conducted to compare the mean scores of mothers and fathers in Groups I and II on the GSI and the nine primary dimensions of the SCL-90-R. The mean GSI T score of fathers ($M = 63.53, SD = 10.47$) was significantly greater ($t = -2.52, p < .05$) than the mean score of mothers ($M = 59.64, SD = 11.49$), indicating that 2 years postdisclosure, fathers were experiencing greater psychological distress than mothers. The only subscale in which there was a significant difference between mothers and fathers was the depression subscale, in which the mean score of fathers ($M = 63.44, SD = 10.97$) was significantly greater ($t = -3.15, p < .05$) than that of mothers ($M = 58.84, SD = 10.82$).

Mean scores obtained on the IES indicate that although an average of 2.2 years had elapsed since the sexual abuse of their child, parents continued to experience intrusive thoughts and images as well as conscious avoidance of ideas and emotions related to their child's abuse. Paired t tests revealed that mothers ($M = 19.52, SD = 12.78$) scored significantly higher than fathers ($M = 15.41, SD = 12.21$) on the intrusion subscale ($t = 2.36, p < .05$). No significant difference was found on the avoidance subscale (mothers, $M = 13.60, SD = 10.21$; fathers, $M = 13.00, SD = 10.77$). A comparison of Groups I and II revealed no significant difference in IES mean scores.

TABLE 1
The Symptom Checklist-90-R Scores of Mothers

Dimensions	Group 1 Sexual Abuse ($N = 32$)	Group 2 Ritualistic Abuse ($N = 33$)	Group 3 Comparison ($N = 67$)
General Severity Index (GSI)[a]			
M	58.16	62.64	44.69
SD	10.85	9.26	9.25
Depression[b]			
M	58.25	61.30	47.24
SD	10.71	8.26	8.90
Interpersonal sensitivity[b]			
M	60.09	61.76	49.68
SD	10.92	10.89	8.10
Hostility[b]			
M	61.09	59.79	49.55
SD	9.86	11.23	7.30
Paranoid[b]			
M	59.29	62.33	46.39
SD	10.79	9.66	6.77
Anxiety[a]			
M	56.81	62.76	45.19
SD	10.99	8.39	8.10
Obsessive-Compulsive[b]			
M	57.06	60.88	46.06
SD	10.83	9.55	8.18
Psychoticism[b]			
M	58.56	60.24	48.27
SD	9.93	9.97	6.56
Somatization[b]			
M	50.56	55.12	43.94
SD	9.11	10.06	7.48
Phobic[b]			
M	54.48	56.85	45.49
SD	9.87	10.59	4.06

[a]Groups 1 and 2 > Group 3**** and Group 2 > Group 1*
[b]Groups 1 and 2 > Group 3 ****
*$p < .05$; ****$p < .0001$

TABLE 2
The Symptom Checklist-90-R Scores of Fathers

Dimensions	Group 1 Sexual Abuse (N = 25)	Group 2 Ritualistic Abuse (N = 21)	Group 3 Comparison (N = 53)
General Severity Index (GSI)[a]			
M	60.68	66.71	47.91
SD	11.05	8.64	7.52
Depression[a]			
M	61.36	65.76	49.00
SD	11.34	9.96	8.68
Interpersonal sensitivity[b]			
M	60.64	65.48	50.06
SD	9.38	7.45	7.36
Hostility[b]			
M	62.52	63.81	48.09
SD	11.15	9.84	7.44
Paranoid[a]			
M	59.16	65.91	46.91
SD	11.19	10.31	7.85
Anxiety[a]			
M	57.84	65.81	48.81
SD	11.31	8.70	7.91
Obsessive-Compulsive[b]			
M	58.92	63.67	49.30
SD	12.03	8.44	8.19
Psychoticism[a]			
M	55.52	62.29	47.55
SD	9.50	8.67	5.69
Somatization[a]			
M	52.96	60.86	47.32
SD	11.67	8.74	9.05
Phobic[b]			
M	54.48	58.05	48.09
SD	9.70	9.30	4.16

[a]Groups 1 and 2 > Group 3 **** and Group 2 > Group 1*
[b]Groups 1 and 2 > Group 3****
*$p < .05$; ****$p < .0001$

Pearson's correlation was used to test for significant relationships between parental stress scores and variables related to the abuse. Parental stress as measured by the GSI was strongly correlated with the IES intrusion subscale, $r = .74, p < .001$, and moderately correlated with the IES avoidance subscale, $r = .53, p < .001$. There was a weak but significant inverse relationship between GSI scores and time elapsed since the sexual abuse, $r = .22, p < .05$, indicating that parental stress decreases with distancing in time from their child's sexual victimization.

Twenty-two percent of mothers ($n = 15$) and 9% of fathers ($n = 6$) in Groups I and II (abuse groups) reported having been victimized as children. The t test for independent samples was used to compare the GSI T scores of abused and nonabused parents. The mean GSI T score of mothers who had been abused during childhood ($M = 64.2, SD = 10.21$) was significantly higher, $t = -1.66, p < .05$ than the mean GSI T scores of mothers without a childhood history of victimization ($M = 59.3, SD = 10.08$). There was no significant difference between GSI T scores of fathers who had been abused and those who had not been abused.

DISCUSSION

The increased psychological distress found in parents of sexually abused children in this study empirically validates the clinical literature which asserts that sexual victimization is a major stressor for parents (DeJong, 1986; Esquilin, 1987; Sesan et al., 1986). The parents of the abused children were found to be highly symptomatic and present strong evidence of experiencing posttraumatic stress disorder. According to Horowitz et al. (1980), posttraumatic stress disorder occurs in reaction to a major traumatic event and is characterized by intrusive ideas and feelings, ideational denial, and emotional numbing, as well as recurrent or prolonged episodes of depression, anxiety, guilt, shame, and hostility. Parents of sexually abused children reported clinical indicators of intrusion and avoidance as measured by the IES, as well as elevated scores on the depression, anxiety, interpersonal sensitivity, and hostility dimensions of the SCL-90-R.

In order to effectively intervene, nurses need to recognize sexual victimization as both an acute and a chronic stressor for parents. During the acute phase, parents are dealing with feelings of shock, anger, denial, and guilt (DeJong, 1986; DeVine, 1980; Finkelhor, 1986; MacFarlane & Waterman, 1986) as well as entanglement in the complex legal, mental health, and social service systems. Sexual abuse is also experienced by parents as a chronic stressor due to the long-term impact on the child, the need for extended therapy, and in many instances, lengthy legal proceedings which may prevent the family from achieving closure on the event. Even when a guilty verdict is rendered, most verdicts end up in a lengthy appeal process which further prolongs the stress reaction. Although, on average, 2 years had elapsed since the discovery of their child's sexual abuse, 52% of parents in the study had psychological distress scores in the clinical range. This persistent symptomatology suggests a chronic form of posttraumatic stress disorder. It is important to note that the psychological distress levels found in parents in this study are comparable to those found in parents 2 years after their child had died from cancer (Moore, Gilliss, & Martinson, 1988).

Despite the fact that two-thirds of the parents in the study received therapy, the majority continued to display persistent psychological distress. Most subjects received less than 6 months of therapy, which suggests that more extended therapy is needed for successful resolution of this traumatic event. The question is whether effective treatment is available to parents in cases of extrafamilial sexual abuse. Studies that examine the efficacy of various intervention strategies for parents in cases of extrafamilial sexual abuse are needed.

The higher distress levels found in fathers in this study are in contrast to the findings of other studies in which the stress responses of mothers and fathers were compared. Moore et al. (1988) found greater psychological distress in mothers than fathers after the death of their child from cancer. Likewise, Klein and Nimorwicz (1982) found greater psychological distress in mothers than fathers of hemophiliac children. Fathers may have been experiencing a delayed stress response, since fathers have been reported as having greater difficulty discussing thoughts and feelings related to their child's victimization (Zimmerman, Wolbert, Burgess, & Hartman, 1987).

The finding that parental stress levels decreased somewhat over time underscores the importance of reassuring parents that the intense psychological distress they initially experience will decrease with time and therapeutic intervention. However, it has yet to be determined how long symptoms persist and a longitudinal study of parental responses beginning immediately after discovery of the abuse with periodic evaluations of psychological distress levels would provide valuable insight into how parents process this stressful event.

The increased psychological distress found in mothers with childhood histories of victimization is of clinical significance. For mothers victimized as children, the sexual abuse of their child may precipitate a twofold crisis in which they must deal simultaneously with their own unresolved trauma as well as the knowledge that their child has been sexually abused. It is therefore imperative to elicit parental histories of childhood sexual abuse when assessing families of child victims and to provide appropriate support to adult survivors of sexual abuse.

Parents of ritually abused children experienced the greatest psychological distress. This finding could be related to several factors including parental knowledge of the severe forms of abuse their child suffered, increased impact associated with ritualistic abuse (Finkelhor et al., 1988; Kelley, 1989), lack of information currently available to parents and professionals on ritualistic abuse, and the skepticism with which some reports of ritualistic abuse are met (Kelley, 1988).

The sexual victimization of a child in day care is a traumatic event for parents which may result in posttraumatic stress disorder, possibly of a chronic nature. Since resolution of the victimization experience by the child can be facilitated or hindered by parental response, professional intervention is imperative for fathers, as well as mothers. Unfortunately, attention in the past has focused almost exclusively on the treatment needs of incestuous families, while overlooking the needs of families who experience extrafamilial abuse. More extensive research needs to be conducted on the effects of extrafamilial abuse on all family members, including nonabused siblings. Factors that may mediate parental reactions to sexual abuse, such as coping style, family dynamics that predate the abuse, cultural and religious influences, and social supports need to be carefully examined.

This study was partially funded by the Theta Chapter (Boston University) of Sigma Theta Tau International.

REFERENCES

Achenbach, T. M., & Edelbrock, C. S. (1983). *The child behavior checklist manual.* Burlington, VT: The University of Vermont.

Anderson, S. C., Bach, C. M., & Griffith, S. (1981). *Psychosocial sequelae in intrafamilial victims of sexual assault and abuse.* Paper presented at the Third International Conference on Child Abuse and Neglect, Amsterdam, The Netherlands.

Conte, J., & Schuerman, J. (1987). Factors associated with an increased impact of child sexual abuse. *Child Abuse and Neglect, 11,* 201–211.

DeJong, A. R. (1986). Childhood sexual abuse precipitating maternal hospitalization. *Child Abuse and Neglect, 10,* 551–553.

Derogatis, L. R. (1977). *The SCL-90-R: Administration, scoring, and procedures manual.* Baltimore: Clinical Psychometrics Research.

DeVine, R. A. (1980). The sexually abused child in the emergency room. In *Sexual abuse of children: Selected readings,* DHHS Publication no. (OHDS) 78-30161 (pp. 11–16). Washington, DC: US Department of Health and Human Services.

De Young, M. (1982). *The sexual victimization of children.* Jefferson, NC: McFarland and Company.

Esquilin, S. C. (1987). Family response to the identification of extrafamilial child sexual abuse. *Psychotherapy in Private Practice, 5*(1), 105–113.

Finkelhor, D. (1986). *A sourcebook on child sexual abuse.* Beverly Hills: Sage Publications.

Finkelhor, D., Williams, L., & Burns, N. (1988). *Sexual abuse in day care: A national study.* Durham, NH: University of New Hampshire.

Friedrich, W. N., & Reams, R. A. (1987). Course of psychological symptoms in sexually abused children. *Psychotherapy, 24*(2), 160–170.

Friedrich, W. N., Urquiza, A. J., & Beilke, R. (1986). Behavioral problems in sexually abused young children. *Journal of Pediatric Psychology, 11,* 47–57.

Gomes-Schwartz, B., Horowitz, J. M., & Sauzier, M. (1984). *Sexually exploited children: Service and research project.* Final report for the Office of Juvenile Justice and Delinquency Prevention. Washington, DC: US Department of Justice.

Gould, C. (1987) Satanic ritual abuse: Child victims, adult survivors, system response. *California Psychologist, 22*(3), 1.

Herman, J. L. (1981). *Father-daughter incest.* Cambridge, MA: Harvard University Press.

Hollingshead, A. B. (1975). Four factor index of social status. Working paper. New Haven, CT: Yale University Department of Sociology.

Hollingsworth, J. (1986). *Unspeakable acts.* New York: Congdon and Weed.

Horowitz, M., Wilner, N., & Alvarez, W. (1979). Impact of event scale: A measure of subjective stress. *Psychosomatic Medicine, 41*(3), 209–218.

Horowitz, M., Wilner, N., Kaltreider, N., & Alvarez, W. (1980). Signs and symptoms of posttraumatic stress disorder. *Archives of General Psychiatry, 37*(1), 85–92.

Kagy, L. (1986). Ritualized abuse of children. *RECAP: Newsletter of the National Child Assault Prevention Project,* Columbus, OH: Winter, 1988, 1–2.

Kaye, M., & Klein, L. (1987). *Clinical indicators of Satanic cult victimization.* Paper presented at the Fourth International Conference for the Study of Multiple Personality Disorder, Chicago, November 1987.

Kelley, S. J. (1988). Ritualistic abuse of children: Dynamics and impact. *Cultic Studies Journal, 5*(2), 228–236.

Kelley, S. J. (1989). Stress responses of children to sexual abuse and ritualistic abuse in day-care centers. *Journal of Interpersonal Violence, 4,* 501–512.

Klein, R. H., & Nimorwicz, P. (1982). The relationship between psychological distress and knowledge of disease among hemophilia patients and their families: A pilot study. *Journal of Psychosomatic Research, 26*(4), 387–391.

MacFarlane, K., & Waterman, J. (1986). *Sexual abuse of young children.* New York: Guilford Press.

Moore, I. M., Gilliss, C. L., & Martinson, I. (1988). Psychosomatic symptoms in parents two years after the death of a child with cancer. *Nursing Research, 37,* 104–107.

Sesan, R., Freeark, K., & Murphy, S. (1986). The support network: Crisis intervention for extrafamilial child sexual abuse. *Professional Psychology, Research, and Practice, 17*(2), 138–146.

Tong, L., Oates, K., & McDowell, M. (1987). Personality development following sexual abuse. *Child Abuse and Neglect, 11*(3), 371–383.

Zimmerman, M. L., Wolbert, W. A., Burgess, A. W., & Hartman, C. R. (1987). Art and group work: Interventions for multiple victims of child molestation. *Archives of Psychiatric Nursing, 1,* 40–46.

UNIT 3

FAMILY HEALTH NURSING CLINICAL PRACTICE

One way to determine whether patterns of family nursing practice are changing is to analyze how nurses are involving the family in practice. This process may be the key to defining and measuring quality family health care. These articles explore implications for family nursing practice. In addition, they form a comprehensive and reliable guide to family health nursing practice based on principles grounded in a wide variety of perspectives and methods. This knowledge can help the nurse organize massive amounts of information and provide a focus for intervention.

CHAPTER 25

Health Promotion, Families, and the Diagnostic Process

Eileen Donnelly

Various health care professionals use the term "diagnosis" to refer to judgments about a client's need for care. Physicians, social workers, nutritionists, and nurses diagnose within their specific disciplines.

For these practitioners, there are diagnostic categories and processes. Physicians use the International Classification of Diseases (ICD) from which to diagnose and to treat. Social workers also use a diagnostic process from which to analyze and to recommend. According to Gordon,[1] a nurse who has done a great deal of analysis regarding the diagnostic process, "diagnosis" refers to both the process of reasoning leading to a diagnosis and the specific judgment made. The diagnostic process entails arriving at a judgment that is based on patterns of behavior. It influences decisions about the subsequent action of practitioners. Practitioners identify client patterns by making observations, collecting data, analyzing data, and then formulating diagnoses.

The American Nurses' Association (ANA) defines nursing as "the diagnosis and treatment of human responses to actual or potential health problems."[2(p9)] Diagnosis is significant to this definition. Although nurses have always made judgments about a client's need for care, the incorporation of the concept of the diagnosis in the definition of nursing is a relatively recent development. Diagnosis is now a critical aspect in the field.

The North American Nursing Diagnosis Association[3] (NANDA) has developed 98 current diagnostic categories that describe the responses to actual or potential health

Reprinted from *Family & Community Health*, Vol. 12, No. 4, pp. 12–20, with permission of Aspen Publishers, Inc., © 1990.

problems and that identify defining characteristics and related etiologic factors. Referred to as Taxonomy 1 and endorsed by the ANA, this formal classification of nursing diagnostic categories represents the thinking of many nurses since 1973 and provides a focus for building clinical knowledge about the phenomena of concern to nursing. These diagnostic categories refer primarily to the ill individual.

Community health nurses working with families and emphasizing health promotion use the same general definition of nursing as other nurses and make diagnostic statements about family relationships. Diagnosis, including the process and ultimate decision, is central to community health nursing practice. Thus the following principles are true:

- *If* nursing diagnosis is central to nursing,
  and community health nursing with the family as client is a part of nursing,
  then nursing diagnosis is central to the family-as-client nursing.
- *If* there is a professional description of the diagnostic process in nursing for the individual client,
  and this description of the diagnostic process is essential to the practice of nursing,
  then the description of the diagnostic process must be made for the family as client in nursing.

The difficulty for community health nurses in performing diagnosis, however, is the essential absence of standardized diagnostic categories that address family and health promotion. The absence of such categories and the need to establish them systematically and comprehensively is the central theme of this article.

Several questions of paramount importance, particularly to family nurse educators and practitioners, have emerged:

1. Is the family as a whole an appropriate unit of analysis for nurses? If yes, why have diagnostic categories been developed to date that predominantly address individuals?
2. To what extent do existing diagnostic categories apply to health promotion with the family client?
3. Can the "diagnostic reasoning process" be used to make decisions about health and health status with regard to the family?
4. If nursing is the diagnosis and treatment of responses to actual or potential health problems, is there a place for health promotion within the conceptualization of diagnosis?
5. Can health promotion interventions directed toward client well-being be incorporated into nursing diagnosis?
6. Is there a need for a counterpart to the existing diagnostic categories to be developed (which applies to the family), or can the existing classification be expanded?

The purposes of this article are to make the case for inclusion of family health promotion diagnoses; to analyze the one standardized family-health-promotion–related nursing diagnostic category and its components so as to gain insight into health promotion with the family client; and to formulate conclusions and to make recommendations for the development of new diagnostic categories and the refinement of existing ones.

The significance of diagnostic categories for community health is tied to the importance of nurses practicing professionally in the field and emphasizing the family as client and a health orientation. This article provides an analysis of these concepts.

CONCEPTS OF HEALTH PROMOTION

Standards for health have been described to a great extent by the Surgeon General's Report, *Healthy People*.[4] In addition, Dunn[5] has identified nine points of attack for promoting high-level wellness. At least two points refer to the family specifically. The first of these points is improvement in conditions in family living and community life; the second is education to assist individuals and families in the application of knowledge to promote health.

Pender[6] differentiates between health-promoting behaviors and health-protecting behaviors. Health-promotion behaviors are activities directed toward developing the resources of clients that maintain or enhance well-being. Health-protecting behaviors predispose individuals toward avoiding illness and disease. Self-initiated activities directed toward the attainment of higher levels of health are reflective of true health promotion. Pender suggests that health focuses on actualization and is an emerging, never-static process characteristic of the entire life span.

The distinction between health-promoting and health-protecting behaviors is critical in that client goals, outcomes, and, ultimately, different patterns of health-related behaviors are determined and developed. This distinction is important to a practitioner because it provides the underlying foundation for the significant difference in orientation between a health focus and an illness, disease focus. Health status is the framework in which health-promotion–clinical decision making is made. Elements constituting health and, implicitly, its promotion must provide the context for diagnosis, including judgment and decisions about subsequent actions influenced by those judgments.

FAMILY CONCEPTS

Friedman[7] maintains that the family is the basic system in which health behavior and care are organized, performed, and secured (ie, the provision of health care is a family function). Duvall[8] describes developmental tasks for families and considers health care to be one of these. Pratt[9] assessed how well families fulfilled the health care function and found that, except for the energized family, families were lacking in their functioning as a personal health care system.

Families are in a fundamental position of defining health and of initiating healthy behaviors and patterns among members. As with the individual client, families differ with respect to definitions of health and health behavior. Curran,[10] a family specialist, surveyed more than 500 professionals who work with families: teachers, family therapists, youth counselors, and ministers. She identified 15 traits commonly shared by families considered by these experts to be "healthy." These traits provide a basis for defining the characteristics of healthy families.

Despite suggestions by some authors that family responsibility for health care functions has been transferred to the hospitals and physicians' offices, families are typically the first to identify signs and symptoms of illness and to decide what subsequent action is appropriate, that is, whether to seek care, where to seek care, and from whom to seek care (eg, physician, practitioner, or, possibly, folk healer). Families, in fact, are the major caregivers of their members. When families make major improvements in maintaining their health through life-style modification and commitments, Pratt[9] asserts that family responsibility for its members' health is strengthened.

Families provide settings in which initial health patterns and behavior are learned. Family patterns of health care influence the development of values and life styles of children with respect to health. The development of health-promotion activities as early in life as possible can result in higher levels of health and longevity for adults as well as children.

Families need to be counseled toward optimizing their health behavior. Presently families that are experiencing increased longevity, rising health care costs, increasing numbers of elderly members, and rising incidence of chronic diseases need to be educated to assume the very crucial role of influencing the health behaviors of their members.

THE DIAGNOSTIC PROCESS

Nurses use a diagnostic reasoning process to make independent judgments about their clients (ie, individuals, family, community) and to determine probable cause.[11] There is a logical sequence that occurs in this process, and it can be explained as follows: The nurse or health care practitioner is an observer of a phenomenon; he or she attempts to describe phenomena in terms of observable signs or symptoms that are indications of some preceding action (or cause). The family health care practitioner attempts to identify the probable cause(s) for the effects or signs or symptoms, thereby arriving at a judgment. This is the logic of the diagnostic process.

The diagnostic process includes the following specific steps:

- collecting information;
- interpreting information;
- clustering the information; and
- naming the cluster.[1]

For practitioners working with families, determining what information is significant and assigning meaning to data depends on a knowledge of baseline data or population norms. Through inferential reasoning the practitioner compares data and determines whether or not cues fall within normal ranges.[12]

The diagnostic process begins with the collection of information in keeping with the concept of the client, in this case, the total family unit. One's conceptual perspective on clients and on nursing goals and outcomes strongly determines what kinds of variables are assessed by practitioners. Health professionals new to this process deal with difficult questions, such as: What information is important? What needs to be assessed and why? How do I select from the vast amount of clinical information and variables that are relevant to family health promotion?

A practitioner needs to develop the capacity to observe health as an effect and to reason out probable causes. What are phenomena regarding health? What are observable health signs? What are reasons for probable causes? How can family health be enhanced?

For the community health nurse, the basis for professional judgments is likely to be shaped in part by the framework provided by the NANDA taxonomy.[3] Such judgments need to reflect uniform standards and must be based on common criteria, as built into the diagnostic categories. Significantly, only seven of the currently approved diagnostic categories address family situations. They are as follows: Family Coping: Potential for Growth; Ineffective Family Coping: Compromised; Ineffective Family Coping: Disabling; Altered Family Processes; Altered Parenting; Potential for Altered Parenting; and Parental Role Conflict. Of further significance is the fact that only one of the family-focused diagnostic categories, Family Coping: Potential for Growth, hints at health-promotion concepts.

The diagnostic process applied to the family as client requires a rethinking about this framework. The integrity of this practice area demands a focus oriented to health and family at each step in the nursing process (assessment, analysis, diagnosis, intervention, and evaluation). Diagnosis is the step in the nursing process that links the observation of a phenomenon to the implementation of an activity. How practitioners conceptualize and implement diagnosis affects both preceding and subsequent steps.

Presently health-promotion intervention strategies with respect to the family are limited and not systematically used by practitioners. There is a need to develop such intervention strategies. Their development can emerge from well-developed diagnostic categories.

As discussed, however, family health is a practice focus about which little has been written in nursing regarding the diagnostic process. The gap in the literature and in nursing practice needs to be addressed by those individuals working in family nursing and family health care. In doing this the diagnostic process applied to family requires an explanation of the bias existing within the current framework—a predominant illness focus—and the development of family health diagnostic categories accordingly.

ANALYSIS OF DIAGNOSTIC CATEGORY

Students, educators, and practitioners using the diagnostic reasoning process with the family as client and health promotion as an orientation are challenged significantly with respect to diagnostic categories. Within the NANDA classification, only one nursing diagnosis (of 98) suggests both a health promotion and family orientation—Family Coping: Potential for Growth. This diagnostic category provides a basis for examining, developing, and applying standardized categories for community health nursing diagnosis.

Three components for each diagnostic category have been outlined: (1) definition, (2) related factors, and (3) defining characteristics. By analyzing the components of this category and how they fit the family versus the individual with a health rather than an illness orientation, practitioners can move toward the use of the diagnostic process with family health promotion rather than health problems.

Definition Component

Of importance is the fact that there are differing conceptual definitions (as well as descriptions of defining characteristics and related factors) for this nursing diagnosis. One definition of Family Coping: Potential for Growth is "the effective management of adaptive tasks by family members involved with the patient's health challenge, combined with readiness for health and growth as a family, individually, and collectively."[13(p921)] Clearly this definition (as well as its defining characteristics and related factors) readily lends itself to a focus on family health and has been so described.[13]

Another definition, less described and the focus of this paper, is "family member has effectively managed adaptive tasks involved with the client's health challenge and is exhibiting desire and readiness for enhanced health and growth in regard to self and in relation to the client."[14(p286)] In this definition the concepts of family as client and health promotion are less clear. The term client is used to refer to an individual family member with a health "challenge." Another family member is referred to; thus this includes at least two members and is considered to be a family.[15] Yet if we think "family," as the concept label implies, the client is the family, the proposed growth is of the family unit, and "adaptive tasks" refer to enhanced family health.

Related Factors Component

The second component of a diagnostic category refers to those factors that contribute to or influence a client's health state. There is one factor identified within the definition being analyzed: readiness for seeking self-actualization. Self-actualization is clearly an individual concept. This etiology makes sense for a family orientation if it is restated as readiness for family-unit outcomes, such as survival (basic needs), continuity (the ability of the family to work together on strengths as well as weaknesses), and growth (the ability to complete tasks and move forward with developmental levels).

Defining Characteristics Component

The third component of a diagnostic category reflects the signs and symptoms of a health condition indicative of a specific nursing diagnosis. The definition being analyzed has three broad, defining characteristics.[14]

On the surface the defining characteristics seem to reflect individual behavior. They could, however, also describe signs of family health behavior by focusing conceptually on the family unit. The "family member" and the "individual" referred to in these defining characteristics, although not specifically explained, are different members of a family. The interpretation is one of health promotion and wellness for the family client.

The one NANDA family- and health-oriented diagnostic category provides a model for developing other family- and health-oriented diagnostic categories. This one category implicitly demonstrates that a diagnosis can be health-promotion oriented and have a family focus. This analysis demonstrates that the NANDA framework can be applied to a health-promoting family focus. Significantly this analysis also demonstrates that the diagnostic process can be used with a family, health-promoting focus.

Moreover, as a result of the analysis this nursing diagnosis has been effectively applied in family- and health-oriented clinical settings. Graduate students working with families throughout three different semesters have successfully used this NANDA category in the manner outlined above—incorporating a family health-promotion perspective. Health-promotion interventions, such as family-health education, have subsequently been planned and implemented.

RECOMMENDATIONS FOR DEVELOPMENT AND APPLICATIONS OF FAMILY HEALTH-PROMOTION DIAGNOSTIC CATEGORIES

The experience of applying the one family health-promotion diagnostic category in a graduate, clinically based family and community nursing health course has pointed out gaps and resulting needs. The primary need is for the development of a set of validated, family health-promotion diagnostic categories. Other needs relate to the need for graduate nursing programs to ensure that a family health-promotion framework is offered even in the absence of NANDA-confirmed categories; the need for NANDA to hasten the development of diagnostic categories; and the need for undergraduate programs to recognize the significance of community-health, family-based orientations, particularly as the practice of nursing moves out of the hospital. There is also the need for family health-promotion practitioners outside of nursing to become involved in the dialogue encompassing the development of family health-promotion diagnoses.

The development of diagnostic categories for community-health nursing emphasizing family must meet professional standards. Yet there is an urgency for the development and use of diagnostic categories. New practitioners are moving into the field and need diagnostic tools to more effectively practice. The time is ripe, since the general population is presently more focused than ever before on health promotion and the family. This momentum should not be lost.

In the field of nursing to date, attention with respect to the NANDA taxonomy has been on the ill individual. Recently a health-promotion nursing diagnosis focusing on the individual client has been accepted.[13]

Diagnostic category labels such as Family Coping: Potential for Growth generally describe a client's health condition but do not indicate whether a problem exists. This particular concept label refers to a family as the client. By assigning meaning to the data collected and comparing cues to normal ranges, a practitioner can determine if a family has a health problem that is dysfunctional or if a family has the potential for growth.

Nursing diagnoses provide a focus for planning interventions. This analysis has demonstrated that the diagnostic process can be applied to "judge" whether a family is healthy or not and then to identify health-oriented strategies. Family health will contribute directly to improved individual health.

The developments over the past two decades have emphasized the importance of nursing diagnosis to the field of nursing as related to illness in the individual. Unfortunately, little attention has been paid to the process of nursing diagnosis as applied to the family with a health orientation.

In analyzing the one NANDA nursing diagnosis referring to family, Family Coping: Potential for Growth, the author describes how a family health-promotion perspective can be incorporated into this diagnostic category. In working with three sections of community-health graduate nurses, successful use of family-health diagnoses has been demonstrated. These diagnoses were then used as a basis for subsequent community-health nursing intervention strategies.

The full development of a comprehensive and systematic set of family diagnostic categories is essential for clinical decision making in family health. Further efforts at generating new family health-promotion–oriented nursing diagnoses are urged.

REFERENCES

1. Gordon, M. *Nursing diagnosis: Process and application.* St. Louis: Mosby, 1987.
2. *A social policy statement.* Kansas City, MO: American Nurses' Association, 1980.
3. North American Nursing Diagnosis Association: NANDA approved nursing diagnostic categories. *Nurs Diagnosis Newslett* 1988; 15(1):1–3.
4. *Healthy people: The surgeon general's report on health promotion and disease prevention.* US Dept of Health, Education, and Welfare publication No. 79-55071, 1979.
5. Dunn, H.L. *High level wellness.* Thorofare, NJ: Charles B. Slack, 1980.
6. Pender, N.J. *Health promotion in nursing practice.* Norwalk, CT: Appleton & Lange, 1987.
7. Friedman, M.M. *Family nursing: Theory and assessment.* Norwalk, CT: Appleton-Century-Crofts, 1986.
8. Duvall, E. *Family development.* Philadelphia: Lippincott, 1962.
9. Pratt, L. *Family structure and effective health behavior.* Boston: Houghton Mifflin, 1976.

10. Curran, D. *Traits of a healthy family.* San Francisco: Harper & Row, 1983.
11. Gordon, M. The nurse as a thinking practitioner, in Hannh, K., Reiner, M., Milla, W., et al (eds): *Clinical judgement and decision making: The future with nursing diagnosis.* New York: Wiley, 1987.
12. Bandman, E., & Bandman, B. *Clinical thinking in nursing.* Norwalk, CT: Appleton & Lange, 1988.
13. McFarland, G., & McFarland, E. *Nursing diagnosis and intervention: Planning for patient care.* St. Louis: Mosby, 1989.
14. Gordon, M. *Manual of nursing diagnosis: 1988–1989.* St. Louis: Mosby, 1989.
15. US Bureau of the Census: *Statistical abstract of the United States: 1986*, ed 106. Washington, DC, 1985, p. 4.

CHAPTER 26

Family-Based Practice: Discussion of a Tool Merging Assessment with Intervention

Cheryl Ann Lapp, Carol Ann Diemert,
Ruth Enestvedt

**FAMILY ASSESSMENT GUIDELINES:
DISCUSSION OF A TOOL FOR
USE WITH FAMILIES**

**Making a Family-Focused Approach a
Reality in Professional Practice**

The family forms the basic unit of our society; it is the social institution that has the most marked effect on its members.[1] It seems logical, therefore, that caregivers should be equipped to use an orientation to the family whenever professional practice claims to serve families. In nursing, for example, the family as a whole has been an early and enduring focus of care. From the very foundation of professional nursing, written evidence can be found of patient care considered within the context of family life. In the 1850s Florence Nightingale's vision of nursing encompassed more than organizing care for patient "soldiers"; she worked to see that the sick wives and children of soldiers were included in her written justification to improve hospital accommodations. She discussed the privacy and financial needs of families when they joined the soldiers at military camp, and she wrote detailed directions to the army for the improved treatment of the women and children in military camps.[2]

Reprinted from *Family & Community Health*, Vol. 12, No. 4, 21–28, with permission of Aspen Publishers, Inc., © 1990.

In keeping with the importance of viewing people in context, a comprehensive family intervention guide has recently been designed for professionals working with families. It uses theory to direct data gathering and explores desired behavior change with family members. In this way family members can be actively engaged in the process of decision making regarding self-health priorities. The family perspective serves to expand the scope of practice, to increase insight, to allow for case finding, and to move health intervention to a more holistic dimension. Empirically, people actively engaged in practice professions have realized that quality of family life is intertwined with the health of its members. However, there has been less clarity among professionals about how to support and to promote such complex interaction.

To carry the nursing example further, despite its historical traditions, practice today frequently deemphasizes the family as the foundational perspective. People are often portrayed as passive recipients of care, completely helpless and isolated from the social context of family, friends, neighbors, or pets. But ironically, now more than ever, nursing practice needs to encompass the family to continue to meet societal needs for a healthy citizenry.

Familism Versus Individualism

Society has a predominant cultural view that minimizes collective need in favor of individualism. Illness-based reimbursement is but one example of the current health care system that directs our practice but that runs counter to public health convictions about serving the public good.

One possible way to improve professional practice is to change the way professionals are being educated. Undergraduate students especially may have difficulty making a connection between giving care to individuals and then viewing these individuals in their relational context as members of families. The problem is how to shift student learning from an individual to a social unit of analysis. The educational process may be flawed when sequenced learning, in which clinical skills are taught in isolation from an early introduction to family theory and contextual information, occurs. Another factor not to be overlooked is the influence of the mainstream cultural orientation in North America that contributes to the perceptual struggle between individualism and "familism," which refers to the deep importance attached to the family by its members.[3] Today's student professionals may acknowledge familism, yet they consistently fall back into an individualistic perspective.[4]

FAMILY ASSESSMENT GUIDELINES: FAMILIES AS PARTNERS

One way to assist students of community health to "think family" was to develop family assessment guidelines (see the box). These guidelines are presented with an emphasis on family as partner in health care decision making, a philosophic position consistent with an interpretation of self-care in which decisional control belongs within the realm of the consumer.[5] In keeping with our interpretation of the self-care perspective, the authors view the primary responsibility for health and life choices as ultimately

---

FAMILY ASSESSMENT GUIDELINES:
INTERVENTION WITH FAMILIES

Family/social network
- Family tradition
- Development stages—life events
- Living environment/household constellation
  1. Space/privacy
  2. Physical safety/comfort/accessibility
  3. Animal companionship/protection
Neighborhood environment
- Stability and direction of change
- Degree of homogeneity
- Proximity and access to essential services
Family health: Family perceived
- Strengths and limitations
- Satisfaction with health behaviors—maintenance/disruption of life patterns

Social and financial resources
- Social support—open v closed system
- Availability and choices regarding leisure time
- Adequacy of income sources of economic stability
- Management of financial, legal, and protective affairs
Life style
- Values/goals
- Communication/decision making
- Role/flexibility
- Use of resources
Priority issues
- Further exploration
- Summary

---

resting with the client family. The authors see the main responsibility of the professional as ensuring that those choices were made on the basis of the most complete information possible while facilitating self-discovery of strengths and resources already existing for a family. With this interpretation of the practice role, these guidelines were designed for use together with families so that all aspects of information gathering would be "family perceived" as well as "professional perceived." The intent of the partnership here is to clarify discrepant views and to discover fresh alternatives for action.

In a partnership context, assessment becomes intervention as new insight and understanding emerge for both the family and practitioner. Active participation is important at every step of the clinical judgment process, beginning with information gathering. But the assessment phase of professional decision making is not a separate preliminary task to be completed before moving to intervention. Rather, assessment and intervention make up a dynamic process that occurs simultaneously.

THEORETICAL CONTRIBUTIONS TO FAMILY ASSESSMENT

Another factor influencing the development of the guidelines was the use of valued content in family theory. After several classical theoretical perspectives had been reviewed and discussed, students were able to apply major relevant concepts in their processing of information. They saw how the theoretical foundations could, at times, assist them in understanding family life in their familiar cultural context. Selected theoretical perspectives that were incorporated into this family assessment included structural-functional theory,[2,6] family developmental theory,[2,7] systems theory,[8] interactional theory,[6] and conflict theory.[9]

While conducting home visits, community nursing students were often able to use each one of these contributing perspectives as they generated their interview questions in an open-ended format. The actual areas of concentration were sequenced to progress from the structural and the least invasive to the more analytic and value laden in recognition of the needed opportunity for family members to establish a trust level on which to base a therapeutic relationship. The guidelines do not prescribe the questions to be asked of families but instead allow for an exploratory and interactional experience in which the content and pace are mutually defined.

Clients benefit by becoming energized and affirmed when actively engaged in a meaningful relationship focused on their own decision making about family health priorities. The "visitor" discovers that a built-in component of validating professional judgment is family perception, a key element providing direction for mutual agreement as to which family goals will be pursued. For both parties the qualitative nature of the information gathering lends to the interaction a richness and depth facilitated by the attainment of trust and rapport. The data itself, true to the strengths of the qualitative style, is dynamic and powerful, in contrast to the limitations of fixed-response format frequently seen in questionnaires and flow sheets.

From the standpoint of educators, this mutual experience engages inductive reasoning.[10] The authors value this approach because students can move from the particular information presented by families to appropriate theoretical perspectives that reflect what examination of the data reveals. The less desirable alternative would be for the student to artificially mold family data to fit a preselected framework.

ASSESSMENT COMPONENTS

Family/Social Network

When considering what constitutes family, in its variety of configurations, family can sometimes be characterized as an "attitude" revealing identification with significant others.[11] One cannot underestimate the importance of social networks of informal support. Particularly for the elderly, friends and neighbors respond to three types of needs: socialization, conducting the tasks of daily living, and assisting in times of need.[12] These closely parallel the classic functions that families are charged with fulfilling for dependent members: social, physical, and affectional.[13] As Peters and Kaiser[12] point out, "there are often cases of long-lived friendships in which the friends actually think of one another as being like relatives and not just as friends."[12(p131)] Although much is yet to be learned about the role of friendship, neighboring, and confidant relationships in social support, research suggests that the role of friendship takes on added importance at certain times in the life course, appears to hold different meaning for women than for men throughout adult life, and may vary with different ethnic group conceptions of friendship.[12]

Once the family boundaries have been clarified, the task unfolds to describe its structure. This is frequently accomplished by using a tool called the family genogram. Its origins are found in the discipline of cultural anthropology, and it usually consists of a three-generational "picture" of a family depicting such things as sex, age, birth order, and lineage.[14] Other basic data can be added to depict such things as religious practices or hereditary conditions. When beginning to explore a family system with family members, the genogram is a "warming" mechanism. As an introductory strategy, it is a relatively noninvasive way to obtain a great deal of information quickly. It is also an activity where participation by family members is frequently enjoyed. Family members tend to ask questions of one another about their parents and grandparents, taking renewed interest in information that has been rediscovered. The structure is diagrammed according to a coded "legend." Such legends may also reveal the existence of family members who are currently absent from the household or those who are deceased but for whom a perceived "presence" is still maintained. The genogram activity is useful for providing insight into cultural factors, acknowledgment of unique family rituals, and family traditions that may be formalized through intergenerational transmission. Usually family members who helped construct the genogram value the experience enough to want a copy left with them.

Once the structural configuration of the family is outlined in genogram form, the developmental stage of the family can be observed and validated with family members. Family developmental theory would direct us to look at the progress of the oldest child or the activity of the breadwinner to discover the positioning of the family in the life cycle. However, in the application of these concepts to assessment and intervention, it is helpful to consider which stages may be occurring simultaneously. Very seldom, if ever, can families progress through the life cycle neatly, completing each task before proceeding to the next. It is important to consider with the family how many of the developmental stages have been successfully completed and for each stage which tasks are considered by the family to be accomplished.

The category "life events" encompasses an area that may not have been logically included in consideration of developmental stages but nevertheless may signify important turning points. One may refer to events that require family accommodation or adjustment, such as a move to a new home or a change in employment. The important feature to keep in mind is the view of family as a social system. General systems theory is based on the premise that all parts are interrelated and that anything affecting one component will influence the family as a whole due to the interdependent and dynamic nature of the system's structure. Therefore if one accepts systems theory, one may project that anything experienced as a significant life event to any one family member will, to some degree, be significant for the family as a whole. In practical terms, this gives us a perspective on the reality that in routine home-visit situations, even though not all family members are likely to be present, the impact of absent members can be felt.

Consideration of living environment and household constellation reminds one to consider the immediate physical environment of the family as it responds to the existing structural-functional configuration. As stated earlier, functional theory holds the family responsible for providing the physical necessities—space, safety, and comfort—for the survival and nurturance of its members. This leads us to assess the internal environment for its safety and support to family members of all ages, offering opportunity for immediate intervention if unsafe situations or conditions are recognized.

Neighborhood Environment

In seeking to work with families, it is important to appreciate the contextual data of the surrounding community. Attention should be given to sociologic features of human group life such as relative stability or transiency and gentrification or deterioration of neighborhoods. The degree of homogeneity, with regard to demographic data and trends toward integration, may give us a clearer picture of such features as ethnic enclaves and how these may serve to enrich or to complicate a sense of the common bond of community life. Especially important environmental factors are perceptions about access to essential services as access is experienced by representative groups such as the elderly.

Family Health: Family Perceived

A major philosophic and practical strength in the intervention guide has to do with the position of family partnership in the decision making regarding self-health priorities. Family perceptions of health are basic, along with professional judgments, to the exploration of any described behavior change in family members. Family strengths,[15] awareness of resources, and satisfaction with health behaviors are explored together with family members.

Social and Financial Resources

Familiarity with the resources available to the family, both material and human, is needed in conjunction with exploration of appropriate and realistic options for intervention. These are increasingly personal areas of data gathering; thus the interviewer would be well advised to review the reasons for requesting such information. For example, insight may be gained regarding the social system's openness to informational exchange. Family choices in the management of resources as they pertain to economic realities and leisure time will reveal the family power structure inherent in structural-functional theory, where role expectations are prescribed and interpreted with the goal of maintaining the unit.

Life Style

The area of life style encompasses decisions over which people have some control. Life-style choices are greatly affected by a family's values as well as by its access to resources.[16] Values expressed are largely determined by cultural background but are mediated by numerous other factors, hence the wide variation in values held among families sharing a common culture. The emphasis on internal dynamics of family life described within interactional theory describes shared meanings and how communication by and within families may be interpreted.[6] Where resources are considered finite, conflict theory focuses on social justice and human nature in its perpetual struggle to balance self-interest against the needs of others. Conflict theory is particularly useful in examining the sexual division of labor in the home and work place, analyzing family life based on social class interests and unequal gender-related access to limited resources.[9]

Priority Issues

Based on information gathered with the family, decisions can be made that incorporate both family and professional perception of need. It is important once again to compare and to contrast these perceptions, for this process may point to the criteria by which priority issues will be decided. For example, the potential for success of any identified goal will largely depend on such things as family commitment to behavior change, awareness of resources, or sources of power within the family. Key issues may be classified as long-term or short-term according to the estimated time frame of action. Some goals established may be amenable to immediate intervention, some may be beyond immediacy and may require consultation or referral, while others may be transferred completely to families within the self-care realm of responsibility.

The guide for family intervention was developed with nursing application as a frame of reference. It has also been tested since 1985 by senior baccalaureate nursing students. In the tradition of public health nursing that primarily serves disadvantaged populations, students have been working with client families who frequently make up vulnerable groups. Many of these are low-income, socially isolated, mentally confused, minority, functionally disabled, or elderly persons. In the authors' experience to date, these family assessment guidelines appear to accommodate culturally and socially diverse groups.

This family assessment perspective need not be restricted to nursing. It may well be that if a tradition of care is enriched by emphasizing mutuality with the family, this contribution could also extend to other professionals, such as social workers, clergy, and counselors/therapists, who strive for a family-based orientation.

REFERENCES

1. Friedman, M. *Family nursing: Theory and assessment*, ed 2. Norwalk, CT: Appleton-Century-Crofts, 1986.
2. Whall, A. The family as the unit of care in nursing: A historical review. *Public Health Nurs* 1986; 3(4):240–249.

3. Friedman, M. Keynote address. International Family Nursing Conference, Calgary, Alberta, Canada, May 25, 1988.

4. Dreher, M. The conflict of conservatism in public health nursing education. *Nurs Outlook* 1982; 30(9):504–509.

5. Levin, L. Patient education and self-care: How do they differ? *Nurs Outlook* 1978; 26(3):170–175.

6. Nye, F., & Berardo, F. (eds). *Emerging conceptual frameworks in family analysis.* New York: Praeger, 1981.

7. Duvall, E. *Marriage and family development.* Philadelphia: Lippincott, 1971.

8. Hazzard, M. An overview of systems theory. *Nurs Clin North Am* 1971; 6(3):385–393.

9. Burr, W., Hill, R., Nye, F., et al. *Contemporary theories about the family*, vol 2. New York: Free Press, 1979.

10. Glaser, B., & Strauss, A. *The discovery of grounded theory: Strategies for qualitative research.* Chicago: Aldine Publishing, 1973.

11. Tufte, V., & Myerhoff, B. (eds). *Changing images of the family.* New Haven, CT: Yale University Press, 1979.

12. Peters, G., & Kaiser, M. The role of friends and neighbors in providing social support, in Sauer, W., & Coward, R. (eds), *Social support networks and the care of the elderly.* New York: Springer, 1985.

13. Murray, R., & Zentner, J. *Nursing concepts for health promotion*, ed 2. Englewood Cliffs, NJ: Prentice Hall, 1979.

14. Starkey, P. Genograms: A guide to understanding one's own family system. *Perspect Psychiatr Care* 1981; 19(5&6):164–173.

15. Otto H. A framework for assessing family strengths. *Fam Proc* 1972; 2:329–339.

16. Steinman, M., Lapp, C., & Mowery, A. Community health nurses battle economic crunch by matching services to needs. *Nurs Health Care* 1985; 6(10):553–557.

CHAPTER 27

The Good Family
Syndrome

Harry J. Satariano, Nancy J. Briggs

Health professionals have tended to classify patients and their families into two
groups: The good families and the families in need of psychosocial evaluation and
intervention.

What is "good family syndrome"? Why are some families classified as "good
families"? How does a family acquire this title? Frequently medical professionals refer to
a patient's family as being a "good family." Yet there is no objective definition available.
However, the term is used formally during case conferences and informally in daily
report. Though screening tools exist for identifying families at high risk for discharge
planning issues, the families at low risk are simply identified as "good families" that
require minimal or no intervention. Often subjective data are used for assessment, and
discharge planning decisions are based upon the category in which the family is placed
by the medical professionals. Also the traditional medical model has reinforced the
attitude of: "The family that has a chronic or critically ill member is probably disfunc-
tional," but somehow a "good family" remains functional. Thus, the medical model
contributes to the myth of "good families." A theoretical reframing is needed to assess
healthy family functioning. Family Systems theory provides the explanation of how
medical professionals are contributing to the "good family" syndrome.

Family Systems is a theoretical framework for psycho-therapy and crisis intervention. It has the following premises: (a) no individual exists in a vacuum; (b) what has an

Reprinted from *Pediatric Nursing, Vol. 15* (No. 3), May/June 1989, pp. 285–286. Used with permission.

effect (result) upon one family member affects (influences) every other family member to a lesser or greater degree (this applies to members of a staff who oftentimes function as a family); and (c) while not all questions of why can be readily answered, it may help to focus upon *what* might help *and how* this might be accomplished.

Family Systems theory has been emerging in the United States mental health field for the past 40 years. In comparison to other medical specialties, it appears to be in its infancy. A major factor to consider is that the Family Systems theory is not a tool of psychoanalysis. In fact, Family Systems has a very different philosophical base in that it is not solely patient focused. Ostensibly, it doesn't readily fit the traditional medical model. Rather, Family Systems assesses strengths as well as concerns of the interactional patterns of a group of individuals. Accordingly, Family Systems is an integrated gestalt model, and is analogous to the view that a patient is more than the sum of his/her anatomical parts. Granted, Family Systems theory is subjective in how it is applied by the clinician. It can, however, provide an objective framework by which health professionals can measure their own biases about the families of their patients.

For instance, when a health professional refers to the behavior of a "good family," might it be inferred that the family handled the recent medical crisis in a manner similar to the way that the health professional would have personally handled the situation? Often a health professional apparently sets parameters by which to monitor a family's interaction or response on a spectrum. That is, the family is not involved enough, either physically or emotionally, and thus the family is dysfunctional. Or the health professional equates the family's degree of expression as appropriate and as "good family." How often has this description been used to cue a colleague? If the family, however, is too involved and asks for additional information, or questions medical procedures beyond the comfort level of the health professional, the family's behavior may be classified as inappropriate and dysfunctional. These parameters are interpreted at various times during critical or chronic care by the health professional as thin lines, lines that a family may inadvertently or blatantly step over. Given that this interpretation is partly human nature, consider that nursing policy can provide guidelines to incorporate Family Systems theory with the health professional's human response.

Many of us as health professionals base a patient's behavior and the behavior of the patient's family upon our own comfort zone of what constitutes appropriate interaction. This may work as long as health professionals are willing to be cognizant of their own biases. This necessitates that health professionals monitor their responses to the differences between how a patient's family and their own families digest information or react to crises.

Perhaps families are neither all good nor all bad. A family's behavior, according to Family Systems approach, is measured on a continuum. Psychosocial interaction at one end of the spectrum is referred to as enmeshed—each member of a group must adhere strictly to the rules and roles that are determined by the power brokers of that group. Consequently, all group members are required to view and interact in a prescribed manner in order to remain a group member in good standing.

Psycho-social interaction at the other extreme of the continuum, the flip side of enmeshment, appears as a behavioral pattern in which a person disengages or isolates self from any association to the prescribed norm. The middle range of this continuum is an ongoing balance of an individual's belief structure, wants, and needs in relation to what is in the best interest of the group's needs and wants.

Another significant element of Family Systems theory is the use of power in psycho-social issues. How power is viewed may determine the latitude to which a patient's family will adapt to parameters of acceptable family behavior established by the health professional. Accordingly, a family who perceives a staff as having power or control over the outcome of a family member's care may adapt to the health professional's definition of "good family." Therefore, good may become relative. Such relative goodness may be assumed to indicate quality of interaction between the health professional and the patient's family. Unfortunately, necessary adjustments in clarification of diagnosis and prognoses may be dispensed, and the health professional may assume a false-positive result.

Family Systems theory questions such blind spots. Is the good family holding up well under the medical crisis? Or is the family so worried about not rocking the boat because of feeling powerless? Regardless, perhaps the family blends into the staff's system of functioning so as not to jeopardize quality of care. How often is a family considered resourceful because one or more family members are also health professionals? Staff members may assume a family to have access to knowledge or an ability to cope with personal medical crisis; this in fact may foster these family members' misinformation, anxiety, and self-doubt.

Yes, interactional dynamics are complicated and perplexing. Responses to crises are not necessarily either black or white. Response may be a process of mixed messages, depending upon the communicators. Too often we as health professionals focus upon the *content* of critical information rather than upon the *process* of information, its impact, level of comprehension, and the degree of short- and long-term ramifications upon the family as well as the patient. Implementing a Family Systems focus may serve as a monitoring device to indicate critical levels of perception in relation to accurate data of what constitutes a "good family."

CHAPTER **28**

Families:
A Link or a Liability?

Barbara J. Kupferschmid, Tess L. Briones,
Carrie Dawson, Cheryl Drongowski

Hospitalization in a critical care setting has multiple effects on patients and their families. For patients, it can be a frightening and dehumanizing experience, while families are confronted with stressors that can disrupt normal family functioning. The nurse is the pivotal figure in the health care system who can positively affect family coping through the support offered. With family needs met, they are then strengthened and able to support their family member. This article examines the roles and relationships of families, social support systems, and nurses. Through the framework of social support, nurses provide emotional, instrumental, spiritual, and appraisal assistances to families. This can potentially positively affect the family's adaptation to a stressful situation, and thus the family's ability to provide support to the patient. A case study analysis is described to illustrate the interactions and interventions through a model of family support (KEYWORDS: families in critical care, social support, critical care nursing).

The event of hospitalization affects both the patient and the family. In addition to experiencing physiologic instability, a patient in a critical care setting also has the potential to be more frightened, lonely, confused, and in many ways, dehumanized than ever before. These effects might be minimized by incorporating family members into the patient's hospitalization experience. Facilitating family support can have a significant impact on the patients' ability to cope, their desire to recover, and even their physiologic state.[1] In actuality, inclusion of the family may help to rehumanize an environment that

Reprinted from *Critical Care Nurse, Vol. 2* (No. 2), May 1991, pp. 252–257. Used with permission.

has become increasingly technologically focused.[2] Many nurses intuitively recognize the essential role some families or social support systems play in the recovery of their ill or injured family member. A widely accepted role of social support systems has been to provide the buffer needed during times of stress. Locke further substantiates this intuition by suggesting that social support systems may actually have a mediating effect upon a patient's immune function, which can be depressed due to nutritional imbalances, stress, or surgery.[3] Consequently, the effect of the family or social support system may not be limited to just psychologic effects. Nursing practice's challenge then is to determine how to actually support the family during this stressful event, meeting their needs so that they in turn are strengthened and able to act as a positive link to the patient. Failure of the nurse to appropriately interact with family members could possibly have deleterious consequences such as heightened anxiety and fear in the family, misunderstanding, mistrust, hostility, and failure to obtain important information about the patient. The family may remain or become dysfunctional and might not regain the natural ability to help care for and support the hospitalized family member. If that occurs the family can actually become a liability requiring more nursing time, showing signs of being needy, and overall, not having a positive influence on the patient.

MODEL FOR IMPLEMENTATION

A model for family-directed nursing care includes several essential elements: nursing, families, and social support systems (Fig. 1). These elements working in synchrony to provide support can potentially affect the outcome of the individual patient's recovery and rehabilitation.[1] Each element will be defined and the role they play in affecting patient outcome will be described. This article will also discuss strategies nurses can incorporate in their practice to provide family support.

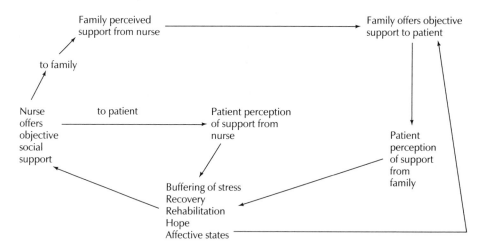

FIGURE 1. A model of family support.

Families

How does the family care for its members? Families have been defined as a human group with significant emotional bonds.[4] They demonstrate caring, commitment, loyalty, and responsibility through the relationships they establish with one another and the communication they engage in. An interdependence helps protect family members in times of stress, through the emotional buffering they provide.[4] Toffler proposes that families are the sanity-preserving constant in human existence, even though as a unit they are very much threatened by the industrialization of our technologic age.[5] If families in our society provide caring, buffer stress, and support their family members, how is that affected or changed in cases of the hospitalization of a family member? Speedling suggests that hospitalization causes an "abrupt rending of the family's social fabric."[6]

Further, he suggests that health care providers fail to incorporate the family members into the therapeutic process. In addition, Speedling observed that another form of family separation resulted from the unit's procedures that emphasized the "here and now."[6] One framework for assessing and intervening with families is proposed by Reutter, who suggests combining family systems theory with Orem's nursing theory.[7,8] Family and nursing theory together would provide a more inclusive and comprehensive framework than either theory individually.

From a systems perspective, the family is viewed as a system with structure and function. When combining Orem's theory with family systems theory, one function of the family member is to meet Orem's self-care requirements of air, food, water, elimination, rest, and activity.[8] A second component is the examination of the effect of both physical and social factors within the environment that can affect the health and health practices of families. Family structure is a third area in family systems theory.

Communication patterns among family members, role relationships, power structure, and value systems within the family are all areas of focus here. Another aspect of family function is its ability to adapt to change. Can the family unit change and grow while continuing as a stable unit? The final area relates to what the family perceives as its strengths and areas for further development.[7] Assessment questions and nursing interventions can be directed toward each of these categories.

Social Support System

Families are also a part of a much broader system, the social support system. Social support is an area that has been increasingly addressed in the literature. Cobb writes that a social support system provides information that leads an individual to believe he is cared for, loved, and valued, and belongs to a network of community obligations.[1] Kahn suggests that social support provides interpersonal transactions that include liking someone, affirming, or giving aid.[9] Still others claim that these systems are ties to other individuals, groups, and the community, each of whom might be accessible to provide support.[10] The role of the social support system is similar to that ascribed to families, that is, attachments among individuals that help improve their abilities to adapt to stress.[11]

The relationship of that network that involves giving and receiving and the relational structure through which assistance is requested and received in that network is called the social support system. Family and friends make up our social environment and their support can be crucial in buffering stress.[12]

Brandt and Weinert wrote that a central emerging theme of the social support system is an individual's "human climate," which plays a significant role in health maintenance and in response to life stressors.[13] A vital aspect of the human experience is a person's connection with or link to others. Families or other social support systems provide that link in the form of social support. The framework for social support was developed by House as a paradigm for stress research.[11] It provides a useful framework for understanding the relationships between social support and adjustment to illness. According to House, the relationship between objective stress and enduring health outcomes is mediated by several factors such as the characteristics of individuals or their social situation, individuals' perceptions of their situations, and the types of short-term responses individuals make to stressful events.[11] Stress occurs when the demands of the situation exceed the ability of people to handle certain events or when the demands are incongruent with individuals' social situations.[14]

Social support is viewed as a characteristic of the social situation that buffers the effect of stress on the health of the individual. Although the specific mechanism through which social support reduces stress is still under investigation, House postulated that social support buffers the effect of stress by enabling the individual to perceive an event as less stressful, facilitating the coping efforts of the individual, or lessening the degree of the individuals' reaction to the stressor.[11]

Social support is not a unitary concept but multidimensional. It can be in the forms of emotional, instrumental, informational, and appraisal assistance.[12] The quality and quantity of social support depend on the social network.

When considering how to actualize the provision of support, one must also consider several factors. First, who provides support and to whom is it given? According to the model illustrated in Figure 1, the nurse acting as a social support system provides support to the patient or, equally important, to the family. The family is then enabled to provide support to the patient. As illustrated, both the nurse and family can have an impact on patient recovery. This system, however, can also produce negative feedback. For example, if the family senses that the patient is depressed or not coping with his situation, this can send a message to the family that more support is necessary or that the support should be modified.

The next question for consideration is, exactly what is provided and how is it provided? Social support as described earlier can be in the forms of emotional, instrumental, informational, and appraisal assistance. Emotional support is described as behaviors that provide empathy, caring, love, and trust. Examples of emotionally supportive behaviors include listening, providing reassurance and encouragement, and providing accompaniment or companionship in a stressful situation.[12]

The second form of support is called instrumental, behaviors that provide tangible or material support or aid. Selected examples include providing suggestions and clarification, buffering the source of stress, and distracting from the problem focus.[15]

Informational support and appraisal assistance are the other two forms of support. Informational support is simply providing a person with information they can use in coping with personal and environmental problems. Reflecting an unconditional access to someone or a readiness to act on their behalf is an example of appraisal assistance.[15]

Another form of support identified frequently through family feedback is that of spiritual support.[12,15] This can be in the form of augmenting an individual's faith or relationship with God or providing them with ties to a pastor or clergy.

Nurses

Implicit in the definition of the social support system is the conclusion that groups other than families can function as a social support system. In case of hospitalization it is possible that nurses can become a social support system for the patient and especially for the family. Nurses are charged to work with the family to strengthen their capacity to care for their members.[16] Nurses reach out to families in their grief and times of emotional despair, share their joys and triumphs as well as their sorrow, and listen and answer their questions.[4] This occurs partly because nurses are available to families through the direct care they provide to patients.

Norbeck proposed that the concept of social support provides a meaningful framework for nursing, incorporating properties of the person as well as situational influences, and is particularly suited to assessment and interventions of families in critical care.[17] Nurses must acknowledge the potentially powerful impact of supportive resources on the family's adaptation to the stressful situation. This premise should underlie theoretical frameworks that enrich the nurses' understanding of the support phenomenon and should be implemented in nursing intervention strategies. According to Stewart, there are several reasons why social support is relevant to the nursing profession.[12] One of these reasons is that as the largest source of health service becoming more oriented to health promotion, nurses have the opportunity to impact health states. Also, in terms of looking at all aspects of patient care, using social support as well as psychosocial-physiologic knowledge can be beneficial, as "unmet needs for support increase human vulnerability to physical disease and prolong recovery from illness."[12] Lastly, nurses can use resources available to them to facilitate their patients' social support network (e.g., pastoral services, social work).

INTERACTIONS AND INTERVENTIONS

Much work has been reported in the literature regarding family needs and sources of stress during a critical illness. These needs have been documented as related to the need for information, emotional support, and proximity to the patient.[18,19] Unfortunately, there is a lack of documentation regarding the appropriateness of nursing interventions designed to meet those needs.[16] For that reason, this article will identify interventions derived from the social support framework using the case study. These interventions have been described in the literature in other contexts (e.g., pregnancy, chronic illness).

CASE STUDY

A 53-year-old male was transferred to the surgical intensive care unit (SICU) from another institution with a diagnosis of pancreatitis. He had been hospitalized for two weeks in a previous institution. His wife described him to be in good health since he had no significant medical problems and had never been hospitalized before. Family and social history revealed that the patient was a university professor with two children in their 20s. He was overweight but denied tobacco use and was described as an occasional social drinker. Within 24 hours after admission to the SICU, he developed respiratory failure, which necessitated mechanical ventilation. He was brought to surgery the next day for partial pancreatectomy secondary to necrotizing pancreatitis. A cholecystectomy was also done and gastrostomy and jejunostomy tubes were inserted. His abdominal wound was left open and packed with sterile dressing. After the first surgery, the patient had multiple trips to surgery for wound debridements and tracheostomy tube placement. Neuromuscular blocking agents such as Pavulon were used to prevent evisceration of abdominal organs, since the wound was left open. During the course of his hospitalization, he developed sepsis and required vasoactive agents for blood pressure support. He also developed acute renal failure and required continuous arteriovenous hemofiltration with dialysis. After the first month of hospitalization, the patient's mental status deteriorated and never improved.

In planning his care, the primary nurse identified the needs of the family and made every effort to meet those needs. Among the identified needs were education and information regarding the patient's illness and hope and religious support.

The plan of care devised by the primary nurse for both the patient and the family was communicated appropriately to the associate nurses to ensure that consistent care was provided. After three months of minimal response to aggressive therapy, a family conference was held to discuss the boundaries of therapy for this patient. A consensus was then reached by the family and the medical staff to withdraw the treatments and make the patient as comfortable as possible. The patient died 48 hours after withdrawing treatment.

Analysis

There is general agreement that social support moderates stress. In the above case study, the nurse first identified the family's social network through the multifaceted analysis that takes into account the structural features of the network, the dynamic features of the relationships, the significant life events affecting the network, and the coping and problem-solving style of the network. This family's social network consisted of the wife, the two children, the wife's sister, and the hospital's chaplain. The dynamic features of the relationships of this family's network are positive, as observed by the primary nurse through frequent contacts with the social network. The influence of significant life events, in this case the hospitalization, seriously disrupted the existing social network of this family. The only consistent support the wife had was the sister and the hospital chaplain because both sons were attending school several miles away from home. Coping behaviors significantly affect the extent of involvement in the network. In this family the coping behavior exhibited was a constant vigil, especially by the wife, at the patient's bedside.

After the family's social support was identified, the nurse helped mobilize support by working with the social network. This was accomplished by reassuring them that they were being helpful, providing them chances to discuss their issues and concerns, facilitating communication among the group, and supporting their efforts to help in the daily care of the patient.

The primary nurse in this case also showed sensitivity to both the strengths and limitations of the network. The nurse recognized that the social network was unable to provide all types of help needed. To ensure that the family received optimal support, the nurse designed the nursing interventions using social support both at the individual level and the dyadic level.[16] On an individual level, the nurse provided emotional, instrumental, and informational support.

The emotional form of support given by the nurse consisted of exhibiting a caring behavior, showing empathy, listening, and providing companionship to the wife in the last few hours before the patient died. The form of instrumental support given by the nurse in this case was to be easily accessible when the family had concerns about medical care. Informational support was given by continuously updating the family with the patient's condition during weekly family conferences with the physicians.

On a dyadic level, the nurse introduced a layperson, which in this case is the hospital chaplain. On this level, support was also provided through the weekly family support sessions conducted in the critical care area.

There are many approaches to assessing and mobilizing social support. The interventions identified in this case were very helpful, as evidenced by the feedback received from the family a month after the patient died. Because a multitude of factors are responsible for the richness and paucity of a family's social support system, it is important to individualize each patient/family system and each situation.

CONCLUSION

In an age when technology abounds in the critical care environment and the focus is on the physiologic condition of the patient, nurses need to realize that the family, the basic unit of society, is also their responsibility. Critical care nurses need to demonstrate a warm, supportive, confident, and competent approach toward the family. Inclusion of the patient's family as recipients of care is not only within the scope of nursing practice but is the expectation for which the nurse is accountable. Nurses need to identify the extent of the family's social support, supplement the support systems for those at risk, and take an active role in providing it. Facilitating family support will potentially strengthen the family in their coping abilities. The family will then be able to demonstrate their support to the patient in his recovery.

REFERENCES

1. Cobb, S. Social support as a moderation of life stress. *Psychosom Med* 1976; 38(5):301–313.
2. Naisbett, J. *Megatrends—Ten new directions transforming our lives.* New York: Warner Books, 1982.

3. Locke, S. Stress, adaptation, and immunity: Studies in humans. *Gen Hosp Psychiatry* 1982; 4(1):49–58.
4. Leavitt, M. *Families at risk: Primary prevention in nursing.* Boston: Little, Brown, 1982.
5. Toffler, A. *Future shock.* New York: Random House, 1970: 258.
6. Speedling, E.J. Social structure and social behavior in an intensive care unit. Patient-family perspective. *Soc Work Health Care* 1980; 6:1–15.
7. Reutter, L. Family health assessment: An integrated approach. *J Adv Nurs* 1984; 9:391–399.
8. Orem, D. *Nursing: Concepts of practice.* Boston: Little, Brown, 1980.
9. Kahn, R. Aging and social support. In Riley, M. ed., *Aging—from birth to death: Interdisciplinary perspectives.* CO: Westview Press, 1979: 77–91.
10. Lin, N., Ensel, W., Simeone, R., & Kuo, W. Social support stressful life events, and illness: A model and empirical test. *J Health Soc Behav* 1979; 20:118–119.
11. House, J. *Work stress and social support.* Reading, MA: Addison-Wesley, 1985.
12. Stewart, M. Social support instruments created by nurse investigators. *Nurs Res* 1989; 38:268–275.
13. Brandt, P., & Weinert, C. Measuring social support with the PRQ. *West J Nurs Res* 1987; 9:589–602.
14. Baille, V., Norbeck, J., & Barnes, L. Stress, social support, and psychological distress of family caregivers of the elderly. *Nurs Res* 1988; 37:217–222.
15. McNett, S. Social support, threat and coping responses and effectiveness in the functionally disabled. *Nurs Res* 1987; 36:98–105.
16. Stewart, M. Social support intervention studies: A review and prospectus of nursing contributions. *Int J Nurs Stud* 1989; 26:93–114.
17. Norbeck, J. Social support. *Annu Rev Nurs Res* 1988; 6:85–109.
18. Molter, N. Needs of relatives of critically ill patients: A descriptive study. *Heart Lung* 1979; 8(2):332–339.
19. Leske, J. Needs of relatives of critically ill patients. *Heart Lung* 1986; 15(2):189–193.

CHAPTER 29

Health Promotion: The Influence of Pets on Life Patterns in the Home

Marlene M. Rosenkoetter

The importance of pets in people's lives has become more widely recognized and the literature has increased considerably over the last several years.[1] Although scientific research is yet insufficient, there is growing evidence to indicate that pets can significantly alter life patterns, emotional and physical responses, and social well-being. Furthermore, the impact of pets is not age-contingent. Boris Levinson,[2] one of the foremost authorities on the subject, has for some time demonstrated that pets can be used in the treatment of childhood behavior disorders, while others have indicated the therapeutic use of pets with the elderly. "For the elderly person who lives alone and is no longer a working and active member of the community, the world can seem a bleak place indeed. An animal friend, however, can do much to provide companionship, love, affection, and a sense of being needed."[3(p176)] Since a pet may act as a source of "constant support [and provide] unconditional joy and warmth"[2(p697)] it may be a supportive adjunct in therapeutic interventions. The pet allows the person to project feelings onto something external without having to interact with another person. Language is reduced to a minimum, and the present and future are emphasized rather than the past.[2]

THE BENEFITS OF PETS

Brickel indicates that "significant emotional needs are satisfied when a pet is felt to be a friend and partner. A pet can also enrich feelings of self-esteem, and act as facilitator

Reprinted from *Holistic Nursing Practice,* Vol. 5, No. 2, pp. 42–51, with permission of Aspen Publishers, Inc., © 1991.

and catalyst for interpersonal relationships."[4(p121)] The pet is not only something to talk *to*, but to talk *about*. Sharing stories about the family cat or dog can spark meaningful conversations, even among strangers. It is a safe, nonthreatening, neutral topic or discussion and one with which nearly everyone can relate. By sharing one's feelings with a pet, a person may be able to cope more effectively with emotional pain and distress. This is particularly evident in the elderly when dealing with the death of a spouse or other loved one. The older person continues to feel important and needed, and the animal "serves a role in preventing social withdrawal and alienating."[4(p122)]

Friedman and colleagues[5] found in a study of patients who had been hospitalized with coronary heart disease that a significantly larger number of the survivors after 1 year were pet owners than were those who did not survive. Pet ownership correlated significantly with survival rate. A variety of reasons have since been suggested for this apparent relationship, including the responsibility of caring for the pet resulting in higher sustained activity levels for the owner. In a study by Corson at Ohio State University, it was found that when pets were used to treat patients who had not responded well to more traditional approaches, there was "improvement in terms of responsiveness, communication, apparent increased self-respect, and independence."[6(p138)] The pet becomes a focus for attention—an accepting, receptive, willing listener.

Pets also facilitate learning. The person learns what to expect from the pet and the pet learns the same in return. More specifically, children and older persons can profit significantly from learning about their pets and pet care. This enhances an understanding of the world for the child and promotes lifelong learning for the older adult. When one observes exchanges between a pet and owner, a number of interactive behaviors may be evident. As a result, the pet becomes a window for insight into the inner feelings and needs of the person. In times of stress, the pet and owner may even share such behaviors as anxiety, malaise, and irritability. These behaviors can be indicators of distress or problems that need further assessment, not only by the nurse, but by the attending physician and even a veterinarian. The nurse may indeed be placed in the position of needing to refer the pet for health care services.

In an article titled "Down on the Farm," Davis[7] reported that a British Children's Aid Team introduced mentally handicapped children to pets and livestock. As a result, the children watched and learned about growth, death, mother's love, and friendship. They learned responsibility from providing care for the animals. Simply by being around animals as they are born, develop, and die, a child experiences the phenomena of growth, separation, and loss, which are a part of life. Animals are also often valued as members of the family. "A pet that provides companionship, safety, a daily routine, and comfort for its owner becomes an integral part of that owner's life."[8(p499)] In home care, the friendship and attention of "furry and feathered friends" have demonstrated that they not only provide someone for the person to care for, but can decrease loneliness while providing security.[9] With sick children, pets can facilitate the therapeutic process between the patient and the nurse.[10] The nurse can learn a great deal about a child's fears, dreams, and thoughts by listening to what is said to and about the pet.

"The introduction of pets into either a long-term care facility, or private home can provide the elderly with continual warmth, companionship, sense of purpose, and the realization of successful accomplishment."[11(p35)] The pet can furnish an incentive to recovery. The animal needs care, the person responds positively to being needed; some structure is added to a life lacking routines. The patient remembers to take an early morning medication at the time the dog goes out,[12] or agrees to have dinner when the cat does. Pets can foster physiologic changes and even significantly alter vital sign readings, including blood pressure.[13] In visits to terminal cancer patients, animals actually lessened feelings of anxiety and despair and assisted the patients in moving through the stages of dying.[14] People no longer felt alone, and as they cared for the animals, they cared for themselves.

According to Beck and Katcher,[15] pets can foster a number of healthful components in a person's life. They

- provide companionship,
- give us something to care for,
- provide pleasurable activity,
- are a source of constancy,
- make us feel safe,
- return us to play and laughter,
- are a stimulus to exercise,
- comfort with touch, and
- are pleasurable to watch.

Pet psychotherapy, or animal-facilitated therapy, has demonstrated remarkable results in changing behavior patterns of a variety of persons including the criminally insane, alcoholics, the elderly, cardiac patients, disturbed children, blind persons, and the mentally disabled.[16] Animals have been found to be helpful for a successful adjustment to retirement. Recently, the Ralston Purina Company began advertising a new program entitled Pets for People, through which they will sponsor matching a pet with a person who is 60 years of age or older and provide initial veterinary expenses as well as some of the other essentials.

Millions of people have companion animals or pets in their homes and consider them integral components of their daily lives. Including the family pet as part of the family health history and assessment is an important part of nursing care that has frequently been overlooked but is essential to the understanding of the complete family system.

PETS, VALUES, AND LIFE PATTERNS— VARIABLES AND APPLICATIONS

When examining the relationship of pets and family members, six areas can be used as a framework for assessing health promotion factors: roles, relationships, self-esteem, use of time, support groups, and life structure.[17] These are used to focus the nursing assessment and facilitate a systematic approach to understanding the pet within a family system. All of these areas are interdependent, dynamic, and influenced by both individual and family expectations as well as sociocultural values.

Roles

At a given moment, each individual has a number of simultaneous roles, but when a pet enters the person's system, there are frequently changes in these roles. The *provider* becomes the caregiver, disciplinarian, surrogate parent, and even exerciser. The individual assumes the responsibility for the nurturing of this creature from the bird or animal world, with or without previous knowledge.

The child learn new roles, while the elderly person may reengage in previous ones. The young person, for example, may have the responsibility for feeding or brushing the family dog and assume the role of caregiver. Children learn about birth and mothering when Tabby has kittens and about the role of a support person when Whiskers dies. The grandfather who now lives alone becomes the sole provider for his pet and once again experiences the role of nurturer.

Pets may be in abusive homes in which not only people but animals are placed in jeopardy. In assessment of the person or family in the home setting, an animal can provide clues to the health of the system, and the nurse needs to be sensitive to these clues. An abused or neglected pet may be evidence of other forms of abuse in the same household (see the box, "Guidelines for Assessment of Roles").

In addition, if problems are noted with individual or family roles and no pet is in the home, would pet placement be an effective intervention to pursue? The type and purpose of the pet need to be thoroughly explored with the client and family members.

GUIDELINES FOR ASSESSMENT OF ROLES

1. Is the pet well fed, clean, and cared for? Is there a relationship between the health of the pet and the health of the individual or family? A well-fed animal and an emaciated elderly woman may suggest that the animal is getting most of the available food. Lack of cleanliness suggests the need for health care teaching.
2. Is there evidence of abuse? Abuse of a pet may indicate that a more in-depth assessment is warranted.
3. Is the pet exercised? If not, this may provide a mechanism to introduce exercise for members of the family. Walking the dog twice a day provides exercise not only for the animal, but for the owner.
4. Does the pet demonstrate poor health? This may suggest the need for health care teaching, including the care of the pet, or referral to other social agencies.
5. Does the pet appear abnormally active or sedentary? Changes in behavior patterns can provide clues to feelings and problems within the family.
6. What clues exist regarding self-care? Is there a relationship between care for the animal and self-care of the client? This may indicate neglect of the client or pet.

Relationships

A pet introduces an additional member to an individual's or family's relationships. The pet becomes a source for caring, affection, humor, companionship, and comfort. It can foster an increased sense of security and an escape from feelings of loneliness. Pets can be calming or exciting, something to caress, and someone to communicate with daily, a willing listener. Fears of being alone are reduced and there is a focus for social interactions. Children fantasize about their pets and play imaginary games with them. Older people talk with pets about new ideas and plans, while nearly every age group is known to "tell them their troubles." Family members share their grief with one another when the pet dies. Many people feel the grief of a deceased pet as strongly as that of a beloved family member. As with any open system, a change in one of the members creates changes throughout the system.

The family pet can fill in for infrequent visits from the children and the inability to get out of the house to see friends and acquaintances. It becomes a topic for conversation and for letters to relatives. It can help to fill the void left by a deceased loved one and even be a link with past friends and family members. A pet helps a person to focus on the present by being a constant reminder of daily activities and needs. With this type of bonding, an animal indeed becomes a member of the family, one which is frequently trusted, cared for, and worried about just like a human being. Consequently, the loss of a pet can create a major emotional crisis that needs direct attention.

A number of animals can now be trained to give special assistance to their masters. Not only are dogs and monkeys available to help the blind, but they can aid the hearing and physically impaired as well. These animals become considerably more than family pets and are trained to fulfill designated services.

Pets can be destructive and, although it is unusual, can inflict harm on their owners or others. Some people are allergic to animals or birds, and this presents health problems. Other people do not like or are afraid of animals and yet are placed in situations where they must be confronted with them daily. This can interfere with what could otherwise be effective relationships in a given home. Likewise, the nurse who has any of these reactions needs to consider them when making home visits, and realize how such reactions are likely to influence assessments and interactions with clients. Parents are sometimes afraid that a small child will injure a pet, that the pet could harm the child, or that the pet will consume too much time or money and be messy. Older persons occasionally fear that they will fall over an animal or will be unable to care for it. Obviously, not everyone wants or should have a pet, and pets are not the miracle solution to relationship problems; however, for many people pets become the most important significant others in their lives (see the box, "Guidelines for Assessment of Relationships").

If there is no pet in the home and the nursing assessment suggests that the person is lonely, needs something to care for, or is looking for this type of relationship, then it may be worthwhile to pursue the feasibility of and interest in pet placement.

GUIDELINES FOR ASSESSMENT OF RELATIONSHIPS

1. What relationships exist between the person or family and pet? How are these healthy or maladaptive? These relationships can provide information on loneliness, lack of security, grieving, alienation, and other feelings that need attention.
2. Does the relationship between the owner and pet suggest that there is a lack of interaction with other people? The pet may be the primary or only source of consistent contact with another being, suggesting that additional alternatives may need to be pursued, if available.
3. If a pet is the primary source for a meaningful relationship, is it working or are needs still unmet? For example, is the person still fearful or feeling alone? If so, are there other means which can be pursued to meet the person's needs?
4. What is the history of relationships with pets? Previous experience may influence present situations and factors.

Self-Esteem

People need to be needed and to feel good about themselves. A person's self-esteem can be directly influenced by owning and nurturing a pet. Pets not only foster a sense of responsibility and are a source for interactions, but they are an excellent opportunity for caring. Because the pet is unable to take care of its own basic needs, a person is needed to fulfill the role of provider. Mutual caring and affection foster a healthy interactional bond. Training focuses on the skills of the owner as a teacher.

A playful kitten is entertaining and a new puppy can be an important distraction from pain and emotional distress. The song of a bird brings cheer to the morning after a lonely night. A guinea pig's squeak can make a small child laugh. Pets foster positive feelings while giving the person an opportunity to be needed. They are accepting of others, no matter what the ailments. A dog does not care if his owner has arthritis, is in a wheelchair, or is dying from an incurable disease. He is there to love, protect, and comfort. People with speech difficulties may feel less embarrassed trying out new sounds and phrases on the family pet than they would by risking humiliation from family members, friends, and even nurses.

People give human qualities to animals, even though they are sometimes embarrassed to acknowledge it. The dog is named Robin or Charlie, and the cat is Sissy or Morris. Muffin sleeps on Jeff's bed at night and Britches gets a hamburger for dinner just like everyone else. Adults frequently talk to their pets as though they are human beings who understand every word. And indeed, at times they listen as though they do! Communication is an important part of the bond between "pet and master," as well as a strong indicator of the impact of the animal on the person's self-esteem (see the box, "Guidelines for Assessment of Self Esteem").

GUIDELINES FOR ASSESSMENT OF SELF-ESTEEM

1. What behaviors exist that suggest the lack of a positive self-esteem? If a pet does not exist, could feelings of self-worth be fostered by having one?
2. What bonding is evident between the client and the pet? Can this be facilitated for a more positive self-esteem? Does the pet, for example, require some special care or feeding that the client could take care of, which would increase feelings of being needed and useful?
3. Where does the pet eat and sleep? What information does this convey about the importance of the pet in this home? There is considerable difference in the human characteristics accorded to the dog who sleeps on the foot of the bed and the one who stays in a house outdoors.
4. What type of communication and affection is displayed between the pet and owner? This may offer insight regarding the person's self-esteem and related needs.

Use of Time

There are two different types of activities for the use of time, meaningful and recreational. Meaningful activities add to one's sense of usefulness and to a positive self-esteem. Recreational activities focus on pleasure and escapism; they may not be at all emotionally useful. How people use their time is an important aspect of health adjustments, especially in such critical developmental stages as older adulthood.[17] Playing golf every day does not necessarily result in a positive contribution to self or society.

Each person has the same amount of time available during a given day, but how it is used varies considerably from one to another and sometimes from one day to the next. For the person who is alone, ill, frightened, or under stress, time can seem considerably longer than it would otherwise. Animals can be a distraction and even a reminder of the time of day and the passing of time. They require care and exercise; they need to be fed; they need to go outside, and some even need medication.

Having an animal in the house provides for a concrete use of time, time that "someone" else needs. It fosters a sense of belonging and usefulness for the older client and suggests productive ways that a child or even an adult can spend time. Care of a pet becomes a "forced activity" for many people in that the bird or animal requires attention and the person feels obliged to provide it. This means the individual *must* get out of bed in the morning, take the dog for a walk, feed the cat, or clean the fish tank. This may be the only impetus for activity in the day, yet it encourages the use of time in a constructive manner. There needs to be time to play with a pet and talk to it about everything that is (or is not) going on. An animal can become a time-consuming activity when there is little else to do or little else that a person is able to do. A "lap pet" can convey such a sense of oneness with his master as to imply that the primary purpose of his master's time and virtual existence is to hold, caress, and love him (see the box, "Guidelines for Assessment of Use of Time").

Support Systems

During the various stages of development throughout life, people have different types of support systems. As children, they derive support from parents and other family members; later they may change to peers, friends, and colleagues. The intent of a support system is to listen and be a caring advocate. Many people, however, have lost their support systems, through death of a spouse or family members, relocation, illness, financial problems, retirement, and even by choice. Animals can serve to fill some of these gaps by being attentive, protective, loving, and nonjudgmental. Animals listen, cuddle, and in effect say, "You're not alone. You have me and I care."

The sick child will often talk freely about an illness or problem to a stuffed teddy bear or rabbit without fear of rejection or harm. A family in crisis will look to the pet dog for constancy and affection. "Well, at least Chipper is still the same." A young college student returns at spring break only to find that old friends no longer have anything in common, but Smokey, the family cat, soothes and reassures her as he climbs into her lap. The widower comes home to an empty house at night but is not alone, because Misty always greets him at the door. Support systems are an important part of many people's lives and when they are missing or inadequate a pet may be able to offer stability and a healthy, caring relationship (see the box, "Guidelines for Assessment of Support Systems").

Life Structure

Throughout life, structure is imposed by both other people and agencies, structure over which the individual person has little control. Parents make decisions for their children, schools determine when students attend classes, and employers decide work schedules. Although there is personal input, there is a considerable degree of external control. When situations change and this life structure is removed, especially with illness and aging, people have new challenges. Depressed, lonely, and elderly people,

---

GUIDELINES FOR ASSESSMENT OF USE OF TIME

1. How does the client spend time each day? Does or could time devoted to a pet foster more meaningful use of time?
2. Does the pet have special needs that one person could perform to help use time and feel needed?
3. Who is the primary person who cares for the pet? Would it be helpful for another member to assume this role?
4. Is the primary care provider able to respond to the care that is needed or does assistance need to be sought?
5. Do both the owner and pet need an exercise routine which they can do together?
6. Is there a schedule for daily activities? Is one needed?

**GUIDELINES FOR ASSESSMENT
OF SUPPORT SYSTEMS**

1. What type of support systems are being used by the client or family? If a support system is available, does the client indicate that it is effective? There may be no support system.
2. What recent events may be indicative that a support system is needed?
3. Is a pet available for support? If not, would facilitating pet placement be an option to pursue with the client?

---

for example, can find it more and more difficult to get out of bed and engage in something productive, to manage activities of daily living, or follow a routine that injects some sense of normalcy into life. Pets can change this loss of life structure, making it more acceptable to the client and helping him or her to feel more useful.

Dogs and cats get up in the morning and want to be fed. This means the owner also needs to get out of bed. Activity is injected into a person's life by virtue of the existence of the pet. Pets need to be walked, played with, brushed, and given attention. This increases mobility in an otherwise inactive person. Walking means exercise and brushing the dog moves a partially paralyzed arm or an arthritic hand.

While taking care of the pet, there is a not so subtle reminder to take care of oneself. Getting-up and feeding activities encourage reality orientation. "Heidi wants out. It must be 6 o'clock." Increased mobility can likewise promote an increased attention to daily necessities such as bathing and household chores. It is essential to remember, however, that if the client is away from the home, through hospitalization or some other unforeseen event, it may be the care of the pet at home that is of more concern than anything else. Concern for the animal may actually be a complicating factor in the person's illness. The owner may worry about the pet much like a much loved family member in distress, even to the point of interfering with his or her own care (see the box, "Guidelines for Assessment of Life Structure").

**GUIDELINES FOR ASSESSMENT
OF LIFE STRUCTURE**

1. What type of life structure does the client have established? Lack of any routine may suggest the need to look for signs of loneliness, depression, or physical impairments.
2. How does the client (or family) describe a normal day, week, month? What kind of affect does the person show when describing these?
3. If a pet is present, how does the pet fit into this life structure?
4. What types of activities seem neglected?

• • •

A necessary component of assessing any client or family system environment is to determine whether there is a family pet and how this pet influences life patterns. People incorporate animals into their personal systems, many times giving them humanlike qualities and showing concern as they would for a human family member. The pet can provide insight into the functioning of the remainder of the system and make alternatives available for care that might otherwise be overlooked or avoided. A systematic history and assessment may suggest that pet placement could be an effective intervention to explore in order to promote healthy life patterns.

REFERENCES

1. Allen, K. *The human animal bond—An annotated bibliography.* Metuchen, NJ: Scarecrow Press, 1985.
2. Levinson, B. Pet psychotherapy: Use of household pets in the treatment of behavior disorders in childhood. *Psychological Reports.* 1965; 17:695-698.
3. Cusack, O., & Smith, E. *Pets and the elderly—The therapeutic bond.* New York, NY: Haworth press; 1984.
4. Brickel, C. A review of the roles of pet animals in psychotherapy and with the elderly. *International Journal of Aging and Human Development.* 1980-1981; 12(2):119-128.
5. Friedmann, E., Katcher, A., Lynch, J., & Thomas, S. Animal companions and one-year survival of patients after discharge from a coronary care unit. *Public Health Reports.* 1980; 95(4):307-312.
6. Patient progressing well? He may have a pet. *Journal of the American Medical Association.* 1979; 241(5):438. JAMA Medical News.
7. Davis, L. Down on the farm. *Nursing Times.* 1986; 82(48):40.
8. Davis, J., & Juhasz, A. The human/companion animal bond: How nurses can use this therapeutic resource. *Nursing and Health Care.* 1984; 5(9):497-501.
9. Dolan, M. Home Rx—Wet nose, soft fur, wagging tail. *Nursing 82.* 1982; 12(10):112.
10. Davis, J. Children and pets: A therapeutic connection. *Pediatric Nursing.* 1985; 11(5):377-379.
11. Twiname, B. Having difficulty meeting your rehabilitation goals? Consider pet therapy? *Rehabilitation Nursing.* 1984; 9(6):34-35.
12. Preshlock, K. Brandy: An incentive to recovery. *Home Healthcare Nurse.* 1985; 3(6):16-17.
13. Baun, M., Bergstrom, N., Langston, N., & Thoma, L. Physiological effects of human/companion animal bonding. *Nursing Research.* 1984; 33(3):126-129.
14. Muschel, I. Pet therapy with terminal cancer patients. *Social Casework.* 1984; 65(8):451-458.
15. Beck, A., Katcher, A. *Between pets and people—The importance of animal companionship.* New York, NY: Putnam; 1983.
16. Serpell, J. Pet psychotherapy. *People-Animals-Environment.* 1983; 1(1):7.
17. Rosenkoetter, M. Is your client ready for a role change after retirement? *Journal of Gerontological Nursing.* 1985; 11(9):21-24.

CHAPTER 30

Comprehensive Assessment of Families of the Critically Ill

Debra J. Lynn-McHale, Ann Smith

The family enters the critical care unit under a significant amount of stress with many diverse and complex needs. During this crisis period, dysfunctional behavior may lead to ineffective coping. This article will present a comprehensive family assessment tool based on Myra Levine's Principles of Conservation. The assessment tool not only will enhance the comprehensiveness of patient and family care, but will provide a method for reassuring families that they are part of their relatives' care and recovery. This tool will also enable the critical care nurse to individually assess and meet the holistic needs of families (KEYWORDS: family, conservation of energy, structural integrity, personal integrity, social integrity, family assessment tool).

Patients are admitted to critical care units at very high acuity levels. Critical care nurses are faced daily with the challenge of meeting the increasingly complex needs of the critically ill patient.

The family enters the critical care unit under a great deal of stress. They are confronted with the fact that their family member is critically ill. They may be uncertain of the patient's condition and prognosis. They may quickly be requested to make important decisions that may affect their family member's outcome. Critical care nurses are in the vital position not only to meet the complex needs of their patients, but also to address the diverse and complex needs of families.

Reprinted from *Critical Care Nurse, Vol. 2* (No. 2), May 1991, pp. 195–209. Used with permission.

FAMILY

Illness in a family member is disruptive not only for the person who is ill, but also for the family as a whole.[1] If family are going to be assisted in coping with the patient's critical illness, it is essential that family are identified, needs assessed, and strategies developed to meet family needs. Often, family is defined as the immediate relatives of an individual. For some patients, this may be true, but often, it is not. Additional consideration needs to be given to non-traditional families. Who do single parents, separated spouses, and the homeless consider their families? Dunkel and Eisendarth define family as anyone related, by birth or not, who is significant to the patient.[2] If the nuclear family alone is used to define family, several significant individuals may not be assessed and included in patient and family care.

Today's society is highly mobile. Extended families no longer live in proximity. Because of this, when an illness occurs, turning to immediate family who live hundreds of miles away may be unrealistic. Additional support systems may be more crucial to the critically ill patient than immediate family.

Who are these support systems? What benefit can they provide to the critically ill patient? What are their needs? How should the critical care nurse assess their needs? How can their needs be adequately met? This article will address these questions.

LITERATURE REVIEW

Numerous studies have been completed regarding families of critically ill patients. The studies clearly demonstrate that families of critically ill patients experience varied stressors and have multiple needs. In an effort to facilitate family functioning, promote family coping, and assist family need satisfaction, it is essential that family stressors and needs be identified. Strategies can then be developed to meet family needs.

Stressors identified by Hodovinic et al. include role changes, isolation from other family members, fear of loss of their loved one, financial concerns, transportation problems to and from the hospital, and heightened emotional turmoil while the family member was hospitalized.[3] Bedsworth and Molen found the greatest stressors reported by spouses of patients having myocardial infarctions were loss of mate, loss of healthy mate, and recurrence of myocardial infarction.[4] It was also found that anxiety and fear were the dominant emotions associated with these stressors. In another study, Potter found that lack of privacy in the critical care unit and inability to perform useful tasks for the critically ill patient were stressful for family.[5]

Several studies have identified needs of families of critically ill patients.[6-11] Family needs can be subdivided into six categories: information, visitation, psychologic aspects significant to the family, institutional support services, personal support services, and environment.

One of the greatest needs identified for families of critically ill patients is the need for information. This includes the need for information about the patient's condition, for explanations family can understand, to be able to talk to the physician daily, and to be called regarding changes in the condition of the patient. Family concerns regarding visitation center around frequency of visits, flexibility of visiting hours, and participation in physical care. Psychologic aspects significant to the family were identified as feeling there is hope, knowing hospital personnel care about the patient, and feeling assured that the patient is receiving the best care possible.

The fourth and fifth categories are institutional support services and personal support services. Family needs identified as important institutional support services include being told about people in the hospital who could help with specific family concerns and being told about available religious services. Personal support system needs identified were receiving friends' support and having another person present when visiting the patient.

The last category of family needs identified in the research addressed environmental needs. These needs included a waiting room near the patient, a bathroom near the waiting room, and a place in the hospital to be alone.

Additional studies have been completed that address family need satisfaction. Dracup and Breu found that when specific nursing interventions were used, families' needs were more consistently and completely met.[12]

Molter found that only four out of 45 needs perceived as important or very important were met less than 50% of the time.[6] These needs were to talk to the physician daily, be told about chaplain services, have a place to be alone, and have someone help with financial problems.

In another study, Rodgers found that 40 out of 46 needs were met for at least 60% of families who perceived them as important.[7] The five needs least satisfied were to be alone, have a bathroom near the waiting room, provide some of the physical care, and talk to the physician daily.

Lynn-McHale and Bellinger found that families' needs were satisfied for 43 out of 46 needs.[11] Those with lower satisfaction levels were to be encouraged to cry, be told about religious services, and be told about hospital services available to help with family problems. The majority of family needs were met by critical care nurses.[6,8,13]

The above studies have expanded our knowledge regarding family stressors and needs. Understanding family needs will assist critical care nurses in planning to meet family needs. It is essential to realize that individualized differences in family stressors and needs can and often do exist. Because of this, it is important that we have a system in place to assess family needs. Unique family needs and concerns can be addressed and intervention strategies can be identified and developed by critical care nurses.

BENEFITS OF FAMILY INVOLVEMENT

Families can be a valuable asset to critical care nurses, physicians, and most importantly, the patient. Many times, the family is the only source of information regarding the patient's past medical history, illnesses, current medications, and level of functioning prehospitalization.

The family can also greatly influence a patient's recovery. The critically ill patient has entered a new and often frightening environment. The patient is cared for by many unfamiliar health team members in a room filled with highly technologic equipment with myriad alarms and mysterious noises. Often, just being able to see their family and hold their hands provides a link to what was normal and can give the patient enormous comfort and support.

If family needs are not identified and met during this period, family anxiety may increase. Families may then place greater demands on critical care nurses, heighten the patient's anxiety, and contribute little to the patient's care and recovery.

A family assessment tool can greatly assist the critical care nurse. Completing the tool together presents the family and the critical care nurse an opportunity to get to know each other. The assessment data will provide the critical care nurse with information about family functioning, weaknesses, and strengths. The assessment data will assist the critical care nurse in planning to meet both patient and family needs.

LEVINE'S MODEL

Using the theory of a holistic being and system theories, Myra Levine describes a person as "a system of systems, and in its wholeness expresses the organization of all its contributing parts."[14] One cannot assess a patient without also exploring the needs of that individual's family. Internal and external environmental aspects affect the patient's adaptation to illness. Levine views the patient's ability to maintain a balance through methods of conservation. These areas of conservation include: energy, structural integrity, personal integrity, and social integrity (Table 1).

These aspects of conservation are easily met for the patient, but not always for the family. Because the patient and family are interdependent, these needs must be met for the family as well. Conservation of energy for a family may involve assessing their understanding of the event to prevent their expending excessive energy worrying over a misperception. Structural integrity relates to additional illnesses within the family, future health needs, and a place to nap, eat, or address personal needs.

Personal integrity for a family may center around past experiences with critical care units, recent life events, and religious and ethnic needs. Conservation of social integrity includes assessing difficulties related to work/career, social support systems for the family, and visitation needs of the family.

Levine describes adaptation as "the process of change whereby the individual retains his integrity within the realities of his environments."[14] While allowing the individual to maintain integrity, the family's integrity must be kept intact. Through the assessment tool using Levine's conservation principles, the principal areas affecting

TABLE 1
Levine's Conservation Model

Conservation of energy
Conservation of structural integrity
Conservation of personal integrity
Conservation of social integrity

families can be examined. The realities for a particular patient may be an element of family dysfunction; however, if recognized by the critical care nurse, efforts at correcting this can be incorporated in the patient's care plan. Strong support exists regarding the relationship between social support and recovery.[15] Levine's model embraces the concepts of person, environment, health, and nursing in an ideal manner for the critical care patient and their family.

FAMILY ASSESSMENT

An assessment tool can facilitate evaluation of family needs. The authors developed a family assessment tool based on Levine's conservation model. As previously discussed, Levine's model includes four models of conservation: energy, structural integrity, personal integrity and social integrity.

Conservation of Energy

Perception of the Event

Often upon entering the health care system, the family is the forgotten group whose needs are not uniformly met. The focus in critical care units is to stabilize an acutely ill patient while the family may pace the waiting room overwhelmed with questions. The nurse cannot begin to fulfill the patient's needs without a thorough family assessment. What the family believes are direct results of the event, chances for recovery, or possible disfigurement have tremendous impact on their perception of the event.

Explanations to the family need to be concise, realistic, and in lay terms. Having the family summarize their viewpoint is beneficial and will provide the health care team with the opportunity to clarify any misconceptions. A heightened level of anxiety may impair the family's ability to establish a realistic perception of the situation. Artinian stresses the importance of congruent nurse-family perceptions.[16]

Coping Mechanisms

Hospitalization creates a crisis for family members, and their ability to be an integral member in their loved one's care revolves around reducing this crisis. Disequilibrium ensues and past coping mechanisms are often relied upon. These mechanisms may be healthy or unhealthy (drug or alcohol abuse, excessive smoking, or poor eating habits) but should be explored with the family members. Individual styles of coping may exist among members as well as different stages of coping. Potter states, "The crisis of acute illness requires a total expenditure of energy for an individual to achieve emotional adaptation."[5] Among other sources, disruption of family routines amplifies stress.

To avoid family neglect, emphasis must be expanded to include the patient's family. Molter has reported that many families feel the nursing staff's responsibility is to the patient and their required care.[6] Ability of present coping skills may be tested during the acute illness of a family member. A family assessment tool may help explore these skills and their successes.

King and Gregor have identified various methods of coping that families may rely upon.[17] Turning to others for support may be one method, whether support comes from friends, relatives, or visitors in the critical care waiting area. Another method King and Gregor describe is that some families maintain vigils at the hospital out of a need to remain near the patient. Review is a method for providing the individual with an emotional catharsis by reexamining the events related to the illness for their family member.

Information-seeking decreases uncertainty for the relative because facts can provide reassurance. Intellectualization, using medical terminology, is a style employed by some families to feel more in control of the situation. This method may offer the family a sense of expertise.

Rehearsal provides the family with a chance to envision certain aspects of their relative's care, the "What if . . . ?" of the situation. Other families may attempt to minimize the situation as a method of eliminating stress or repeatedly ask for the same information from every staff member, which may be a method of avoiding more painful concerns.

Hope repeatedly is cited as a key need of families to cope with the crisis of a critical illness. The ability to assist the family in maintaining a balance of reality and optimism is often difficult for nurses to accomplish.

Review of present coping methods provides an opportunity to assess the family's defense mechanisms and examine what they are relying on. Possible frustration, guilt, and loneliness should be explored and the family assisted with dealing with the impact these emotions have on their physical and emotional health. Sense of humor may be an additional method of coping. Often families will use humor, diversionary activities, or increased smoking or eating to vent or reduce stress.

Logistics

Families may experience unique logistic issues that influence their needs. Logistic issues may include distance from the hospital, transportation to and from the hospital, and lodging. Often, patients are transported to hospitals for specialty services, thereby compelling families to commute long distances. In addition to this, patients may have become critically ill while out of town for business or vacation.

It is important to assess the effects that traveling distance has on the family, such as fatigue and the time available for visitation. Special consideration of these concerns is essential in adapting visitation hours to facilitate family functioning.

Family often are reluctant to leave the hospital when a family member is critically ill, a concern that may be intensified if families have a long distance to travel. They may be afraid that, should the patient's condition change, they would be unable to return to the hospital quickly. Families may need hospital services, such as available rooms for lodging or discounted parking rates, explained to them. Families may also need information on local motels or hotels close to the hospital.

Some families, because of distance and other obligations, may visit infrequently and need to communicate by telephone. These families will rely greatly on the critical care staff to keep them apprised of the patient's condition and when their presence is most needed.

Conservation of Structural Integrity

Acute Versus Chronic Illness

It is very important to assess the patient's illness as acute or chronic, as well as whether the illness was expected or unexpected. Consider a healthy family easily able to meet its day-to-day responsibilities; a sudden, critical illness of one of its members will be a significant shock to the family and most likely disrupt family functioning. Additional issues are confronted by families if the patient was involved in a traumatic incident of violence. The family may be in more disarray as they deal with the critical illness and the fact that the illness may have been self-induced or intentionally inflicted by another. Mixed feelings of anxiety and anger may be experienced by the family.

If the patient prescheduled coronary artery bypass surgery, both the patient and family may have had plenty of time to physically and psychologically prepare themselves for the surgery. If, conversely, the patient is admitted to the critical care unit experiencing an acute evolving myocardial infarction, little if any time may be available for the patient and family to prepare themselves.

During the admission of the patient to the critical care unit, information needs to be obtained from the patient or family regarding the patient's past and present health. If the patient has a chronic illness, it is especially important to assess how the patient and family were coping with the illness.

If the patient's condition has been chronic, an acute exacerbation may be a frustrating setback. An example is a patient with progressive heart failure for whom an acute episode of pulmonary edema may be a major blow. The patient and family may be frustrated by the disease and the difficulties they have experienced in managing it. The patient and family may experience increased anxiety and fear because the acute episodes are more frequent and that the disease may be worsening.

Families accustomed to assisting with care at home need to be questioned about the level of involvement they would like to have while the patient is acutely ill. They may want to continue to provide some patient care and maintain as many of their preestablished routines as possible. On the other hand, family may welcome a needed rest from care-giving responsibilities.

Family Functioning

Each member of a family plays different roles, the fulfillment of which facilitates family functioning. A critical illness requires reallocation of a patient's roles to others in the family.[18] This can place additional stress upon the remaining family members.[18]

It is important to assess whether there are any roles the family will need assistance with. The critically ill patient may have been the financial manager for the family, the child care provider, or the cook. Family may need help with roles they are not accustomed to. The family may be able to divvy up roles between other family members. Family may also be able to call on additional support systems (friends, extended family) for assistance. If the patient's illness is prolonged, the family will need to further develop certain skills in order to accomplish new role responsibilities and reestablish stable family functioning.

An assessment of the family's ability to maintain family functioning is crucial. According to Fife, families that have maintained adequate and functional relationships prior to a crisis will return to a state of functional stability after the crisis.[19] On the other hand, if family functioning was not optimal prior to the crisis, the family may experience further disruption.

Assessment data may be obtained that reflect whether the family adequately relate with each other. If problems are identified, the critical care nurse may be better able to anticipate family needs and understand family concerns. Specific interventions may be identified to assist family coping and family functioning.

Current and Future Health Needs

From admission to discharge, health needs of both patient and family need to be identified. Alterations in the patient's appearance or cognitive function may be very disturbing to the family. Initially, information related to prognosis may be limited due to uncertainty of recovery, thereby making it difficult to project health needs. Families may ask, "What will we need at home?" or "How can we care for him at home?"

The altered health status of their relative may cause tremendous changes in activities of daily living within the family. Honest descriptions of the patient's abilities or disabilities should be presented to the family and their acceptance of this should be assessed. Programs for brain injury, substance abuse, cardiac rehabilitation, or outpatient physical therapy may be among the outreach programs necessary to assist with patient care. Various support groups through the American Cancer Society, the American Heart Association, the American Thoracic Society, and others offer emotional support to patients and families and interest in these groups should be elicited.

In situations such as sudden cardiac death or trauma related to alcohol abuse, families often fear recurrences. Exploring this in the initial assessment is helpful to provide an open forum for discussion to assist the critical care nurse with initiating referrals and establishing discharge plans.

The family is the patient's link to society, and to achieve a supportive transition from the critical care unit to home, needs for future health must be assessed upon entry into the health care system. However, many critically ill patients will not survive the hospitalization. For their families, assessment must address the grief experience and how this will affect the family's future health. Services such as "Parents without Partners," "Mothers against Drunk Drivers," and religious organizations need to be suggested to these families.

Patients who will survive need discharge plans addressed upon admission to the critical care unit. Preventive measures to be taught, such as wearing seat belts to reduce the chance of motor vehicle injuries, not drinking and driving, not omitting important cardiac medications, and abiding low cholesterol diets may be crucial to lower recurrences. Inspection of the home environment for safety is another method to anticipate the patient's future needs prior to discharge, but the necessity for this can be part of the initial assessment.

Many past studies addressing family needs focused on the critical care unit cardiac patient group or the traditional medical-surgical critical care patient. Entering this new decade, the patient population has changed with the increased number of transplant patients, trauma patients, and homeless individuals. Their future health needs may be quite complex and require creativity in planning.

Conservation of Personal Integrity

Past Experience with Critical Illness

In order for critical care nurses to better understand and meet family needs, it is important to assess past experiences family have had with critical illness. What were the past experiences? What was the patient outcome? What factors helped or hindered family coping with the past experiences?

If families have had no experience with critical illness, they will need a complete orientation to the critical care unit and what to expect. Clarification may be necessary regarding why the patient needs to be in a critical care unit. Families may believe that a critical care unit is a place to go before death. Family may need to know that patients often are admitted to a critical care unit for extensive monitoring to prevent complications or provide earlier detection of problems.

Families with past experiences with a critical illness may need to be reoriented to the reasons patients are admitted to a critical care unit. Families may have specific questions or concerns regarding the current illness of a family member.

According to Williams, more experiences of loss and coping certainly help individuals and families face a similar situation again.[20] Although the outcome of the family's past experience may have been death of the patient, the family may have developed new coping skills or strengthened family bonds. Whether the patient's outcome was positive or negative, it is key to assess what the family found most or least helpful when involved with critical illness in the past.

Life Events

According to the systems theory, Yoder believes a family is a system of networking relationships.[21] Williams states that every illness has a family component and the family must be assessed individually according to their positions in their life cycles.[20] The interdependence of patient and family cannot be denied and the impact of the patient's illness may vary if the family has a stable group of relationships among members versus the family in transition confronted with a multitude of problems.

In the assessment of the critical care family, the nurse must observe for the nuances of each family as well as family members. Besides the crisis of their loved one being a patient in the critical care unit, the family will respond based on any recent life events that may have affected them.

Life events may be positive such as the birth of a child, a graduation, a member receiving a career advancement, or a family member moving or buying a house. Negative life events may be loss of employment, a death, a miscarriage, the birth of a child with a health problem, or financial debts. The individualized meaning for every family with regard to the impact of these events needs to be assessed. Who in the family is most affected and what the various family members' roles are in these events need to be discussed. There may be changes occurring in family relationships secondary to painful transitions, and the family may be more receptive to interventions during crisis than at a time of stability.

Ethnic/Religious

It is important to assess ethnic customs considered essential for the family to maintain. For instance, the family may have specific dietary preferences they may need assistance in meeting. The hospital may be able to help facilitate family functioning within their culture.

Religion can be an additional source of support for families experiencing crisis. Members of the family may have different religious beliefs. Assessing family's religion and intervening to assure religious concerns are addressed may facilitate family coping.

Additional Family Needs

Family routines are disrupted, intimacy is removed, and relationships are tested when a relative is admitted to the critical care unit. The patient belongs to the family, not the hospital staff, but many times families may wonder whether this is true. They may have to linger in waiting rooms for visiting hours designed by the hospital, they may feel distanced from their loved one by all of the equipment, and they may lose the support of family members and friends if the hospitalization is prolonged. "Providing comprehensive care to the relatives of the critically ill patients begins with the identification and assessment of their needs."[9]

In this period of adaptation, uncertainty ensues related to the family altering its structure, rules, roles, and responsibilities.[22] The major capabilities available to families are their resources and strengths and their coping behaviors and strategies.[22] Reviewing these with families may provide the critical care nurse with an overview of the strengths and weaknesses of the family and how they may be assisted in this crisis period.

Comfort needs and emotional reassurance may be areas the family needs help with but is hesitant to seek assistance with. Exploring with the family their needs for privacy, information sharing, and communication allows them to have their unique needs met. Family conferences on a daily basis may be crucial for one family, whereas another family prefers minimal information to avoid being overwhelmed. The need for a family to participate and interact with their relative may be crucial for one family, but another family may be too nervous to kiss or hold hands with their hospitalized loved one.

Reassuring the family that their individual needs are important is essential to convey caring to the family and diminish their sense of aloneness in the hospital environment. Daily accessibility of the primary nurse, clinical nurse specialist, and physician should be explained to the family to provide them with opportunities for discussion of their needs and concerns.

Conservation of Social Integrity

Support Systems

It can be difficult to deal with the critical illness of a family member when one is alone. Families spend many hours in critical care waiting rooms. Some family members feel it is a weakness to need help from others[18] and will often wait alone rather than call someone to be with them.

Often families merely need encouragement to call additional family members or friends. Many times, family may need to feel in control or that they can handle it. Suggestions such as "It's OK if you call someone" or "Why don't you give a friend a call" prompt a family to ask for assistance. Having someone to talk with or be with provides not only support, distraction, friendship, and assistance with coping, but also can strengthen relationships and build bonds.

Visitation

For families, waiting outside the doors of the critical care unit between visits can seem eternal. Being able to talk with, sit with, touch, or just see their family member can be comforting. If the patient cannot respond, family can still talk to the patient and keep the patient informed of family activities and current affairs.

It is important to assess what families expect during visitation. Family may expect time to be alone with the patient, which may or may not be possible depending on the acuteness of the patient's condition. They may also expect changes in the patient's condition each time they visit and will require ongoing assessment of their understanding of the patient's condition.

Family may also expect to assist with some aspects of patient care. They may want to help with bathing, feeding, or range of motion. Families may believe that, by participating in care, they are helping the patient and can make a real difference.

The critical care nurse is in an ideal position to assess family functioning during visitation and to foster family interactions. The critical care nurse can also assess when the patient and a family need time for rest. Family may need encouragement to take walks, go for meal breaks, or participate in diversionary activities.

Work Pattern

Economic stability is paramount to family members in order to meet the financial strain of hospitalization. During the crisis of an acute illness, families may encounter problems related to their occupations. An employer may be intolerant of the need for a family member to leave the job site during work hours for visiting or an emergency. Families may work shifts not conducive to established hospital visiting policies and may be hesitant to negotiate the need for flexibility with employers or hospital staff. There may be a need for family members to attend educational sessions at the hospital to learn aspects of care for their relative and this may create stress in their work environment.

The hospitalized individual may be the major economic source for the family, and the family members may be stressed by a diminished source of income. Family members often report inability to concentrate on their work related to increased apprehension from not being with their relative. Employers may be adding additional pressure by finding deficiencies in the family member's work.

In the case of closed head injury, patients' families may face the realities of the patient not returning to their career and requiring extensive rehabilitation, further exacerbating economic difficulties.

APPLICATION OF THE TOOL

The family assessment tool can be used in the critical care setting upon admission of the patient and completed within 48 hours. The primary nurse or clinical nurse specialist should interview the family in a conference room setting to provide privacy and enhance open discussion. An initial introduction to the critical care unit should occur as an adjunct, providing the family with a degree of orientation to the critical care unit. At the time of the family assessment interview, an introduction of staff may also be helpful to family members and may decrease their anxiety.

By using this tool, the critical care nurse can assess the discharge planning needs of the patient and family. The family should be provided with an explanation that the tool is to assist in individualizing their relative's care and providing holistic care for them as a family unit. Information from this assessment can be incorporated into the nursing care plan, as well as shared with other disciplines. The tool will assist with conveying important information to the unit the patient is transferred to and may serve as a resource on subsequent readmission to the hospital.

The assessment tool will not only enhance the comprehensiveness of patient and family care, but provide a method for reassuring families that they are a vital part of their relative's care and recovery. A tool such as this will provide time for clarification of misconceptions and provide a means for strengthening the nurse-family relationship. Intricacies of family patterns can be assessed and interventions provided before family dysfunction escalates.

CONCLUSION

It is essential to assess needs of families of critically ill patients during their crisis period. Levine's model of conservation provides a framework for holistic family assessment. Only with a thorough understanding of the family will the critical care nurse be able to develop intervention strategies to meet families' diversified needs.

REFERENCES

1. Ganglione, K.M. Assessing and intervening with families of CCU patients. *Nurs Clin North Am* 1984; 19:427–432.
2. Dunkel, J., & Eisendarth, S. Families in the intensive care unit: Their effects on staff. *Heart Lung* 1983; 12:258–261.
3. Hodovinic, B.H., Reardon, D., Reese, W., & Wedges, B. Family crisis intervention program in the medical intensive care unit. *Heart Lung* 1984; 13:243–249.
4. Bedsworth, J.A., & Molen, M.T. Psychological stress in spouses of patients with myocardial infarctions.. *Heart Lung* 1982; 11:450–456.

5. Potter, P.A. Stress and the intensive care unit—the family's perception. *Missouri Nurse* 1979; 48:5–8.
6. Molter, N.C. Needs of relatives of critically ill patients: A descriptive study. *Heart Lung* 1979; 8:332–339.
7. Rodgers, C.D. Needs of relatives of cardiac surgery patients during the critical care phase. *Focus on Critical Care* 1983; 10:50–55.
8. Daley, L. The perceived immediate needs of families with relatives in the intensive care setting. *Heart Lung* 1984; 13:231–237.
9. Leske, J.S. Needs of relatives of critically ill patients: A follow-up. *Heart Lung* 1986; 15:189–193.
10. Norris, L.O., & Grove, S.K. Investigation of selected psychosocial needs of family members of critically ill adult patients. *Heart Lung* 1986; 15:194–199.
11. Lynn-McHale, D.J., & Bellinger, A. Need satisfaction levels of family members of critical care patients and accuracy of nurses' perceptions. *Heart Lung* 1988; 17:447–453.
12. Dracup, K.A., & Breu, C.S. Using nursing research findings to meet the needs of grieving spouses. *Nurs Res* 1978; 27:212–216.
13. Bouman, C.C. Identifying priority concerns of families of ICU patients. *Dimensions of Critical Care Nursing* 1984; 3:313–319.
14. Levine, M.E. *Introduction to clinical nursing*, 2nd ed. Philadelphia: FA Davis; 1973.
15. Dockters, B., Black, D.R., Hovell, M.F., et al. Families and intensive care nurses: Comparison of perceptions. *Patient Education and Counseling* 1988; 12:29–36.
16. Artinian, N.T. Family member perceptions of a cardiac surgery event. *Focus on Critical Care* 1989; 16:301–308.
17. King, S.L., & Gregor, F.M. Stress and coping in families of the critically ill. *Critical Care Nurse* 1985; 5:48–51.
18. Roberts, S.L. *Behavioral concepts and the critically ill patient*. Englewood Cliffs, NJ: Prentice Hall; 1976.
19. Fife, B.L. A model for predicting the adaptation of families to medical crisis: An analysis of role integration. *Image* 1985; 17:108–112.
20. William, P.R. *Family problems*. Oxford: Oxford University; 1989.
21. Yoder, L., & Jones, S.L. The family of the emergency room patient as seen through the eyes of the nurse. *Int J Nurs Stud* 1982; 19:29–36.
22. Figley, C.R. *Treating stress in families*. New York: Brunner/Mazel; 1989.

APPENDIX A
FAMILY ASSESSMENT TOOL

Contact person(s):

Name _____ Telephone # _____

Name _____ Telephone # _____

Significant others:

_____

_____

_____

ASSESSMENT OF ENERGY

I. Perception of the Event

A. What does the family know about the patient's condition?

_____

_____

B. What does the family think caused the patient's condition?

_____

_____

II. Coping Mechanisms

A. How has the family coped with past crises?

_____

_____

B. What helped the most during past crises?

_____

_____

C. What helped the least during past crises?

_____

_____

D. What activities helped the family cope?

_____ Drugs/alcohol   _____ Exercise

_____ Sleeping   _____ Smoking

_____ Overeating   _____ Undereating

E. Who in the family may have the most difficulty coping with the patient's current illness?

_____

_____

_____

III. Logistics

A. What is the average distance the family needs to travel to and from the hospital?

_____

_____

B. Does the family have any transportation problems?

_____

_____

C. Does the family need assistance with transportation and/or lodging?

_____

_____

ASSESSMENT OF STRUCTURAL INTEGRITY

I. Acute Versus Chronic Illness

A. Was the patient's illness:

_____ Acute   _____ Chronic

_____ Expected   _____ Unexpected

B. Was the family involved in care-giving prior to the patient's hospitalization?

_____

_____

C. Does the family want to participate in specific aspects of patient care?

_____

_____

II. Family Functioning

A. Who is taking care of home affairs?

Finances _____

Children _____

Parents _____

Pets _____

B. How was the family functioning prior to the patient's admission to the critical care unit?

_____

_____

C. How has family functioning been affected by the patient's admission to the critical care unit?

_____

_____

D. How close is the family?

_____

_____

E. How does the family best communicate?

_____

_____

F. Does the family anticipate any role adjustments?

_____

_____

G. Are the family resources adequate to meet family needs?

_____

_____

H. Are any referrals needed?

Social services _____

Home care _____

Business office _____

Patient representative _____

Other _____

III. Current and Future Health Needs

A. Are family members meeting their own health needs?

Sleep/rest _____

Nutrition _____

B. Does the family anticipate any need for:

Health teaching _____

Prevention education _____

Home safety assessment _____

Rehabilitative services _____

Substance abuse referral _____

ASSESSMENT OF PERSONAL INTEGRITY

I. Past Experiences

A. What past experiences has the family had with critical illness? (Type of unit, circumstances, outcome.)

_____

_____

B. What factors helped the family cope with past experiences of critical illness?

_____

_____

C. What factors inhibited family coping with past experiences of critical illness?

_____

_____

II. Life Events

A. Has the family experienced any recent health problems?

_____

_____

B. Has the family had any additional stressors in the past year?

_____

_____

C. Have there been any additional disruptions in family routines?

_____

_____

III. Ethnic/Religious

A. Are there any ethnic customs the family may need assistance with?

_____

_____

B. What is (are) the family's religion(s)?

_____

_____

C. Would the family like the clergy contacted?

_____

_____

D. Does the family know where the chapel is located and have information regarding nursing services?

_____

_____

IV. Additional Family Needs

Does the family know:

A. Where they can go to be alone?

_____

_____

B. Who they can go to for answers to their questions?

_____

_____

C. How to contact the critical care nurse?

_____

_____

D. How to arrange a meeting with the physician or clinical nurse specialist?

_____

_____

ASSESSMENT OF SOCIAL INTEGRITY

I. Support Systems

A. Are family support systems available?

_____

_____

B. Who are family support systems?

_____

_____

C. Are there additional resources that family depend on for support?

_____

_____

II. Visitation

A. Who will be visiting?

_____

_____

B. Are there any visiting restrictions?

_____

_____

C. What does the family expect during critical care visits?

_____

_____

D. Are there any special requirements for visitors? (Chair or support needed at bedside.)

_____

_____

E. Does the family have any concerns related to visiting times?

_____

_____

III. Work Patterns

A. Whose income supports the family?

_____

_____

B. Are additional family members employed?

_____

_____

C. What type of work schedules and/or patterns do the family members have?

_____

_____

D. Does the family have any flexibility in work schedules and/or patterns?

_____

_____

CHAPTER 31

Preventive Work with Families: Issues Facing Public Health Nurses

Linda J. Kristjanson, Karen I. Chalmers

This paper examines the issues that nurses experience when entering the family system to work preventively. The theoretical basis of family-centred nursing is analysed and the need for empirical work is identified in order to develop a knowledge base for this practice. Some unique characteristics of the public health nursing role are discussed with emphasis on territorial issues, power relationships, and accountability problems. The need for public health nurses to function as advanced generalists across different system levels is recommended and family skills necessary for effective family nursing are examined. The authors identify the unique role of public health nurses because they have access to healthy families and families dealing with early stages of health concerns. The authors support the general structure of public health practice as of value for preventive work with families. However, clarity regarding referrals, contracting and the rights of clients is called for to facilitate collaborative family-centred nursing.

INTRODUCTION

For years public health nurses have recognized that 'community' care is usually 'family' care and that the family is the primary unit of health care. Over the past decade there has been an increasing emphasis in the literature on 'family-focused care,' 'family-centred nursing' and 'family interventions' (Barnes 1985, Garrett 1985, Gilliss *et al.* 1989, Pesznecker & Zahlis 1986, Sullivan 1982, Wright & Leahey 1984). These writings have

Reprinted from *Journal of Advanced Nursing, Vol. 16*, 1991, pp. 147–153. Used with permission of Blackwell Scientific Publications, Ltd., and the authors.

been helpful in understanding how families contribute to or restore health and prevent illness. This literature has widened the conceptual lens through which health problems are assessed and managed.

A second theme in the public health literature is the need for preventive health care (Breslow 1978, Pender 1987). The aim of reducing and eliminating health problems through early detection and intervention is recognized by many health professionals as a priority for health care (Canada Health Survey 1981).

This paper is designed to contribute to the understanding of how public health nurses can work preventively with families to promote their health. Although we agree with the 'expanded lens' approach to community health care that includes the family, we share concerns about the methods used in this care, the theory base for this practice, and obstacles to family-centred care that may be inherent in some traditional public health practices. As well, discussion regarding family-focused nursing can become confusing because of different viewpoints about who constitutes the family and when and how to use family-focused interventions.

This paper will argue the following points:

1. That the nursing literature, to date, lacks a theory base to direct family health-care practice. Most literature currently used by nurses has been 'borrowed' from the social sciences and family therapy and has not been tested for its 'fit' within family nursing contexts.
2. That much of the family theory used by nursing is based upon a male-dominated systems view that does not recognize that the majority of family health care is given by women.
3. That there is a related need to develop an empirically based theory to explain and predict effective public health nursing with families.
4. That there are unique features of the public health role that are both an advantage and disadvantage to the nurse interested in providing family-centered nursing. Some of these influences come from the historical public health role and the power relationship between public health nurses and their clients.
5. That the most appropriate level for public health nursing intervention may vary. It is recommended that in some instances greater benefit might be attained from intervening at the macro-system level rather than at the family level.
6. And finally, that the skills required by public health nurses who work preventively with families are varied and complex, requiring that these individuals are prepared as advanced generalists.

THEORY BASE OF FAMILY NURSING

There is a lack of clearly documented theory related to how to nurse families in the community. The knowledge that does exist includes authors' opinions or anecdotal experiences about individual family nursing incidents. Community health textbooks describe the importance of family-centred nursing and identify key times to include the family in health care, but are rather non-specific about actually how to work with families.

In a search for a theory base to guide practice, nurses have often looked to other disciplines for assistance. This is not unusual, as many disciplines share aspects of theoretical knowledge. However, to adopt a body of theory from a neighbouring field without careful analysis and testing of its 'fit' to nursing practice is a serious error (Fawcett 1984, Hardy 1978). Using theory from another discipline may be entirely legitimate; but nurses must evaluate the conditions unique to nursing practice which alter other disciplines' generalizations. As well, nurses may also find that they need to expand the original theory.

These theories were developed by social scientists to explain and predict patterns of family functioning (Ackerman 1938, Bateson *et al.* 1956, Bowen 1976, Duvall 1971). In recent years, nurses have looked to the field of family therapy as a theoretical source of direction. Much of this theoretical writing originated from the work of family therapists who developed their theory from clinical work with specific population groups. For example, Minuchin's structural theory was developed from his work with low-income families with disturbed adolescents, and was later expanded and tested with families with anorexic members (Minuchin *et al.* 1967, Minuchin *et al.* 1978). Indeed, the reference population of most family therapists is families with entrenched patterns of dysfunction.

The population that public health nurses encounter, however, is not the same population from which family therapists developed their theories. Many family issues that public health nurses encounter involve families considered to be generally healthy. Some might be experiencing health concerns in the early phases of a problem, requiring more straightforward preventive and supportive interventions. As well, the context in which public health nurses work is quite different from that of family therapists. For the most part, family therapy is conducted in the health professional's territory for a recognized family problem. In public health nursing, family-centred care occurs in the family's territory, most often initiated by the nurse for a health concern that may or may not be obvious to the family. Public health nurses need a theory base that helps them understand how to approach families in their territory, how to assess potential or actual health concerns from a family perspective, and how to intervene most effectively with families to prevent and manage health concerns. Although some family theory developed in other disciplines may be appropriate to community nursing contexts, such as family developmental theory, more research is needed to test these theories in family nursing settings and isolate important theoretical constructs and propositions that may be unique to family health care nursing.

Nursing Women in Families

Although the literature in public health nursing frequently refers to family nursing, the majority of this health care is directed at women as the recipient of services such as maternal health care, preventive paediatric care, and management of home care for the elderly and chronically ill. The family caregiving literature documents that much of the nurturing and health care provided to children, elderly and the chronically ill is provided by wives and daughters (Brody 1981, Brody & Lang 1982, Burke 1987, Mace & Rabins 1981, Heckerman 1980, Smoyak 1987).

In addition, family theory has been criticized for presenting a male-dominated definition of the family. This criticism has been directed particularly at structural-functional family therapy because of the emphasis on the importance of conventional family roles and boundaries. Feminist critics of family theory literature (Bogdan 1984, Braverman 1986, Goldner 1985, 1987, 1988, Oakley 1980) have been quick to argue that the concept (gender) influences family dynamics in relation to power, privilege and fairness and is of profound importance to effective intervention with families. These authors point out that an analysis of gender issues is notably absent in the theoretical writing about families, limiting understanding by the practitioner who employs these theories. Public health nurses who adopt or borrow this body of literature without careful examination of the biases inherent in the work, may be applying theory inappropriately in client contexts. The fact that women form the major group of family caregivers, and are most frequently the recipient of public health nursing services, necessitates careful attention to these issues.

The Need for a Research Basis for Practice

Another issue related to the theory basis of family-centred community health nursing is the research base that underlies the theory and direct practice. With some exceptions, nursing's current theory is rationally or deductively arrived at, with few empirical verifications. It is essential in the development of a scientific theory base that these modes of inquiry interface so that logical explanations are rooted in observed phenomena (Gortner 1983).

> Nursing has a mandate from society to use its specialized body of knowledge and skills for the betterment of humans. The mandate implies that knowledge and skills must go in such a way as to keep up with the changing health goals of society.
>
> (Hardy 1978)

There has been a tendency to base nursing actions on tradition, routine and intuition (Hamilton & Bush 1988). According to Hardy (1978), these sources of knowledge may give nurses a sense of security in what they do but they remain in the realm of myth and non-scientific knowledge.

A particular example of the need for research in family community health practice relates to the timing and amount of nursing intervention provided. A popular assumption in health care is that early intervention will prevent later health problems. For example, early detection of cancer will lead to longer survival rates. The literature related to child abuse describes the importance of preventive work to decrease the likelihood of abuse (Campbell & Humphreys 1984). However, it is also known that some health care interventions are more effective if applied later in the dysfunctional process. Cataracts, for instance, are best treated when sufficient lens damage is present that the person is almost blind. It may also be true that certain family problems are more effectively managed when intervention is applied late in the course of the problem, making preventive efforts inappropriate. At present, there is little empirical knowledge in the community health nursing literature related to the success and timing of interventions with families. Research is needed to test the effectiveness of the application of different strategies at various points in the development of family problems.

As well, the 'dosage' or amount of intervention is another variable that may require study. The current practice in public health is to visit families according to a routine schedule, the nurses' sense of completion of goals, or, in some cases, according to a nurse–client contract. How often do nurses need to visit families to prevent or intervene in family health problems? Effective use of nursing time and energies could be enhanced by evaluative research that addresses this issue. As well, it might be important to ask if there is such a thing as an 'overdose' of family nursing interventions? To assume that nurses enter family systems and effect only benevolent results is naive and professionally arrogant. Therefore, clinical research is required to explore these important questions.

It appears that the study of preventive interventions with families has been particularly neglected. Part of the reason for the paucity of research in this area is that evaluative research related to family work is fraught with complexities. It is difficult to control the multiple variables that impinge on a family and simply measure the effect of the timing or type of preventive nursing interventions. However, despite the challenges of this type of research it is important to evaluate systematically the process of nursing care to community health families in order to build a scientific knowledge base to direct practice.

WHAT MAKES PUBLIC HEALTH NURSING WITH FAMILIES UNIQUE?

Public health nurses are in a unique position because they are the professional group that has the opportunity to visit families in their own homes to detect health concerns and prevent problems before they become serious. This role is not performed by other health or social service professions. In other instances, families seek out health professionals because a health or family problem is of sufficient severity to prompt families to find external resources. If a family does not comply with or follow through with ongoing interventions the helping relationship, in most instances, dissolves.

One exception might be the social worker who visits families in their homes to assess family functioning with respect to child welfare concerns. In these instances, however, there is a specific risk in the family's mind of the child being apprehended or some mandatory intervention or treatment being imposed. The relationship here occurs in the family's territory, but the professional clearly holds the balance of power and the reason for contact is not a positive health-promoting one. In contrast, the public health nurse is the ambassador of the health care system who enters family territory to promote health and prevent problems. The nurse is a 'guest in the house' and offers a service that may or may not be received by the family.

In any professional–client relationship, the issue of power emerges as a potential block. Public health nurses enter family territory often as uninvited guests. For example, they often initiate contact with families because of a routine visiting requirement to postpartum families. Families' receptiveness to the nurse will vary depending upon their previous perceptions of public health nurses and their understanding of the reason for the visit. Some families may be influenced by notions of public health nurses that arise from historical public health practices.

Public health practice was based on the public health model developed in the nineteenth century, when the major threats to health were communicable disease and malnutrition. For a nurse practising within this model, the focus was on screening the population for early detection of disease or detection of individuals at high risk for developing problems (Pender 1987). Case finding was carried out so that interventions could be applied early and the disease process arrested or slowed down. With the passage of time, and as many communicable diseases were brought under control, public health nurses have addressed the prevention of chronic illness, often through lifestyle risk reduction, and the social health problems of high-risk families. The predominant interventions, however, have remained active case finding through assessment and screening procedures, and ongoing surveillance and monitoring. The public health model places strong emphasis on the nurse as the definer of the health problem. The nurse frequently detects the problem, seeks out the family and attempts to intervene. The client may or may not be aware or interested in the health concern as the nurse defines it, and may not be wanting service. The nurse appears to justify her attempts to engage the client based on her concept of health (Chalmers 1984).

Problems

The influence of the earlier public health role may result in a number of problems related to family-focused community-health nursing today. The historical stereotype of a public health nurse may be held by families who see the nurse as someone coming to 'check' on them and report them to some unknown authority. Indeed, recent experiences with public health nurses may have led families to expect nurses to perform in this way. Although a more collaborative approach to working with people is being used to some extent currently and is recommended in the more recent public health literature (Baum 1988, Kickbusch 1987, Labonte 1989, Martin & McQueen 1989), some nurses may see themselves as authority figures who can define the family's problem and give advice and teaching. This may be perceived as unhelpful or intrusive and also may not be aimed at concerns that families may be experiencing.

Public health nurses need to be aware of how some perceptions of the public health role may disadvantage them in their work with families. On the other hand, the preventive perspective and concern for health of groups that this history also emphasizes are aspects that should be retained and fostered. However, in family-focused community nursing there may need to be more specific efforts to establish collaborative relationships with families and communicate purposes for contact and establishment of mutual goals for health. In these ways, counterproductive 'ghosts' that represent a more authoritarian style of public health protection may be erased in nurse–family interactions.

Another control-related issue is the nurse's accountability. The nature of public health work makes the nurse accountable to the community as a whole, as well as to the individual or family being nursed. This responsibility to the aggregate may be in conflict with the nurse's responsibility to the professional ethics by which he/she practices. Codes of ethics of nursing practice emphasize the individual's right to autonomy, self-determinism, privacy and the nurse's requirement to respect these rights (Canadian Nurses Association 1989, Fry 1983). These rights may be violated under existing public health practices such as universal follow-up of all postnatal clients, or discussion of children with school officials without parental consent, or seeking out special groups for assessment and teaching.

Although policies are set by public health administrators, it is the nurse in the field who must resolve this conflict of initiating contacts with clients who have not requested service. Clients may react with anger, indifference or passivity, all difficult positions on which to base a collaborative working relationship. When adults alone are involved, nurses may resolve this dilemma more easily and remove themselves from unwanted client interactions. However, when young children in high-risk families are involved, nurses find themselves in deeper conflict. Should nurses press for involvement with unwilling families and risk intruding on rights to autonomy and self-determination, or withdraw and live with the uneasiness that these children may at some point be abused or neglected (Chalmers 1984)?

In these instances, public health nurses' primary responsibility is to protect the health of the children. Here, the purpose of the visit may not be made explicit to parents. This may be necessary and prudent. However, in the majority of instances this vagueness is not appropriate. A large part of the difficulty associated with effective family nursing stems from a lack of clarity about the reason for public health contact. In general, much more attention needs to be given to the process of referral to the community and nurses' entries into family systems. Mechanisms need to be developed so that clients are aware of the rationale for nurses' contacts by referring sources. Sometimes, families are unaware of the referral source or reason for referral to public health nurses. When concerns exist, the referring person needs to articulate clearly these to clients, and some level of consensus for follow-up needs to be reached prior to initiation of the referral to the nurse. This clarity would facilitate entry of the nurse into the family territory and set the stage for a collaborative relationship based on a more balanced and clearer understanding of the purpose of the contact.

LEVEL OF INTERVENTION

An additional problem exists concerning the application of current family theory to nurses' work with families. It could be argued from a systems perspective that the family's problem is based at the macro level (e.g. poverty) rather than within the family system. While system theory may be used by public health nurses in their work with families, interventions usually are aimed at family processes rather than at external stressors. This may be helpful and appropriate. However, nurses working with families in the community also often need to work at the macro system level with the external stressors, as an advocate for families. For example, a problem that might be identified by a public health nurse would be poor nutritional practices of a low-income family. A nurse could work with the family to increase their knowledge of good nutrition and help them plan their budget to allow for nutritious meal planning. However, upon further analysis the nurse might also decide to use a macro system approach to address the problem by advocating for an increased food budget for the family at the welfare office, or working with an Anti-Poverty Coalition to improve the standard of living for those on low fixed incomes.

It is argued that to be effective in dealing with many potential health concerns, public health nurses need to be able to work at various levels of the system. This notion is exemplified well by the story of the nurse standing by the river who sees a man floating face down in the water (McKinlay 1979). She quickly pulls the man out of the water and begins to resuscitate him, when she notices a second man floating face down in the water and then sees a third and a fourth person floating downstream. The nurse becomes so busy pulling nearly drowned bodies out of the river, that she has no time to run upstream and see who is pushing the people into the river.

This story illustrates that over-attention to one level of action may limit effective management of a problem. Nurses are usually less confident at intervening at macro or sociopolitical levels of the system and feel more comfortable 'downstream' dealing with individuals/families who are in distress. Yet they often express frustration that they are performing 'band-aid' types of interventions that do not really address the sources of family health concerns. Nurse educators and public health administrators are encouraged to examine ways that are helpful in preparing and supporting public health nurses to intervene at this level. As a collective, public health nurses could play a much more active role at this level.

Necessary Skills

Nurses require special skills to 'enter' a family. Usually the family has not sought the nurse's services and therefore may not welcome the nurse easily into their territory. Nurses need to have 'engaging' skills or social skills that convey interest in and acceptance of the family. Authoritarian or heavy-handed approaches that presume automatic entry into the family will more than likely result in passive if not active rejection of the nurse.

Usually, nurses enter the family system because of a recognized health concern. The concern is most often focused on one individual family member. Upon further assessment, the problem may be identified by the nurse as rooted in the family and therefore successful work on the problem necessitates a shift from an individual to a family level. The family may not see the need for the nurse to meet, let alone work with, the whole family. Therefore, access to the entire family may be limited, as nurses find themselves talking to mothers and babies only. Tangles of contracting to work often begin here.

Nurses need the skills to be able to contract with families clearly and openly in order to clarify the purpose of visits and the usefulness of family involvement in discussion of health concerns. Nurses need to meet families to assess the impact of one family member's health on the other members, and vice versa. Once a family assessment has been conducted, nurses have the further task of helping families explore actual and potential health problems, learning new ways of dealing with situations, or changing potentially hazardous health behaviours. This is when the ability to contract is essential. The problem or potential problem must be mutually recognized and the family should be included in determining their own goals for health. It is evident that communication skills are central to effective family work, as nurses need to negotiate and interact with a variety of families who may have different perceptions and expectations of the nurse's role. Nurses also need to examine their own value systems and look critically at their styles of practice. Do they hold on to power and control? Do they like to be the authority and the expert? Can they work in a non-judgmental way with different families? To work effectively and collaboratively with families, nurses must be willing to be a 'guest in the house.' They must accept that although they have expert power in terms of their general knowledge base, there is much that they do not know about the uniqueness of the particular family they are visiting.

This combination of knowledge and abilities is extensive and many public health nurses would identify these skills as part of the usual repertoire of a competent generalist. However, based upon our own practice experience, observations of nursing students and research with community health nurses (Kristjanson & Chalmers 1987, 1990), it appears that the complexity of community situations and family dynamics in this context requires that the public health nurse be prepared as an advanced generalist. This would require a clinical major in advanced community practice with families, either as an internship or elective, or advanced study at the master's level of community health practice.

CONCLUSION

Public health nurses could choose to go the route of many other helping professions and have the system within which they work restructured so that families come to them, thus eliminating the frustrations of working with families who may not wholeheartedly welcome nurses into their homes. On the other hand, if this restructuring were to occur, nurses would miss opportunities to see health problems early, offer anticipatory teaching and support to families and help a family mobilize resources that they might not otherwise locate. The risk of intruding into family territory is still present, and nurses must be sensitive and cautious so as not to invade. However, the potential benefits to families and to society appear to warrant this risk. The important issue is that nurses acknowledge that a risk exists and make efforts to minimize it. In most instances, except for the few health problems that legally require the nurse to contact the family, the family should be in control as to whether or not the nursing service is accepted. Prevention of health problems in families is an important role for public health nurses to assume. Waiting for a family to recognize a health problem may be too late in the process to work preventively. Therefore, the 'door-to-door' approach of public health nursing fills an important void in the family health system.

The literature indicates that several factors influence a person's decision to seek preventive health services (Murray & Zentner 1979, Pender 1987, Pratt 1976, Ramsay 1985). First, the person may seek health care because of family encouragement. Second, patterns of using preventive services are learned in the family. Third, expectations of friends are powerful motivators to seek preventive health care. Fourth, information and respectful care from health professionals also increases the readiness to engage in preventive health behaviour, especially if the health professional is seen as knowledgeable and caring.

Further empirical research is needed to clarify the processes that public health nurses carry out that lead to improved health outcomes with families. However, in the meantime nurses need to analyze and assess their day to day work with families. Family-focused community nursing provides an excellent opportunity to promote health practices, understand family processes that affect health, and intervene in a meaningful way at a preventive level. Public health nurses can be strong influences in promoting positive health outcomes for families by helping them make knowledgeable choices about their health.

REFERENCES

Ackerman, N. (1938). The family as a social and emotional unit. *Archives of Pediatrics, 55*, 51–61.

Baum, F. (1988). Community-based research for promoting the new public health. *Health Promotion, 3*(3), 259–268.

Barnes, A. (1985). The continuity of care in the family. *Nursing, 36*, 1051–1054.

Bateson, G., Jackson, D.D., Haley, J., & Weakland, J. (1956). Toward a theory of schizophrenia. *Behavioral Science, 1*(4), 251–264.

Bogdan, J.L. (1984). Family organization as an ecology of ideas: an alternative to the reification of family systems. *Family Process, 23*, 375–388.

Bowen, M. (1976). Theory in the practice of psychotherapy. In *Family Therapy* (Guerin, Jr., P.J., ed.), New York: Gardner Press.

Braverman, L. (1986). Beyond families: strategic family therapy and the female client. *Family Therapy, 8*, 143–152.

Breslow, L. (1978). Prospects for improving health through reducing risk factors. *Preventive Medicine, 1*, 449–458.

Brody, E.M. (1981). 'Women in the middle' and family help to older people. *Gerontologist, 21*(5), 471–480.

Brody, E.M., & Lang, A. (1982). 'They can't do it all': Aging daughters with aging mothers. *Generations, 7*, 18–20.

Burke, S. O. (1987). Assessing single-parent families with physically disabled children. In *Families and chronic illness* (Wright, M., & Leahey, M., eds), Springhouse, PA: Springhouse.

Campbell, J., & Humphreys, J. (1984). *Nursing care of victims of family violence.* Reston, VA: Reston.

Canada Health Survey. (1981). *The health of Canadians: Report on the Canada health survey* (No. 82-538E). Health and Welfare Canada, Ottawa.

Canadian Nurses Association. (1989). *Code of ethics for nursing.* Canadian Nurses Association, Ottawa.

Chalmers, K.I. (1984). Family nursing: the need for clearly defined frameworks for practice. *Proceedings of the conference 'Expanding the Scope of Nursing Practice: Development of Theoretical Frameworks'.* College of Nursing, University of Saskatchewan, Saskatoon, pp. 276–287.

Duvall, E.M. (1971). *Family development.* Philadelphia: J.B. Lippincott.

Fawcett, J. (1984). *Analyis and evaluation of conceptual models of nursing.* Philadelphia: F.A. Davis.

Fry, S.T. (1983). Dilemma in community health ethics. *Nursing Outlook, 31*(3), 176–179.

Garrett, G. (1985). Family care and the elderly. *Nursing, 36,* 1061–1063.

Gilliss, C., Highley, B., Roberts, B., & Martinson, I. (1989). *Toward a science of family nursing.* Don Mills, Ontario: Addison-Wesley.

Goldner, V. (1985). Feminism and family therapy. *Family Process, 24,* 31–47.

Goldner, V. (1987). Instrumentalism, feminism and the limits of family therapy. *Journal of Family Psychology, 1,* 109–116.

Goldner, V. (1988). Generation and gender: normative and covert hierarchies. *Family Process, 27,* 17–31.

Gortner, S.R. (1983). The history and philosophy of nursing science and research. *Advances in Nursing Science, 5*(2), 1–8.

Hamilton, P., & Bush, H. (1988). Theory development in community health nursing: issues. *Scholarly Inquiry for Nursing Practice, 12*(2), 145–160.

Hardy, M.E. (1978). Perspectives on nursing theory. *Advances in Nursing Science, 1*(1), 37–48.

Heckerman, C. (1980). *The evolving female: Women in psychosocial context.* New York: Human Sciences Press.

Kickbusch, I. (1987). Issues in health promotion. *Health Promotion, 1*(4), 437–442.

Kristjanson, L.J., & Chalmers, K.I. (1987). Nurse–client interactions in community based practice. Unpublished research report.

Kristjanson, L.J., & Chalmers, K.I. (1990). Nurse–client interactions in community based practice: creating common meaning. *Public Health Nursing, 7*(4).

Labonte, R. (1989). Community health promotion strategies. In *Readings for a new public health* (Martin, C., & McQueen, D., eds), Edinburgh: Edinburgh University Press, pp. 235–249.

Mace, N.L., & Rabins, P.V. (1981). *The 36-hour day.* Baltimore: Johns Hopkins University Press.

Martin, C., & McQueen, D. (1989). Framework for a new public health. In *Readings for a new public health* (Martin, C., & McQueen, D., eds), Edinburgh: Edinburgh University Press, pp. 1–10.

McKinlay, J.B. (1979). A case for re-focusing upstream: the political economy of illness. In *Physicians and illness,* 3rd ed. (Jaco, E.G., ed.), New York: The Free Press, pp. 9–25.

Minuchin, S., Montalvo, B., Guerney, B.G. Jr., Rosman, B.L., & Schumer, F. (1967). *Families of the slums: An exploration of their structure and treatment.* New York: Basic Books.

Minuchin, S., Rosman, B., & Baker, L. (1978). *Psychosomatic families.* Cambridge, MA: Harvard University Press.

Murray, R.B., & Zentner, J.P. (1979). *Nursing concepts for health promotion.* Englewood Cliffs, NJ: Prentice-Hall.

Oakley, A. (1980). *Women confined: Towards a sociology of childbirth.* Oxford: Martin Robertson.

Pender, N.J. (1987). *Health promotion in nursing practice.* Norwalk, CT: Appleton-Century-Crofts.

Pesznecker, B.L., & Zahlis, E. (1986). Establishing mutual-help groups for family-member care givers: a new role for community health nurses. *Public Health Nursing, 3*(1), 29–37.

Pratt, L. (1976). *Family structure and effective health behaviour: The energized family.* Boston: Houghton Mifflin.

Ramsay, J. (1985). Health behavior and compliance. In *Community health nursing in Canada* (Stewart, M., Innes, J., Searl, S., & Smillie, C., eds), Toronto: Gage, pp. 437–461.

Smoyak, S.A. (1987). Assessing aging families and their caretakers. In *Families and chronic illness* (Wright, M., & Leahey, M., eds), Springhouse, PA: Springhouse.

Sullivan, J.A. (1982). *Directions in community health nursing.* Oxford: Blackwell Scientific.

Wright, L., & Leahey, M. (1984). *Nurses and families: A guide to family assessment and intervention.* Philadelphia: F.A. Davis.

CHAPTER 32

Support for
Family Caregivers
in the Community

Susan R. Jacob

Family caregivers provide services to elderly relatives in the home, usually without the benefit of formal training. According to Horowitz,[1] research on families and
older adults has consistently documented that families, and especially adult children,
are the predominant health care providers for the impaired elderly. In the past, unmarried daughters were expected to care for their aging parents. Today, primary caregivers
in family settings are spouses, daughters, sisters, daughters-in-law, nieces, and friends.
Caregiving is primarily seen as women's responsibility; 85% of caregivers are female.
Women, viewed as nurturers and natural supports for the family, often find themselves
in a caregiving role.[2] Family caregivers enable older persons to remain in the community
and avoid institutionalization. However, they have been a neglected and invisible group.

The chances of developing chronic illness and severe disablement requiring help
in personal care activities increase with age. In 1985, approximately 5.2 million persons
aged 65 years or older were estimated to need assistance to remain at home in the
community. This figure is expected to reach 7.2 million by the year 2000, 10.1 million by
2020, and 14.4 million by 2050.[3] More people, therefore, will spend a part of their lives as
caregivers. In the past, even though the role of family caregiver was not uncommon, it
was still unexpected. It now has become so common that Brody[4] has suggested that the
caregiver role (particularly "parent care") be considered a normal and predictable life
course experience.

Reprinted from *Family & Community Health,* Vol. 14, No. 1, pp. 16–21, with permission of Aspen Publishers, Inc., © 1991.

CAREGIVER STRESS

Because of the increase in life expectancy, more older partners may end up caring for each other. Sixty percent of primary caregivers to older people are wives of disabled, often older husbands. Increasing numbers of the "old old" (aged 75 years and older) need assistance from spouses or children who are themselves aging. For older adult caregivers, the responsibilities associated with caregiving are compounded by their own physical disabilities and financial burdens. The stress may be even greater for recently married older couples with blended families.

A family caregiver faces a multitude of daily stresses, including the following:

- physical strain of assisting the patient in activities of daily living,
- isolation and loneliness,
- loss of privacy and personal control of time,
- lack of sleep,
- emotional reaction to the physical decline and anticipated death of a loved one,
- expense, and
- family distress.

Although there are major differences in how caregivers adapt to these stresses, when adults assume caretaking tasks for aging relatives they may feel overwhelmed. Support for families facing this task may be minimal or nonexistent.[5]

ASSESSMENT

Health care professionals who work with caregivers must understand the caregivers' burden to intervene effectively and promote healthy adaptation to the stress. They must evaluate family strengths and weaknesses when the initial assessment of the care receiver is made. Health care professionals must observe the family unit to determine the strength of established relationships. The health care team must get to know not only the older adult client, but also the caregiver and extended family, including likes and dislikes and burdens and joys. The team must make an effort to understand the family's organization and coping style and the impact of the illness or dependency on the system. Having to care for or be cared for by a family member can threaten the status and role of the older person and can create anger, resentment, and other negative feelings.[6]

Even in the most favorable family situations, guilt exists, and health care professionals need to take measures to counteract it. In addition, they need to communicate the normalcy of guilt, which results from feelings of helplessness and ambivalence. People like to feel needed and helpful; caregivers feel frustrated when, for example, the older adult has a poor appetite and the caregiver cannot entice him or her to eat. Health care professionals must communicate with families to help them understand and deal with the guilt that results from helplessness.[7]

Ambivalent feelings regarding caregiving also can surface and lead to guilt, especially when the caregiver's life goals are interrupted. The daughter who must retire early to care for an aging parent or the retired wife who can no longer look forward to traveling because of the disability of her husband may experience such feelings.

Health care professionals must assess the relationship between the family caregiver and the older adult to discover unresolved issues and negative feelings as well as sources of strength and resilience. It is very important to acknowledge and affirm the caregiver's efforts.[8] Plans can then be made to offer support, provide information, mobilize resources, and strengthen family weaknesses.[9]

When an older adult becomes unable to function independently and a family member agrees to serve as a caregiver, changes in the family's accustomed structure, patterns, and roles occur. These changes call for a reevaluation of old rules and a new flexibility. The health care professional should assess the family's financial and emotional roles and adaptation patterns by observing and talking with the family about the diagnosis and its impact on roles and relationships.

The primary needs of caregivers can be categorized as education or support. Health care professionals must accurately assess the family's educational and support needs before planning interventions to meet individual specific needs of the caregiver and the older adult and thus preserving the integrity and optimal functioning of the family system. Ultimately this process will result in quality health care of the older adult and caregiver.

EDUCATION

Health care professionals must educate caregivers about ways to promote an optimal level of functioning in the older adult. Demonstration, repetition, explanation, and question answering will guide caregivers as they become informed consumers.[10] Basic medical information about the older person's condition, disease course, symptoms, treatment, and medical management should be presented to the caregiver. In addition, health care professionals must provide information about behavioral problems and their management, the aging process, common family responses to caregiver stress, and available supportive community resources. Health care professionals who work with clients and caregivers in the home should help them compile a list of questions for their physicians to assist them in gathering appropriate information.[11]

The caregiver must be included as part of the team to enable him or her to better support the patient and work toward mutual goals. Information about the older adult's disease process must be shared. When the disease responds to treatment, the hope of a cure or remission should be shared. When disease appears to have escaped control, the family caregivers should also be informed. When the older adult and caregiver are not informed on the same level, the gap between their insights can become difficult to bridge and distancing in the relationship will most definitely occur.

There are several areas in which a caregiver can be essential in preventing additional disability and preserving the independence of the older adult. These include prevention of falls; prevention of acute illness, especially colds and influenza; special attention to any behavioral change that could indicate an undetected illness; and attention to drug interactions or intoxication.

Preventing falls reduces the risk of serious injury and disability. Caregivers must be educated in the evaluation of safety hazards in the home. Exposed cords, loose rugs, and improperly arranged furniture can be rearranged to lessen the risk of falling. Caregivers also need information and guidance in obtaining necessary medical equipment and assistive devices, such as handrails for the bathroom, walkers, bedside commode chairs, hospital beds, and bedside rails.

Education in the area of medications is vitally important. The home care nurse is often the most appropriate team member to instruct the caregiver in the organization and administration of medications. To ensure safety, the caregiver must be instructed in the desired effects and possible side effects that might occur.[12]

Health care professionals must also educate family caregivers about available community resources. In addition to the formal agency resources, the caregiver should also be instructed to evaluate untapped resources in the extended family and the informal network of friends and neighbors. Northouse[13] stressed the importance of teaching family caregivers to enhance the quality of care for the older adult by using both formal and informal support systems.

SUPPORT

Physical and emotional stress can lead to burnout if not dealt with effectively. For example, health care professionals can assist family caregivers by supporting care decisions made mutually with the older adult. Well-meaning friends and uninvolved family members may question the wisdom of caring for the older person at home with the support of home health or hospice services rather than hospitalizing him or her. Health care professionals can help caregivers feel positive about the decisions they have made.

Caregivers also must be reassured that feelings of guilt, anger, and resentment are neither uncommon nor bad. They should be cautioned that other people may offer well-meaning advice with an abundance of "shoulds" and "oughts" regarding the treatment of the older person. Caregivers need a larger dose of empathy than judgment from health care professionals.[6]

Support can also take the form of allowing caregivers to ventilate feelings. They often have a strong need to tell their story, and the importance of being able to communicate openly with someone who understands the situation is immeasurable. Caregivers need to feel that someone is available to talk with without having to wait 3 weeks for the next available office appointment.[11]

The role of the family caregiver is very challenging. Time off, even for a few hours a week, can enable the caregiver to continue providing care. Brief periods of emergency relief or prescheduled respite from the physical and emotional strain can reenergize a caregiver and renew his or her dedication to the role.[12] A wide variety of respite care solutions is available, but some caregivers are hesitant to arrange such services because they fear that others may not be able to "do it right." Health care professionals must help caregivers explore the range of options for relief. Whether the choice is in-home supportive service, day care, or a temporary overnight facility, such respite is vital to the caregiver's well-being.

Relief from emotional distress can also prevent elder abuse. Family members and caretakers may express their frustration in subtle ways, such as frequently reminding the patient that he or she is impaired and is a burden, talking to others about the older adult as if he or she were not in the room, and arguing with the older adult about unimportant issues.[11] The potential for elder abuse is greatest when caretakers have no relief from the constant burden of care. Visiting with friends, attending church or social gatherings, or simply spending time alone will promote relaxation and lower anxiety levels in the caregiver, leaving him or her refreshed and better able to cope with the caregiving burden.

Self-help groups have emerged as a popular source of support to cope with caring for an elderly relative.[14] The self-help process enables the caregiver to explore emotional, social, and financial issues faced by the family; to learn practical home care and behavior management techniques; and to gain access to formal and informal resources to relieve the burden of caregiving. Problem-solving is also a key skill learned and practiced in the groups.[15] Health care professionals should link the caregiver with such groups and provide a trained volunteer to stay with the older adult in the absence of the caregiver.

The caregiver's needs are as vital as the care receiver's needs, and the responsibility that the primary family caregiver has assumed for the care should be recognized. Health care professionals must become partners with the caregiver of the older adult to develop specific care plans involving an accurate assessment of the unique situation and individual intervention in the areas of education and support. This teamwork can help preserve this essential part of the caregiving network, ultimately resulting in the maintenance of the older adult in the home.

REFERENCES

1. Horowitz, A. Sons and daughters are caregivers to older parents: Differences in role performance and consequences. Presented at the 34th Annual Scientific Meeting of the Gerontological Society of America; November 1981; Toronto, Ontario, Canada.
2. Sommers, T. Caregiving: A woman's issue. *Generations* 1985; 10(1):9–13.
3. Stone, R., Cafferta, G., & Sangl, J. *Caregivers of the frail elderly: A national profile.* Washington, DC: US Dept of Health and Human Services; 1986.
4. Brody, E. Parent care as a normative family stress. *Gerontologist* 1985; 25:19–29.
5. Ebersole, P., & Hess, P. *Toward healthy aging.* St. Louis, MO: Mosby, 1985.
6. Eliopoulos, C. *Gerontological nursing.* Philadelphia: Lippincott, 1987.
7. Van Wormer, K. Guilt feelings in the spouse of the terminally ill. *Home Healthcare Nurse* 1985; 3(5):21–25.
8. Bernstein, L., Grieco, A., & Dete, M. *Primary care in the home.* Philadelphia: Lippincott, 1987.
9. Ward, B. Hospice home care programs. *Nurs Outlook* 1978; 26:646–649.
10. Archer, S., & Fleshman, R. *Community health nursing.* Belmont, CA: Wadsworth, 1985.
11. Cutler, L. Counseling caregivers. *Generations* 1985; 10(1):53–57.
12. Bould, S., Sanborn, B., & Rief, L. *Eighty-five plus.* Belmont, CA: Wadsworth, 1989.
13. Northouse, L. Who supports the support system? *J Psychiatric Nurs* 1980; 18(15):11–15.
14. Reever, K., & Thomas, E. Training facilitators of self-help groups for caregivers to elders. *Generations* 1985; 10(1):50–52.
15. Lieberman, M. Self-help groups. *Generations* 1985; 10(1):45–49.

CHAPTER 33

Nurses and Families: Partners in Care of the Patient with Alzheimer's Disease

Fay W. Whitney, Dorothea C. Pfohl

An explosion of interest in the needs, roles, and concerns of informal, family caregivers has occurred. As society grapples with the changing future demographics in which more elderly and fewer fiscal or human resources coexist, informal caregivers are becoming vital to the future health of the nation. Studies[1] describing chronic illnesses and disabilities among the elderly have grown in number, and increasingly, studies[2-7] concerning the value and effectiveness of caregivers and support groups among the elderly are appearing. Common problems among caregivers[8-10] and feasible methods for covering costs caregivers assume[11] have also been explored. Perhaps nowhere is the attention targeted toward this group more important than among families of patients with Alzheimer's disease (AD).

It is rare to find a person with AD whose illness affects solely that person; as T.S. Eliot so eloquently stated,

> It is often the case my patients are only pieces of a total situation which I have to explore. The single patient who is ill himself, is rather the exception.[12(p101)]

Nurses, too, soon learn that it is impossible to care adequately for people with AD unless the whole family is viewed as "the patient." This broader view of the patient requires a highly interactive process between nurses and families when the person with AD is admitted to the acute setting. Yet, the resources necessary to form a "caregiver partnership," where needs of the ill person, the family, and the nurse are met, are not

Reprinted from *Journal of Advanced Medical-Surgical Nursing, Vol. 1* (No. 2), March 1989, pp. 55–66, with permission of Aspen Publishers, Inc., © 1989.

always available. The purpose of this article is to identify special needs of people with AD, common family concerns, human needs of caregivers, issues related to caregiving, methods for assessing family needs, and some useful resources to help in laying groundwork for a successful caregiver partnership.

CHRONIC DEMENTIA IN THE ACUTE CARE SETTING

With economic incentives to shorten lengths of stay, there is increased external pressure on nurses and patients to truncate the recovery process and hasten discharge from the acute care setting. Chronic dementia in an acutely ill person adds greatly to the burden of mobilizing individual and institutional resources in a timely way. What often occurs is that little attention is paid to managing the chronic disease, yet all efforts to "cure" the acute illness seem to be impeded. The patient gets labeled as difficult, uncooperative, and noncompliant. Families become involved negatively and add to the burden of professional caregiving. In the extreme, the admission may end in unnecessary long-term institutionalization and leave behind a nursing staff convinced that elderly, demented people are impossible to care for in an acute care setting.

Special considerations need to be given to people with chronically altered mental states. The major chronic cognitive, expressive, and behavioral deficits AD patients exhibit preclude efficient and effective adaptation to new environments and situations. Small disruptions, even as small as an earache, can tumble the shaky structure upon which their functioning rests:

> The wife of one patient with AD emotionally recounts a trip to the emergency department (ED) following an episode at home in which her husband was suddenly incoherent, raging, and unable to stand or walk. She thought he was having a stroke. The ambulance crew had difficulty keeping him on the stretcher. Once at the ED, he was examined and found to have "only an ear infection." The physician prescribed antibiotics and discharged him, apparently oblivious to the fact that the wife could not control his behavior, had no transportation, could not be reimbursed for ambulance travel with this diagnosis, and was faced with a person whose acute episode of fever and pain had destroyed his fragile self-control, making him nearly impossible for her to manage. Admission was not even considered to stabilize him, and social services were not mobilized to aid her. She was finally able to recruit several neighbors to help her get him home, but was faced with several days of his sleeplessness, heightened wandering, and irascibility. He refused medication and believed that his wife had meant to abandon him at "that place." All of this inhibited his recovery from the ear infection and from regaining balance in his daily life with his chronic illness.

The fragility of this situation exemplifies what may happen to the chronically ill patient with AD and the family caregiver in any acute care setting. The very tenuous balance between function and nonfunction and between coping and noncoping is ever present. The diagnosis and the incapacity caused by it often do not correlate. The acute illness may be the "straw that breaks the camel's back," and the disproportionate inability of both the ill person and the family to cope requires alert, knowledgeable interventions. They are best served by cooperative planning between the nursing staff and the family that incorporates the usual daily activities and habits into the acute care plan.

COMMON FAMILY CONCERNS

Among caregivers to the ailing elderly, common problems that place them at risk for poor outcomes include (1) unremitting needs for supervision of and assistance to the elderly person; (2) tension caused by never knowing what will go wrong, or when; (3) inflexibility of scheduling; (4) financial burdens; (5) physical care of the dependent person when ill; (6) family differences over care of the family member; and (7) general environmental barriers to social outlets for elders.[13]

In addition, families caring for patients with AD must also deal with episodes of agitation and restlessness; apathy and helplessness; depression; aggressive, combative, and hostile behavior; suspicion and chronic mistrust; chronic negativism and defenselessness; and increasing loss of communication and recognition as the illness progresses. Often, the method used to cope with these difficult behaviors is to routinize activities, maintain fairly rigid schedules, and move toward changes slowly and deliberately. It is not surprising, then, that families who are suddenly faced with placing their relative in an acute care setting have enormous, immediate fears about what will happen to their loved one and to themselves. The family worries about how they can protect their relative from the results of so many changes. They wonder what will happen to the daily care plan they have worked out at home, whether or not the patient will die, whether the patient will ever go home again, and if the patient returns home, what life may be like when discharge occurs. Nurses who are alert to family needs and fears, and who spend the time to make the family members partners in care, can bring great comfort and speed recovery.

SHARED PERCEPTIONS

Glick gives some insight into the idea of sharing between professional and family caregivers:[14(p241,242)]

> Just as there is a person within every patient, there is behind every patient an "idea of person" that is the special preserve of family and friends. . . . These perceptions can only be shared in the most limited way by those who did not know the person. . . . This difficulty faced by health professionals and other strangers is compounded when the first encounter takes the form of a crisis in which the needs of the patient as a biological organism are paramount. From this disparity of perspectives emanates not only problems in patient management, but profound difficulties in communication with family and friends.

In communicating with formal caregivers about the patient with AD, families talk about what their loved one used to be like and try to convey an image of the better qualities of character that have been lost. It may seem as if family members are denying reality or that they are convincing themselves that things will be the same again. More often, however, families are trying to present a picture of the "whole person" that nursing staff cannot help but lack, and to engage the staff in looking at their relative as more than an "old, sick person."

Most families do *not* feel relieved of their primary responsibility to the family member simply because he or she is now housed in a different place. Studies[5,6] show that caregivers of the institutionalized spend as much time with their relatives as do those who have them at home, except for sleep hours. Nurses complain that they are unable to get family members to go home and rest, yet it is not uncommon to see the patient physically or chemically restrained in the acute care hospital when family members are not present to deal with the agitation or wandering that is probably inevitable. Strumpf and Evans[15] found that cognitively impaired patients vividly describe anger, discomfort, resistance, and fear in response to physical restraints. Obviously, the fears of the family are not unfounded. Allowing family members to participate realistically in care gives great peace of mind and helps them accept the need for different types of care when they are not available. Given the situation, staff and families need shared perceptions of what is safe, necessary, and appropriate.

MAJOR FAMILY NEEDS

Although these families have many needs, three main areas of concern repeatedly arise: the need for information about the diagnosis and the disease process,[3,6,10] financial help,[16,17] and legal advice.[16,18]

Diagnosis and Information Needs

Expanding public and professional awareness about AD and other dementing illnesses has encouraged earlier recognition of signs and symptoms, as well as interventions. Families seeking early assessment may now confront the implications of an incurable, fatal, and degenerative disease while the affected member is still functioning at a relatively unimpaired level. For some victims and their families, diagnosis explains the ambiguous and frightening state where there was noted decline, but where the cause had been attributed to failed relationships, mental illness, or other equally devastating life events. The diagnosis is the first step toward resolution of this fear and ambiguity. However, for others, diagnosis is the first step toward despair and dissolution of "normality."

There are a growing number of centers specializing in evaluation and diagnosis of the elderly and persons with concern about mental decline. Advances in neuropsychologic testing and sophisticated imaging techniques such as magnetic resonance imaging (MRI) and computed tomography (CT), as well as research options such as positron emission tomography (PET), allow professionals to assess patients more precisely and provide tentative diagnoses earlier in the course of the disease. CT and MRI have revealed[18] that there is cortical atrophy with ventricular enlargement in many cases of AD; PET scans show reduced metabolic rates, especially in the parietal-temporal areas, signifying decreased blood flow and oxygenation.[19] Neurotransmitter activity (such as decreases in somatostatinergic, catecholaminergic, and cholinergic activity) has also been studied in living humans using PET scans.[18] Lack of this type of evidence does not preclude AD, but its presence, in conjunction with appropriate clinical examination, allows some measure of certainty regarding the diagnosis.

Despite the growing availability of improved evaluation and diagnosis, many health care practitioners remain unaware of the importance of a comprehensive investigation to rule out secondary, treatable causes of dementia. One family reported in a group meeting that their doctor's response to the request for a full medical assessment was, "Why put her through it?" Yet this attitude may not only cause a misdiagnosis of a treatable dementia, it may preclude appropriate management of concurrent yet undiagnosed medical (ie, cardiac, endocrine) or psychologic problems (ie, depression, anxiety) that further compromise the AD patient when untreated. The needs of these people challenge the nurse to intervene compassionately, knowledgeably, and effectively with the afflicted person and the family in crisis. Part of that intervention may be advocacy for appropriate diagnosis.

It is best that families participate in the diagnostic evaluation process. Regardless of the response evoked by "labeling the disease," family members report that inability to gain knowledge about the disease and interact effectively with professionals about issues relating to management and prognosis of the disease are among their greatest caregiver burdens.[3] The areas of concern most often noted are lack of knowledge about etiology, the relationship to genetics and heredity, treatment alternatives, and everyday management routines. Until recently, there has been a paucity of information, but cellular pathology of the dementing diseases, the relationship to other diseases, and epidemiologic study of familial trends (eg, Down's syndrome, Parkinson's disease) are among the most active neurobiologic and clinical research areas[19,20] providing new information.

At the cellular level, more information about the neurofibrillary tangles and plaques that appear in greater numbers among patients with AD is now available. The tangles, made up of highly insoluble cross-linked peptides, have specific and distinct crossover patterns that may be related to the dynamic properties of neurons whose dysfunction and death are important to clinical expressions of the disease.[19] The symptoms of memory loss and behavioral changes, followed by personal withdrawal and clinically significant neurologic deficits, are probably due to a profusion of polypeptide plaques in the amygdala, hippocampus, and neocortex and changes in neurotransmitters produced there. Changes in the axons, myelin sheath, and nerve terminals in these particular brain centers probably account for dysfunction and change in the major somatostatinergic, catecholaminergic, and cholinergic systems that produce imbalances in integrating the mental system.

Etiology

Concern over etiology is associated with anxiety and guilt about how this disease might have been prevented, whether it is communicable, and what the link to other family members might be. Environmental and life-style precursors to the development of AD have been implicated (ingestion and metabolism of aluminum; slow virus infection) and are under study, but it is not generally believed that AD can be "caught" or prevented by avoiding any particular environmental conditions or life style. The guilt of not having done enough for the family member prior to the onset of the disease can be debunked and a great deal of mental stress relieved with this information.

Heredity and Genetics

In studying chromosome 21 in Down's syndrome,[20,21] researchers are exploring autosomal dominant genetic links to AD. Families watching the mental deterioration of a loved one fear that either they or their offspring will have a similar fate. It is important that families understand that there is evidence that AD is familial. Scientists[21,22] have determined that first-degree relatives (parents and siblings) of patients with AD have approximately 12% incidence of carrying the gene and that the mathematical probability of getting the disease is 4.3 times greater than the general public. Researchers stress, however, that these numbers do not reflect the *penetrance* (how many cases actually result) of AD in the adult population. There are generations in which no cases result that can be directly tied to a first-degree relative or the onset of the disease is so late in life that other diseases are the cause of death. Thus, it is more a possibility rather than a probability that first-degree relatives will also become AD victims,[21] and if they do, they are often five years or more older than the affected family member when it occurs.

Parents and siblings of Down's syndrome children have a higher risk; parents have the highest risk in this group. Still, Heston and colleagues[21] found that a third of all families in their study who had symptoms of dementia had secondary causes rather than familial causes. Their work corroborates the notion that both Down's syndrome children and patients with AD have a significant number of deaths from other causes, and for many, the onset of the dementia is very late in the normal life span of either group.

Nurses need to be cognizant of the latest data regarding familial tendencies and of the great toll that this information has on the caregiver's emotional well-being. The "facts" are not entirely clear as yet, but it is imperative that relatives of patients with AD receive competent genetic counseling because this information will have an impact on their childbearing decisions and on their concerns about their own susceptibility. Nurses can provide this resource by referring family members to medical colleagues with experience in this area, or to the Alzheimer's Disease and Related Disorders Association (ADRDA).

Financial Concerns

Dementing illness may create an overwhelming financial burden across several practical dimensions. A common and early complication of AD is the inability to perform normal work, with a resultant loss of employment. If the afflicted person is the primary wage earner, a significant means of support, as well as health insurance coverage, may be compromised at just the time when health care is most needed for hospitalization or diagnostic evaluation. Inability to manage financial affairs is also common even in early stages of the disease. If the caregiver is dependent financially and inexperienced in money matters, and if savings and investments have not been carefully managed, that caregiver may suddenly be forced to undertake financial management responsibilities under the most trying circumstances. The strain of worrying about immediate finances and future resources is thereby added to the burden of caregiving.

The wage earner who becomes the caregiver faces the dilemma of enduring escalating performance pressures in both roles. As the family's primary means of support, the caregiver/employee feels the strain of juggling time and energy to provide direct care, while knowing that failure to keep up at work could jeopardize income and health benefits, resources crucial to the long-term management of maintaining an impaired loved one. Even caregivers whose employment supplements family income (part-time workers or children of the impaired, for example) must grapple with the choice of whether to continue working and pay someone else to care for the family member or to stop working and take on the caregiving role directly.[2]

Further financial problems arise as the patient's ability to make financial decisions about his or her own resources decreases. For example, family members may become embroiled in "estate fights," arguing about how to protect the patient's funds set aside for heirs, while money for care is forgone or misspent. As legal and financial issues are often intertwined, family members, who are often inexperienced in these matters, are compelled to seek legal advice while avoiding exploitation by unethical professionals. Thus, beyond the physical management of the patient and the attendant feelings of loss and grief, family caregivers confront tremendous life-style adjustments related to financial changes and setbacks.

LEGAL CONCERNS

Because of the inevitable decline in cognitive and functional ability over the course of the disease, the major legal considerations for patients with AD and families are competence and guardianship.[16] Gottleib and Reisberg[16] make the following points: (1) Until recently, most competency legislation in the United States had an "all or nothing" approach to determining competence, with only 10 states providing for regular review of the need for continued guardianship. (2) Competency hearings are rarely attended by the individual in question, yet appointment of a guardian is frequent. (3) Because AD has been primarily a diagnosis of exclusion, the assessment and definition of competency has been inadequate to accommodate the changing needs of the individual over time and to allow maximal function where possible.

Caregivers, who have difficult emotional choices to make regarding competency, have not been well served by past statutes; however, some changes are occurring. In 1984, the National Institute of Neurological and Communicative Disorders and Stroke and the Alzheimer's Disease and Related Disorders Association (NINCDS-ADRDA) Work Group recognized the need for a better method of objectively assessing these patients and developed preliminary criteria for use as guides in categorizing probable, possible, and definite diagnoses for patients with AD.[1] Helpful as these changes are, there are still major difficulties to be faced regarding the compromised loved one. For instance, many families are faced with the question of whether to prolong a relative's life with elective procedures, forced-feeding, or experimental drugs and procedures. These families, regardless of their legal standing, may need to make such decisions based on their best guess of "what the patient would have wanted." Nurses can help patients and families face the inevitable need for such decisions early in the disease, when cognitive impairment has not yet rendered patients unable to make their own decision on whether to prolong life through technological means. Durable power of attorney with a health care clause[18] may not be useful in some states, but it can inform decisions in the future by representing the then incompetent patient. It is useful in helping families sort through differences between their opinions and the wishes of the AD victim, and to work through ethical dilemmas that will inevitably occur.

HUMAN NEEDS OF CAREGIVERS

Despite the challenge and heartbreak of dementing illness, despair and hopelessness do not automatically overcome caregivers. In fact, there are many reports of positive outcomes related to increasing caregiver burdens.[17,23] Some families draw closer together to mount the needed effort to support the afflicted family member. Spouses find new strengths and bonds in fulfilling caregiving roles. This is exemplified in one wife's statement, "I never knew that I could manage so well. . . . [taking care of my husband] has made me more appreciative of how he spent all those years trying to provide for us and how much it must have cost him. That, too, is a kind of loving."

Nevertheless, caregivers cannot always manage, and it is difficult for nurses who have only brief glimpses of the caregiver and family to know what may be the most pressing needs. Although it is true that each situation is unique, caregivers of AD victims have surprisingly similar problems and needs.[3,10] In discussing caregiver distress, several authors[9,23,24] agree that the severity of cognitive dysfunction or loss of functional ability in daily care are not the major variables. Instead, it is the AD victim's disruptive behavior, increasing withdrawal, apathy, and poor physical self-maintenance that cause social isolation and loneliness for the caregiver that are responsible for the greatest personal distress. A comment overhead at a conference for caregivers—"a sure way not to get invited to dinner parties is to get Alzheimer's disease"—hints at the pain once socially active people feel when friends withdraw. But, it does not represent the depth of anger, disappointment, fear, and grief felt by socially stigmatized caregivers who must invest scarce energy in building new networks at a time when they are on the verge of social and financial bankruptcy. Gwyther[6] suggests that organized family support groups are of great importance in

- establishing new social bonds;
- defusing fear, anger, guilt, and despair;
- helping to manage the concept of stigmatizing responses;
- providing collective advocacy; and
- decreasing the trauma and loneliness associated with grief and loss.

Participants in support groups such as ADRDA chapters routinely show courage that gives testimony to the everyday heroism in the human spirit, creating an environment described as "inspirational, intensely emotional, and never boring." Support groups empower families to cope by substituting for lost social opportunities, legitimizing the caregiving role, and providing useful, applicable information. Nurses need to be aware of the support groups available in their area, and if there are none, they should start one!

In an excellent review of the literature, Clark and Rakowski[3] categorize caregiving tasks in three areas, each containing several items:

1. task of providing direct services (14 items),
2. personal tasks (19 items), and
3. familial (8 items) and societal tasks (4 items).

Among those tasks noted as especially stressful or difficult, only the task of providing care required for activities of daily living was noted in the first category.

In the second category, seven of the 19 items emphasized feelings of guilt and disappointment over the caregiver's ability to provide safe, appropriate care, general need to keep up physical and emotional strength in the face of constant demand, decreased personal time, and lack of knowledge about the disease. The third category includes managing feelings of those family members who are not involved in caregiving and balancing other family roles; among societal problems, dealing with professionals involved in care of the loved one was the top issue. Already burdened family caregivers must often act as their own case managers in a system that apparently provides them with little information, contact, or support and that makes them feel abandoned.

Ware and Carper[24] and George[5] corroborate the need of caregivers for relief from mental and physical demands; opportunities for guilt and grief resolution; help in time and energy management for other family demands; need for increased social interaction to decrease isolation and loneliness; and recognition and treatment of depression, anxiety, and exhaustion. Most caregivers studied did not suffer from increases in poor physical health[5] as much as mental health problems. However, nurses know empirically that health problems are rampant among people burdened with relentless life stresses. The welfare of informal, family caregivers is of prime importance, and the development of preventive, health-promoting, and supportive measures should be a priority of health care workers.

ISSUES RELATED TO CAREGIVING

Neglect and Abuse

The unceasing stress associated with caring for a demented patient creates opportunities for excesses and abuses. Copstead and Paterson[13] identify signs and symptoms of incompatibility among family members who have generally healthy aging relatives. Signs of possible neglect or abuse by the family may be seen in open hostility, distancing from and avoidance of the elder, negative criticism, and noticeable poor hygiene or nutrition in the elder. The elder may show fear, withdrawal, cognitive changes, depression or paranoia, or hostility toward the family.

Frustration, fatigue, depression, and anger may lead to neglect or abuse of the dependent and debilitated patient with AD, but it may be more difficult to detect, since some of the warning signs in the elder may appear to be part of the disease process. Elder abusers need help. If abuse is suspected, adult protective services are responsive and can advise professionals or caregivers who are not involved. Area agencies on aging (AOA) can provide some of the support services that may be needed to relieve the caregiver's stress (eg, home health aides, Meals on Wheels, transportation). Physical and verbal abuse may also be directed at the caregiver by the demented person who may still be capable, however unknowingly, of cruelty. Even devoted caregivers express guilt about not being able to personally provide all that the loved one needs. Some blame themselves for the abuse they receive, while others are willing to accept the behavior saying, "He isn't himself. He doesn't know what he's doing." Nonetheless, abuse breaks the spirit, and nurses should be alert to its manifestations in both the caregiver and the patient.

Substance Abuse

Both the patient and the caregiver may have had active or historical substance abuse before onset of the illness. Caregivers may seek relief or escape through food, drugs, or alcohol. They may use any of these to "calm" the disruptive patient with AD or inadvertently leave those items in easily accessible areas where the AD patient can ingest them indiscriminately. Substance abuse in the patient may be precipitated by the memory loss associated with the disease. AD patients may forget that they have a drink already, or a bowl of ice cream, and will proceed to have another, and another. Whatever the cause, substance abuse by either the caregiver or the AD victim only complicates the problems they have and serves to destroy an already tenuous situation.

These two issues serve to remind nurses that AD patients and their families are subject to the same difficulties as families without an AD relative. More important, both types of families have many of the same strengths. It is equally important for nurses to be knowledgeable about the major problems of caregivers as it is to view the patient and caregiver as a positive, dynamic unit.

RESOURCES

It is impossible to know of or have access to all resources that families will need to deal with individual problems. However, access to knowledge is important, and a list of recent, readable references is included (see Suggested Readings). This list includes books that are useful for either the family or the professional with limited experience with patients with AD.

A frequent question put to nurses is: "Who do I ask about how to deal with this disease?" Fortunately, in most cases, nurses can refer family members to ADRDA, a strong and reliable network. The national office can direct the family to local chapters; their own resources; or direct the family to local organizations, lawyers, and health resources that are familiar with AD patient problems.

Information about diagnostic centers, day-care centers, respite care, legal advisors, and other services vary among regions. Guidelines for choosing these services are offered by ADRDA, by the American Association of Retired People (AARP), in some books,[25] and through local chapters of other rehabilitation and disability support groups. An important ingredient that nurses bring to the informal caregiver is providing access to networks and a caring attitude that allow family caregivers to maximize their external and internal resources.

Family caregivers who care for aging and disabled relatives are among the nation's most valuable resources. Nurses and families who care for patients with AD can become partners in caregiving through sharing of burdens, resources, and understanding. It is a road fraught with curves, potholes, and long hills to climb, but along the way, there are incredible glimpses of courage, love, and humor. In describing the combined efforts of professional and family caregivers to help brain-damaged people travel along this difficult road, Glick says,

> Even if the person should never emerge to embody the idea of the person that the family has cherished, even if the campaign that the staff has waged on behalf of the patient should never succeed, the process of shared commitment is important for those survivors, both family and staff, who have cared greatly.[14(p245)]

REFERENCES

1. Ory, M.G., Williams, T.F., Emr, M., et al. Families, informal supports, and Alzheimer's disease: Current research and future agendas. *Res Aging* 1985;7:623–644.
2. Brody, E.M. Testimony on the effects of Alzheimer's disease on caregiving families. Presented to the Committee on Energy and Commerce, Subcommittee on Health and the Environment, and the Select Committee on Aging, Subcommittee on Long-Term Care, Washington, DC, August, 1983.
3. Clark, N.M., & Rakowski, W. Family caregivers of older adults: Improving helping skills. *Gerontologist* 1983;23:637–641.
4. Deimling, G.T., & Bass, D.M. Symptoms of mental impairment among elderly adults and their effects on family caregivers. *J Gerontol* 1986;41:778–784.
5. George, L.K. The burden of caregiving: How much? What kinds? For whom? in *Center reports on advances in research.* Durham, NC: Duke University Center for the Study of Aging and Human Development, 1984, vol 8, pp. 1–7.
6. Gwyther, L. Caring for caregivers: A statewide family support program mobilizes mutual help in *Center reports on advances in research.* Durham, NC: Duke University Center for the Study of Aging and Human Development, 1982, vol 6, pp. 1–8.
7. Zarit, S.H., & Zarit, J.M. Families under stress: Interventions for caregivers of senile dementia patients. *Psychotherapy* 1983;19:461–471.
8. Kahan, J., Kemp, B., Staples, F.R., et al. Decreasing the burden in families caring for a relative with a dementing illness. *J Am Geriatr Soc* 1985;35:664–1985.
9. Greene, J.G., Smith, R., Gardiner, M., et al. Measuring behavioral disturbance of elderly demented patients in the community and its effects on relatives: A factor analytic study. *Age Ageing* 1982;11:121–126.
10. Barnes, R.F., Raskind, M.A., Scott, M.A., et al. Problems of families caring for Alzheimer Patients: Use of a support group. *J Am Geriatr Soc* 1981;29:80–85.

11. Arling, G., & McAuley, W.J. The feasibility of public payments for family caregiving. *Gerontologist* 1983;23:300–306.
12. Eliot, T.S. *The cocktail party.* New York: Harcourt Brace, 1954, p. 101.
13. Copstead, L., & Paterson, S. Families of the elderly, in Carnevali, D.L., & Patrick, M. (eds): *Nursing management for the elderly.* Philadelphia: JB Lippincott, 1986.
14. Glick, T.H. *The process of neurologic care in medical practice.* Cambridge, MA: The Harvard Univ. Press, 1984.
15. Strumpf, N.E., & Evans, L.K. Physical restraint of the hospitalized elderly: Perceptions of patients and nurses. *Nurs Res* 1988;37:132–137.
16. Gottleib, G.L., & Reisberg, B. Legal issues in Alzheimer's disease. *Am J Alzheimer's Care Relat Disord* 1988;3:24–36.
17. Zarit, S.H., Reever, K.E., & Bach-Peterson, J. Relatives of the impaired elderly: Correlate of feelings of burden. *Gerontology* 1980;20:649–655.
18. We rage against it, but being prepared helps relieve the darkness when saying final goodbyes. *Modern Maturity* June-July 1988; 29–33, 88–92.
19. Price, D.L., Kitt, C.A., Struble, R.G., et al. Neurobiological studies of transmitter systems in aging and in Alzheimer-type dementia. *Ann NY Acad Sci* 1985;457:35–51.
20. Sinex, F.M., & Merrill, C.R. (eds). Alzheimer's disease, Down's syndrome, and aging. *Ann NY Acad Sci* 1982;396.
21. Heston, L.L. Alzheimer's dementia and Down's syndrome: Genetic evidence suggesting an association. *Ann NY Acad Sci* 1982;396:29–37.
22. Larsson, T., Sjogren, T., & Jacobsen, G. A clinical, sociomedical and genetic study. *Acta Psychiatr Scand* 1963;167(suppl):1–259.
23. Lebowitz, B. Families, informal supports and Alzheimer's disease. Position paper submitted to the National Institute on Aging, September, 1983.
24. Ware, L.A., & Carper, M. Living with Alzheimer's disease patients: Family stresses and coping mechanisms. Presented at the meeting of the American Psychological Association, Los Angeles, 1981.
25. Mace, N., & Rabins, P. *The 36-hour day.* Baltimore: Johns Hopkins Univ. Press, 1981.

SUGGESTED READINGS

Brown, D.S. *Handle with care: A question of Alzheimer's.* Buffalo, NY: Prometheus Books, 1985.
Burnside, I.M. (ed). Alzheimer's disease: An in-depth report/1982–1983. *J Gerontol Nurs* 1983;9:1–68.
Carnevali, D.L., & Patrick, M. *Nursing management for the elderly,* ed 2. Philadelphia: JB Lippincott, 1986.
Cohen, D., & Eisdorfer, C. *The loss of self: A family resource for the care of AD and related disorders.* New York: Norton, 1986.
Gwyther, L.P. *Care of Alzheimer's patients: A manual for nursing home staff.* Durham, NC: American Health Care Association and ADRDA, 1985.
Heston, L.L., & White, J.A. *Dementia: A practical guide to Alzheimer's disease and related illness.* New York: WH Freeman, 1983.
Mace, N.L., & Rabins, P.V. *The 36-hour day.* Baltimore: Johns Hopkins Univ. Press, 1981.
Powell, L.S., & Courtice, K. *Alzheimer's disease: A guide for families.* Reading, MA: Addison-Wesley, 1983.
Reisberg, B. *A guide to Alzheimer's disease.* New York: Free Press, 1981.
Roach, M. *Another name for madness.* Boston: Houghton Mifflin, 1985.
Terry, R.D., & Katzman, R. Senile dementia of the Alzheimer type. *Ann Neurol* 1983;14:497–506.
Wells, C.E. *Dementia.* Philadelphia: FA Davis, 1977.
Zarit, S.H., Orr, N.K., & Zarit, J.M. *Caring for the patient with Alzheimer's disease: Families under stress.* New York: New York Univ. Press, 1985.

CHAPTER 34

Assessing and Intervening with Dysfunctional Families

Sue P. Heiney

The pediatric oncology nurse often is faced with assessing and supporting families who are coping with a chronic, yet life-threatening illness. To differentiate families with significant psychopathology from families experiencing situational stress related to the impact of the illness, the nurse needs a framework for accurately assessing the family's ability to function. The concepts, emotional system, differentiation, and triangling are from Murray Bowen's theory of family functioning. Also discussed are specific intervention strategies, such as supporting the executive subsystem, promoting the family's mental health, reframing negatives, and modeling positive communication. This paper cites examples of situations in which these strategies are effectively employed and discusses guidelines for a referral.

The pediatric oncology nurse often is faced with assessing and supporting families who are coping with a chronic, yet life-threatening illness.[1] The chronic nature of the illness contributes to internal conflict due to medical, personal and social stresses.[2] Research findings documenting the effects of these stresses have been conflicting.[2-6] Although these stresses do not affect the divorce rate, for example, they may "pile up" and decrease the quality of the marital relationship.[2,3] The nurse is challenged to screen families at risk of developing difficulties while supporting healthy family adaptation.[6]

Reprinted from the *Oncology Nursing Forum* with permission from the Oncology Nursing Press, Inc. Heiney, Sue P. Assessing and Intervening with Dysfunctional Families. *Oncology Nursing Forum 15* (5):585–90, 1988.

To identify families with significant psychopathology, the nurse needs a framework for making an accurate assessment of the family's functioning. The many hours spent caring for the patient provide an opportunity to observe and interact with the family, and to identify possible dysfunction by using a theory of family functioning. The difficulty in assessment is being able to temporarily ignore responses to stress and instead to become adept at focusing on family interaction and characterizing these dynamics as either functional or dysfunctional. To validate the accuracy of this assessment, the nurse may want to consult with other team members. The social worker, chaplain, psychologist, or mental health clinical nurse specialist may add insights and aid in assessment. Using this framework and a team approach to assessment, the nurse can determine whether the family needs emotional support from the health care team or needs referral to a mental health professional.

Bowen's theory of family functioning is one framework the nurse may use in assessing a family's mental health. This theory describes three concepts regarding family interaction that may assist the nurse in assessment: the emotional system, individual differentiation, and triangling.[7] See Figure 1 for a summary of these three concepts.

EMOTIONAL SYSTEM

In Bowen's theory, the emotional system of the family refers to the force that motivates the family system and describes patterns of emotional functioning in a family. These patterns are expressed through relationships formed within the family system.[7,8] In the healthy family, these relationships foster growth and development in children and encourage independence and positive self-esteem in all family members. Additionally, healthy families are flexible and can adapt to change.[9] For example, in one family with three children, the mother was three months pregnant when the two-year-old son's cancer was diagnosed. Even though this was another major stressor and a major life change, the parents still managed to both work and adapt to the illness and a new baby. They often rotated bringing the sick child for therapy so neither was overburdened.

In the dysfunctional family, three patterns may emerge indicating that individuals are having difficulty with conflict resolution and problem-solving: excessive marital conflict, over-adequate/inadequate reciprocity, and the projection process.[10] Looking for these patterns is part of the assessment for dysfunction.

Bowen's Family Concepts for Assessment

Emotional System: Patterns of emotional functioning.
Differentiation: A sense of individuality and separateness among family members.
Undifferentiation: "Stuck togetherness" or fusion; an excessive sense of emotional closeness in family members.
Triangling: A pattern of interaction among family members when two people are emotionally very close and a third family member is emotionally very distant.

FIGURE 1. A summary of Bowen's family concepts.

In excessive marital conflict the parents cannot resolve issues or work through problems. Arguments are repeated over and over and may escalate into abuse.[8] The nurse may be alerted to this if both parents, at separate times, want to discuss a decision that needs to be made. The nurse may wonder why the parents have not discussed this at home. This same pattern may be noticed over several successive clinic visits. For example, in one family with numerous children, the parents were unable to develop a plan to assure that siblings were kept abreast of the sick child's status. With each diagnostic test or change in the child's treatment, the couple argued about what to tell the siblings, when to talk to them, and who should talk to them. They usually were unable to agree. If an agreement was reached, no actual follow-up occurred. Consequently, the other children were kept in suspense about the brother's illness, intensifying the distress with the family system.

The second pattern is *over-adequate/inadequate reciprocity* which occurs when one spouse functions at the expense of the other or seems to draw energy from the other.[7] For instance, this pattern of functioning may be suspected when one parent calls the treatment center frequently with trivial questions or continually asks the same questions. The other parent, however, is either never heard from or always seems calm and competent in any interactions with staff. In this example, the extremely anxious parent appears inadequate and unable to cope. This overt observation may be inaccurate. Upon further observation, the other spouse, while appearing excessively competent, is just as insecure. For example, during a support group meeting, the husband, who previously seemed unemotional and to be coping well, begins crying and sharing his fear that this son will not live. This behavior contradicts his usual calmness, in spite of the fact the staff perceived the frequently tearful wife as the only family member having difficulty coping.

Bowen's third observable pattern is the *projection process.* This pattern occurs when the parents' anxiety and conflict spill over and are manifested in the child's behavior. The "acting out" child, through his misbehavior, gives the parents an alternative focus for their energy instead of their own conflict. By misbehaving, the child helps to maintain peace between the parents and "saves" their relationship.[8] For example, during an outpatient appointment, the nurse and a mother discussed the mother's concern about her son's temper tantrums. The nurse practitioner advised her to use limit setting and "time-out" as consequences to the tantrums. This plan was discussed at length, and the importance of the father's participation was stressed. During the next clinic visit, the mother related that she "just never got around to trying the technique." However, the mother continued to talk about the tantrums and how the parents spent all their time trying to satisfy the child.

The occurrence of any of these three patterns in the family's emotional system— *excessive marital conflict, over-adequate/inadequate reciprocity,* and *projection process*—may appear temporarily in healthy families experiencing high stress. When these processes occur repeatedly and to the exclusion of other coping mechanisms, they usually indicate a dysfunctional family. Positive coping strategies in healthy families include having a cognitive understanding of the illness, communicating about the illness to the immediate and extended family, expressing appropriate feelings concerning the illness, and emphasizing the positive.[6,10] Prior to intervening with the family, further assessment into other aspects of the family's functioning should be completed.

DIFFERENTIATION

The second major concept from Bowen's theory of family functioning, individual differentiation, describes the amount of emotional maturity in an individual within the family system.[7] Individuals with poor differentiation have a great degree of fusion between their emotions and thoughts. Such people have behavior patterns that seem automatic and preset; their emotions seem to drive their intellectual systems. They form dependent relationships that are very susceptible to stress, become dysfunctional easily, and have difficulty recovering. Conversely, individuals who are able to separate thoughts from feelings, who are able to choose between intimacy and purposeful activity, and who can derive pleasure and satisfaction from either state, are differentiated.[11]

When undifferentiated individuals marry, they appear to be stuck together or fused to one another. This sense of fusion continues when children are born and pervades most aspects of family life. The family exhibits several common characteristics related to the fusion or undifferentiation. In assessing for differentiation, the nurse may observe either individuals within the family or the family as a unit. If assessment indicates that the characteristics discussed below are present in a family, the nurse may infer that the family is undifferentiated, which is another indicator of dysfunction.

First, undifferentiated individuals do not have a clear sense of themselves as separate from other family members. In such families, individuals may describe themselves as very close to one another. They may be "up" when the patient is doing well and "down" if the patient does poorly. For example, in discussing the patient's illness, the mother may use the word "we" frequently, and may speak for the patient by saying such things as "we are losing our hair." In a healthy family, the parents might express concern that the hair loss is causing the teenager to feel depressed. They would relate how the teenager had behaved and what he/she had said when the hair started falling out. In a healthy family, the nurse would be able to discern between feelings of the parent and those of the teenager.

Second, undifferentiated family members may seem so connected that only one set of beliefs or ideas is acceptable. The issue of discipline will frequently elicit conflict. The mind-set that there is one "right" way to manage the child's behavior will be voiced. Each parent may think that his or her method is the best and should always be used by both parents. For example, the father will want to spank, and the mother will want to talk to the child. Each will claim that the other's method is ineffective and not what the "experts" recommend. Both parents seem unwilling to objectively evaluate the other's method.[12] In a healthy family, several solutions might be possible. For example, the parents might compromise and agree that spanking is appropriate for some offenses and then would clearly define these offenses to the child. When the child misbehaved, either parent would willingly carry out the agreed upon punishment. In this situation, the parents are able to communicate and problem-solve.

Finally, undifferentiated family members react emotionally to one another without any attempt to think through issues or situations. This reaction is obvious during situations of high anxiety such as bone marrow aspirations or biopsies. During the procedure, the child seems to sense the parent's fright and reacts by being extremely uncooperative. The tearful parents stand by helplessly while the child kicks, screams, or bites the staff. The parents are unable to support the child because they cannot separate the child's feelings from their own. In a functional family, the parents would be able to discuss their own anxiety and seek ways to manage their fear so that they could support the child.

TRIANGLING

The family should be evaluated for the presence of triangling, a third component of Bowen's theory. Triangling occurs when individuals respond to high stress by automatically interacting with family members in a fixed rigid pattern.[7] This pattern, two people close and a third one distant, can be visualized by thinking of a triangle with two long equidistant sides and one short side (see Figure 2). An absence of triangling in families could be diagrammed as an equilateral triangle.

Triangling in families is inferred from observation of family interaction (particularly during periods of high stress), descriptions of family relationships, and discussions about conflict resolution. Typically, two family members will distance themselves from each other by pulling in a third person in order to avoid overt conflict. Interaction might include instances when one spouse sides with a child against the other spouse, when

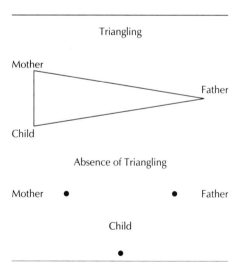

FIGURE 2. Diagrammatic representation of triangling, a concept of Bowen's theory of family functioning.

the couple may talk about each other to a third person, or when an issue rather than their conflict is discussed.[11] For example, the mother may state that she is very close to the sick child. The father may infer that another child is his favorite and that they are very close. Or the sick child may be referred to as the mother's child and another child referred to as the father's child.

Each parent may bitterly criticize the other parent to the nurse. The nurse may be pulled into the family's emotionalism and may feel impelled to react to whatever situation the family is confronting. The nurse should be alert to being aligned with one family member against another. Such alignment could be an indication that the family has triangled the nurse into their conflict.[13]

ASSESSMENT SUMMARY

Family assessment is not an exact science. Therefore, the nurse is encouraged to be as objective as possible when assessing the family and making observations about the emotional system of the family, the differentiation of the family members, and the presence of triangling. The frequency and intensity of all three should be identified and described in the family assessment. Table 1 outlines contrasting functional and dysfunctional characteristics.

TABLE 1
Assessment Summary for Functional Versus Dysfunctional Family Characteristics

Functional	Dysfunctional
Emotional System	Emotional System
Independence is encouraged	Dependence is encouraged
Positive self-esteem promoted	One person is "identified" as "problem"
Positive conflict resolution	Negative conflict resolution
Adapts to change	Repetitive, rigid use of ineffective coping
Differentiation	Lack of Differentiation
Relationships foster emotional maturity	Emotional immaturity encouraged
Thoughts separated from feelings	Thoughts and feelings are enmeshed
Sense of separateness among family members	Sense of fusion
Differences of opinion are allowed and encouraged	Differences of opinion are unacceptable
Problem-solving to generate solutions to concerns occurs	Family members do not think through alternatives to problems
Absence of Triangling	Triangling
Patterns of interaction among family members are flexible and adaptive to the situation	Patterns of interaction among family members are fixed and rigid

The nurse should note the amount of conflict and the way in which conflict is handled. Additionally, the nurse should ascertain if coping styles are congruent and if one parent seems to overcompensate for the other. The nurse should observe how the children fit into the family and whether they serve as a buffer to dull the parents' feelings toward each other. The nurse should assess for high levels of dependence and decreased self-esteem and whether the family is concerned about the lack of initiative in family members. Finally, the nurse can assess for excessively rigid relationships among family members. These examples of family functioning are indicators of an unhealthy family system, especially when they are fixed and rigid.

Through these observations, the nurse obtains a composite picture of family functioning. Noting negative processes would alert the nurse to possible psychopathology. This dysfunction is differentiated from a reaction to situational stress by the intensity and duration of the processes and by the type of processes. Assessment of healthy families experiencing stress or a crisis may show some of the dysfunctional processes described above, but these occur only on a sporadic basis. The more typical picture of a reaction to crisis or acute stress shows a short period of cognitive disorganization and emotional lability followed by attempts to master the situation. In contrast, the dysfunctional family continues to exhibit negative processes within the family along with inflexible responses to stress. A pattern, not just the presence of a particular process, is the greatest indicator of psychopathology.[9] A picture of dysfunction is not always easy to identify; even experienced mental health professionals do not always agree on dysfunction. A nurse should strive to understand family functioning and to improve assessment skills so that judgments are as unbiased and as accurate as possible.

FAMILY INTERVENTIONS

When a family appears to be either dysfunctional or experiencing temporary disequilibrium, the nurse needs to develop a plan for supporting the family and/or make a mental health referral. Interventions derived from family therapy strategies also can be used to help the healthy family adapt to stressful situations, such as situational stress, or improve family functioning.

Parents as a Primary Focus

Targeting the parents as the primary focus for alleviating anxiety is an intervention based on two premises. First, children experience and express anxiety within the context of the family. Parents may communicate anxiety to the child and may reinforce anxiety felt by the child.[14,15] Second, parents are the executives of the family and determine how the family will cope. Therefore, it is doubly important to support the parents so they can give age-appropriate comfort to the child or adolescent.[15] The purpose of this intervention is to stop the cycle of anxiety by alleviating parental anxiety thereby promoting parental functioning. The natural tendency may be to support the child and decrease his/her anxiety. However, efforts should be directed toward decreasing parental anxiety and involving them in the process of supporting the child to increase their sense of competence. Supporting the child is a short-term approach that temporarily may alleviate the problem but, without parental involvement, is less likely to achieve desired long-term results.

The parents should be supported by identifying the source of their anxiety. For example, a five-year-old was usually very difficult to examine. His mother appeared extremely upset as the nurse practitioner tried to get the child to cooperate. During the examination, the nurse practitioner learned that the mother had dreamed that the examination would reveal that her child had relapsed.

Parents also can be supported by ascertaining what concerns they have about clinical issues. The nurse then can offer information about procedures, tests, or the child's illness. The nurse also could demonstrate stress management techniques that help the child to be more cooperative during procedures. For example, parents could be taught and encouraged to practice relaxation techniques and could coach the child in learning these techniques.

The developmental age of the child should be considered. The nurse must recognize the emerging independence of the adolescent while attending to the influence of the family system on the patient. With the older adolescent, the nurse may want to discuss clinical issues and concerns with both the teenager and parent. For example, when discussing the need for a bone marrow, the nurse practitioner gave both the parents and the teenager time to ask questions.

Promoting Mental Health

A second intervention is to promote the family's mental health,[16] aiming toward long-term support of the child by strengthening any positive dynamics that occur in the family. The nurse first should focus on positives rather than negatives so the family will respond to the positive reinforcement the nurse is providing. For example, one mother displayed excessive amounts of denial in coping with her child's illness. This denial did not interfere with the mother being rational about her child. The denial allowed the mother to spend time with her other children and to appropriately discipline the sick child. When the staff began to focus on the positive aspects of the denial, they could relate to the mother with less disapproval. This mother subsequently took part in several parent groups and was able to help other parents see the need to attend to the needs of other children in the family. As the nurse shifts to a more positive perspective on the family's methods of coping, the family exhibits positive dynamics in response to the expectation of the nurse. In this same example, the mother became more open with the staff.

Reframing Negatives

Another technique that can promote family mental health is changing the environment in which the family functions.[16] Reframing involves changing a negative label for a behavior into a positive one. To reframe a negative behavior, the nurse must identify a positive counterpart to the behavior. This does not mean the nurse is positive about the negative behavior or projects a positive attitude hoping that the behavior will improve. Instead, the nurse highlights some aspect of the behavior which, if enhanced, could become a positive force. For example, when patients exhibit uncooperative and belligerent behavior, they may evoke a defensive reaction from parents, friends, and staff. If this behavior could be relabeled as efforts toward independence, parents and others could provide situations that would promote growth toward maturity.

Positive Communication

Another intervention is to *model positive communication,* providing the family with a behavioral example of appropriate communication by the manner in which interactions occur. Positive communication includes strategies, such as assertiveness and active listening skills, to maintain an effective relationship with the family while improving family interaction.[17] Modeling is particularly important to use when working with dysfunctional families who seem to thwart efforts to interact with them. The nurse's instinctive response is to avoid these families because of their resistance to interventions.

One way to integrate the technique is to ask family members what they think about a particular issue rather than how they feel about it. This strategy is particularly effective when used in the presence of both parents. By asking each parent the same question, listening to their thoughts, then summarizing them, the nurse has shown the parents how to decrease their emotionalism. As each parent listens to the other, a new pattern of communication can emerge. For example, a nurse listened while a couple discussed terminating therapy. The nurse noted that the conversation was strained, that both parents were very anxious, and that neither parent was hearing the other's perspective. They suddenly turned and asked the nurse's opinion. The nurse responded first by asking the mother, then the father, what they thought about terminating therapy. Using this strategy the nurse prevented the family's usual anxious argument. By decreasing their emotionalism and creating a situation where they were able to listen to each other's thoughts, the family has moved toward problem solving.[12,18]

The nurse can further model effective communication by maintaining an "I" position in talking with the family. For example, the nurse can use such phrases as "I know, I think, I am not sure," when discussing a problem. This approach demonstrates the nurse's differentiation from the family while showing family members how to express their own thoughts. Additionally, the nurse can encourage family members to clarify and discuss their views without interruption from others. Such a strategy supports developmental differentiation of family members and furthers positive family dynamics.[8,12]

SELF-AWARENESS AND NURSING INTERVENTION

Family therapy strategies are particularly appropriate for nurses practicing in pediatric oncology. Because of the long-term nature of the therapy protocols, nurses often develop intense personal relationships with the child and family. These relationships involve emotionally intensive interactions with families during the course of the child's treatment.[19] The nurse experiences the family's feelings of fear, sadness, anger, and despair. The nurse may become a part of the "psychological" family of the patient and have much influence on the family's dynamics. Conversely, the dysfunctional family also can influence the nurse. The dysfunctional family makes attempts to absorb others into their psychopathology, especially during times of conflict or stress.[20,21]

To prevent the nurse from being pulled into the family's dysfunctional system, the nurse must maintain a sense of separateness from the family's emotional system. The nurse can remain detached without rejecting the family by being objective and conveying a sense of concern and empathy for the seriousness of the problem.[8,12,13]

REFERRAL GUIDELINES

If strategies fail to stabilize the family's functioning, the nurse should consider making a referral to a mental health professional. Interventions should begin as soon as possible after the nurse assesses that the family seems dysfunctional. The best time to initiate the referral is during the crisis period when people are more open and amenable to help.[22] To be most effective, interventions should be initiated within the first six weeks following any crisis point, including diagnosis, relapse, or terminal illness.[23]

How the referral is presented to the family may have a great influence on their acceptance of counseling. A referral should be framed in a positive way so the family does not lose face and feel worse when counseling is recommended. One approach is to tell the family that even strong families use support to increase their coping ability. This technique emphasizes the positive aspects of counseling. Another approach is to tell the family that having a child with cancer is a very stressful situation difficult for all families. By emphasizing the highly stressful nature of the diagnosis, the family doesn't feel inadequate for coping ineffectively. By using these techniques when making the referral, the family is more likely to comply.[24]

CONCLUSION

Bowen's theory of family functioning[7] provides the nurse with a theoretical framework for assessing psychopathology in families by identifying dysfunctional interactions. The nurse can employ strategies from family therapy to help stabilize the dysfunctional family and improve their interaction. If these strategies are ineffective, the nurse should consider making a referral to a mental health professional.

The author wishes to acknowledge George Bush and Ronnie Neuberg, MD, for their critique and recommendations regarding this manuscript.

REFERENCES

1. Hammond, G. The cure of childhood cancers. *Supplement to Cancer,* 58(2):407–413, 1986.
2. Lansky, S., Cairns, C., Hassaein, R., Wehr, J. & Lowman, J. Childhood cancer: Parental discord and divorce. *Pediatrics,* 62(2):184–188, 1978.
3. Hurley, P. Childhood cancer: A pilot study of parental stress. *Oncol Nurs Forum,* 11(5):44–48, 1984.
4. Chester, M., & Barbarin, O. *Childhood cancer and the family meeting the challenge of stress and support.* New York: Brunner/Mazel Publishers, 1987.

5. Barbarin, O., Hughes, D., & Chesler, M. Stress, coping and marital functioning among parents of children with cancer. *Journal of Marriage and the Family, 47*(5):437–480, 1985.
6. Kupst, M. J., Schulman, J., Maurer, H., Honig, G., Morgan, E., & Fochtman, D. Coping with pediatric leukemia: A two year follow-up. *Journal of Pediatric Psychology, 9*(2):149–163.
7. Bowen, M. Family therapy and family group therapy. (In) Olson, D. (ed): *Treating relationships.* Lake Mills, IA: Graphic Publishing. 1976:219–274.
8. Miller, S., & Winstead-Fry, P. *Family systems theory in nursing practice.* Reston, VA: Reston Publishing Company, Inc. 1982.
9. Cain, A. Family therapy: One role of the clinical specialist in psychiatric nursing. *Nurs Clin North Am, 2*(3):483–491, 1986.
10. Kaplan, D., Brobstein, R., & Smith, A. Predicting the impact of severe illness in families. *Health and Social Work 1*(3):72–82, 1976.
11. Cain, S. Assessment of family structure. (In) Miller, J., & Janosik, E. (eds), *Family focused care.* New York: McGraw-Hill Book Company, 1980:115–131.
12. Dashiff, C. Coaching developmental differentiation. *Topics in Clin Nurs 1*(3):11–20, 1979.
13. Sills, G. Bias therapists in family therapy. (In) Smoyak, S. (ed), *The psychiatric nurse as a family therapist.* New York: John Wiley and Sons, Inc. 1975:13–23.
14. Alexander, D., White, M., & Powell, G. Anxiety of non-rooming in parents of hospitalized children. *Children's Health Care 15*(1):14–20, 1986.
15. Sargent, J. The family and childhood psychosomatic disorders. *General Hospital Psychiatry 5*:41–48, 1983.
16. Minuchin, S., & Fishman, C. *Family therapy techniques.* Harvard University Press, 1981.
17. Satir, V. *Conjoint Family Therapy.* Science and Behavior Books, Inc. 1983.
18. Morrison, E. Functional family intervention. (In) Miller, J., & Janosik, E. (eds), *Family focused care.* New York: McGraw-Hill Book Company, 1980:346–369.
19. Trygstad, L. Professional friends: The inclusion of the personal into the professional. *Cancer Nursing 9*(6):326–332, 1986.
20. Fialkov, M., & Miller, J. Severe psychosomatic illness in children: Effect on a pediatric ward's staff. *Clin Pediatr 20*(12):792–796, 1981.
21. Marten, G., & Mauer, A. Interaction of health-care professionals with critically ill children and their parents. *Clin Pediatr 21*(9):540–544.
22. Caplan, G. *An approach to community mental health.* Orlando, FL: Grune and Stratton, 1972.
23. Christ, G. A psychosocial assessment framework for cancer patients and their families. *Health and Social Work 8*(1):57–64, 1983.
24. Hodas, G., & Honig, P. An approach to psychiatric referrals in pediatric patients. *Clin Pediatr 22*(3):167–172, 1983.

CHAPTER 35

Family Recovery
from Alcoholism:
Mediating Family Factors

Constance Captain

One stone cast into a pool of water causes ever widening ripples around it. In the same way, alcoholism in one family member resonates through the family system touching the lives of its members in countless ways. Ten million Americans are alcoholic. For every alcoholic, at least four others are intimately affected by the disease, primarily the family. In a 1982 National Gallup Survey, one-third of persons interviewed said alcohol had caused problems in their families.[12]

Managing alcoholism affects family life in numerous ways. "Getting by" replaces growth, "duty" replaces love, and life in general seems out of control and unsatisfying. For many families, life is at an impasse, "a predicament affording no obvious escape."[40] Dissolution of the marriage seems the only recourse for some families. Divorce and separation consistently have been found to be more prevalent in problem drinkers than other comparison groups.[25,41] Evidence suggests that the rate of divorce and separation for alcoholic families is seven times that of the general population.[31] Some families remain intact but continue to contribute to the statistics on dysfunctional families. Alcoholism has been linked to family violence,[13] teen pregnancy, adolescent substance abuse, delinquency,[18] child neglect,[30] incest,[11] and psychological disorders.[33]

Fortunately, growing numbers of families are seeking treatment as a way to move beyond their impasse. This trend can be expected to continue. Recent clinical reports and research studies have begun to direct increased attention toward the importance of

Reprinted from *Nursing Clinics of North America, Vol. 24* (No. 1), March 1989, pp. 55–67. Used by permission of W. B. Saunders Company and the author.

the family's involvement in successful rehabilitation from alcoholism. With alcoholism identified as a family illness, clinicians indicate that recovery is partially contingent upon a family's ability to renegotiate patterns of interacting and functioning without alcohol. The degree to which a family is able to make these necessary adjustments may determine the extent to which rehabilitation will be maintained by the alcoholic. Moreover, it may have a bearing on the health and survival of the entire family system.

Given the prevalence of alcohol abuse, it is highly probable that nurses will be working with patients and/or families managing this disease. To assist nurses in assuming a therapeutic role in these contacts, the purpose of the article is to: (1) summarize what is "known" about family functioning during recovery from alcoholism, and (2) suggest nursing interventions aimed at helping families manage the recovery process.

While the importance of family factors and their effect on recovery have been recognized, empirical testing has been limited. Current knowledge and understanding derive primarily from clinical reports, theoretical papers, and a few exploratory research studies. This work can best be described as enthusiastic and promising. However, interpretations far outdistance substantiated findings.[38] For this discussion, the available information has been organized within the context of family theory. This approach argues for integrating available information into a framework that can guide nursing practice with families in recovery.

THEORETICAL FRAMEWORK

While alcoholism is most often explained from a systems theory perspective, family response to alcoholism also has been conceptualized and researched from a stress theory perspective.[6,16,26] Because each approach adds a dimension to our understanding of family recovery, each will be addressed.

Systems Theory

Systems theory provides us with a conceptual framework for examining the alcoholic family in two ways: from an organizational perspective and from an operational perspective. Organization describes the "who" and "what" by defining the basic structure of family membership and system boundaries, which consist of family rules, member roles, and communication patterns. The operational dimension addresses the "how" by identifying the on-going process of changing relationships among members and the manner in which homeostasis strategies are enacted to achieve family goals. In system theory terminology these two dimensions are labeled "structure" and "function." Operationally, they are interdependent. How a family functions will eventually affect family structure, and in turn, structure determines function. The Robertson family, a clinical example, exemplifies the distinction between structure and function.

Mr. Robertson spent little time with his family during his drinking years. As a result, his wife and children aligned as a separate subsystem (structure). Mr. Robertson engaged in few parental activities, thus relinquishing these to his wife (function). The children learned to look to their mother for direction, seldom seeking counsel from their father (function). With sobriety, Mr. Robertson expected to resume his parental role (structure) and was disappointed when his children did not readily respond to his interest in them (function). The reciprocal causal relationship between family structure and function is apparent. In working with families, it is important for the nurse to carefully assess how each dimension is contributing to overall family functioning. Understanding this relationship is a significant initial step in planning interventions.

From a systems perspective, other properties considered important to understanding family function during recovery include wholeness, homeostasis, and feedback mechanisms.

Wholeness refers to the relationship between the total system and its parts. A system as an integrated coherent entity is highly sensitive to a change in one member. Sobriety in the alcoholic represents a major change and necessitates a redefinition of family members' relationships if this change is to be maintained. This principle underlies the recent emphasis on including the family in the alcoholic's treatment program.

Homeostasis refers to the dynamic balance of a system. Prior to treatment, alcoholic families are perceived to have been maintaining an alcohol-governed homeostatic system. Generally, alcohol abuse is considered dysfunctional. However, several investigators have identified adaptive consequences as well. According to Steinglass et al,[37] drinking may satisfy unconscious needs of family members, and it may represent an integral operating aspect of family relationships. According to this viewpoint, families develop repetitive complementary responses to the drinking behavior, which over time serves to maintain homeostasis. A study by Davis et al[8] of communication styles in alcoholic marriages demonstrates this. The investigators examined the differences between sober and intoxicated interactions. It was noted that when the alcoholic husband was drinking, the wife related to him in a more congenial, attentive way. They concluded that although a wife may complain about her husband's drinking, she may in fact be reinforcing it by the attention she gives him when intoxicated. Dynamics such as these support the adaptive aspects of alcoholism in a marriage. In recovery these established dynamics are altered. Since most families are primarily unaware of how they have accommodated to the drinking, they are puzzled by the tensions they experience with sobriety. Jackson,[16] in an early study of family adjustment to alcoholism, observed that spouse expectations for a life without alcohol were unrealistic. Often alcohol abuse had been blamed for all the family difficulties. The wives in the study assumed that when the drinking stopped the marital problems also would. When this did not occur, these women were unprepared to meet the demands of family reorganization that recovery necessitated.

From a systems theory perspective, family reorganization is the result of feedback processes. Changes in family functioning are made through positive feedback, whereas the goal of negative feedback is to resist change and maintain the status quo. As theorist David Speer[35] has pointed out, while seemingly dichotomous, these two feedback processes are actually complementary. Both processes are needed for family system survival. Too many or too few changes produce the same outcome—a negative effect on family functioning. The optimal situation during recovery is for a family to balance negative and positive feedback mechanisms. Helping families work through manageable changes is an important focus for nurses involved in after-care programs.

Family Stress Theory

More than three decades ago Jackson[16] introduced the concepts of stress and crisis into alcoholism research. She claimed the progression of alcoholism in a family member precipitated a cumulative crisis for the family. Similarly, Hill[15] classified alcoholism as an intrafamily stressful event involving disturbances in role patterns, family demoralization, and eventually family crisis. Hill combined systems theory and concepts of family stress theory in his formulation of how stress becomes crisis. He cited several possible outcomes when a family is faced with a situation of sufficient magnitude to bring about a change in the family system. When family demands equal capabilities, minimal stress is experienced and homeostasis is maintained. When family demands exceed capabilities, stress results and the family must make minor changes in the system to restore equilibrium. However, in the case of continued demand-capability imbalance, the family experiences a crisis. Stress becomes crisis when stability cannot be restored without making major changes in how the family functions.

Clinical accounts document this progression. In the early stages of alcoholism, the family adjusts by denying the problem or explaining it away. As alcohol abuse increases, alcohol-related demands on the family exceed adjustment capabilities, stress is experienced, and the family is required to make minor changes in the system to restore equilibrium. At this point families recognize the problem is alcoholism and make attempts to eliminate it from within. Family roles and relationships are altered; compensatory changes in family functioning characterize family dynamics. For example, family members cover for the alcoholic, enact home remedies to control the alcoholic's use, and shift the alcoholic's roles and responsibilities to other members in an effort to keep the family intact. Continued alcohol abuse with increased alcohol-related problems eventuate in family disorganization. At this juncture the family is in crisis. They realize internal capabilities are insufficient to manage the magnitude of demands; major changes are needed to restore system equilibrium. This is when some families seek treatment.

Research from a family stress theory perspective seeks to identify what factors may be important to family reorganization. The Double ABCX model[23] represents one approach (Fig. 1).

The primary variables in Hill's[15] original ABCX Family Crisis model, reformulated by McCubbin and Patterson in the Double ABCX model, include Aa (family "pile-up" of life events and added stresses over time), interacting with Bb (existing and new resources), interacting with Ce (family perceptions of pile-up demands *and* resources), mediated by coping, produces Xx (family adaptation). Hill's model focuses on pre-crisis variables, whereas McCubbin and Patterson address post-crisis family factors. According to these authors,[22] the central goal of family stress investigations is to determine "how much and what kinds of stressors; mediated by what personal, family, and community resources, and by what family coping responses; and what family processes shape the course and ease of family adjustment and adaptation over time" (p 7).

The model is used to organize the research findings about family factors and recovery.

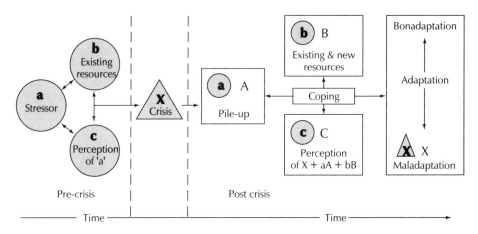

FIGURE 1. *From* McCubbin H.I. and J. Patterson (1983). "The Family Stress Process: The Double ABCX Model of Adjustment and Adaptation." In H.I. McCubbin, M.B. Sussman, and J.M. Patterson (Eds.) *Advances and Developments in Family Stress Theory and Research.* New York: Haworth Press.

Pile-Up of System Demands (Aa Factor)

The concept of "pile-up," or cumulative stress, aptly describes alcoholic families. Some of these stressors have been investigated. The most consistently studied area has been normative and non-normative life change events. In accordance wtih the psychosomatic tradition, the focus is on change rather than any direct measure of stress. As the magnitude of changes increases, family vulnerability increases, and the family's capacity to adjust may become depleted. Studies of factors that precipitate relapse highlight the importance of stressful life situations. Negative life events have been demonstrated to adversely impact on family functioning,[28] lead to relapse in male alcoholics,[26] and continued alcohol abuse in females.[20] A high proportion of relapse occurs within the first 90 days after treatment and is often triggered by interpersonal conflicts, social pressure to drink, and skepticism about the alcoholic's ability to maintain sobriety.[6]

Most families bring to the recovery experience residual stress from prior alcohol-related hardships such as family conflict, sporadic work records, financial deficits, drunken driving charges, and arrests. These are circumstances not easily rectified. The on-going effects contribute to marital dissatisfaction during recovery[16,19,43] and demonstrate a negative effect on sobriety.[29] Conversely, multiple hardships have been associated with treatment compliance.[6,27] While seemingly contradictory, these findings support the clinical observation that many alcoholics do not seek treatment until alcohol-induced problems have seriously complicated their lives. At this stage in the progression of alcoholism, denial is no longer tenable.

Recovery itself is a major stressor as multiple destabilizing pressures confront the family. Families enter treatment with unrealistic expectations,[16] face exposing unresolved marital problems,[24] are expected to confront sensitive issues and make attitudinal and behavioral changes,[38] and soon realize that sobriety does not necessarily improve family functioning.[6,16,43]

Resources (Bb Factor)

The Double ABCX model suggests that adequate resources may mitigate the effects of high system demands. In an alcoholic family, existing resources often have been seriously compromised. Alcohol abuse exhausts the reservoir of good will within both the family and community (for example, because of unkept promises, bad debts). Accordingly, many families begin recovery with high demands and less than adequate resources.[6] Recent treatment studies have attempted to identify those resources necessary to family recovery. Researchers indicate that family environment factors may constitute the most important resource in recovery.

Billings and Moos[4] in a study comparing community controls and relapsed and recovered alcoholics over a 2-year period identified several salient family characteristics. Families of recovered patients evidenced higher levels of cohesion, expressiveness, and greater involvement in recreational and religious activities; showed decreased conflict and control; and jointly engaged in more household tasks. The importance of family cohesion has been supported in other studies,[29,36] suggesting that this dimension of family health is most affected by alcoholism and may be the best predictor of better function after treatment.

Investigation of social support, a resource generally considered important to managing stress and adaptation to life crises, has been limited to the benefits derived from attending Alcoholics Anonymous and Al-Anon.[39]

As stated earlier, family involvement in treatment represents a critical resource in recovery. Studies on family therapy, while sparse, consistently report positive outcomes such as improved marital satisfaction,[34] maintenance of sobriety,[9] improved problem-solving skills,[7] and more satisfactory family communication.[24]

Perception (Cc Factor)

This concept refers to a family's subjective appraisal of a situation, in this case, the recovery process. McCubbin and Patterson[22] report that family coping is facilitated when a family can define a situation as a challenge (versus a threat) or can endow difficult circumstances with significant meaning. Other stress theorists view perception as a critical organizing factor to all subsequent responses.[5,32] From this perspective, a belief that sobriety is possible may contribute to positive treatment outcomes. In support of this, positive perceptions for recovery differentiated between relapsed and abstinent patients at 4 months after treatment.[6]

Coping (Bridging Variable)

Functional coping responses mediate the effects of stressors and can directly influence family functioning during recovery. Pro-active coping strategies have been identified as more helpful than avoidance responses or passive acceptance of circumstances. For example, "reframing," the ability to define a problem in more positive terms, was a distinguishing characteristic of couples in whom the alcoholic husband maintained abstinence. Relapse, on the other hand, was associated with passive responses, for example, waiting for problems to go away. Alcoholic families, by nature of their situation, do not bring to recovery a sense of confidence in their ability to cope. Previous coping behaviors are seen by the family as ineffective. The alcoholic drank and family members were unable to alter this. The outcome of this coping was more family tension, crises, and a sense of defeat. Recovery fosters hope and renewed interest in learning effective coping strategies—a situation nurses need to capitalize on.

Adaptation

Traditionally, treatment success has been judged primarily by one criterion, the drinking status of the alcoholic. This was congruent with individual/symptom-focused treatment approaches. Recent inclusion of the family in treatment and application of family systems concepts have expanded the range of outcome variables to include factors important to healthy family functioning.

THEORETICAL IMPLICATIONS FOR NURSING

Two theoretical approaches to the relationship between alcoholism and the family have been set forth in the literature. Systems theory, as a holistic paradigm, seeks to understand the complex interaction of change and stability mechanisms operant when a family is faced with a shift in established homeostasis, as in recovery. From this perspective, nursing interventions are directed toward helping the family renegotiate family roles and patterns of interacting and functioning. The family stress model serves to explain variability in family adaption by identifying critical stress-regulating factors that may be important in buffering the effects of a family crisis. Therapeutic efforts by the nurse are aimed at restoring the balance between family demands and capabilities. Combined, these theoretical perspectives provide a comprehensive, yet practical, paradigm to direct family assessment and interventions for nurses practicing at the generalist level in varied clinical settings.

NURSING INTERVENTIONS

Nurses working with alcoholic families provide care within the context of family-centered nursing or function as a family therapist. Nursing interventions presented here address family-centered practice. Issues and techniques of family therapy are beyond the scope of this article. Moreover, nurses who function as family therapists have completed specialized training programs and hold advanced degrees. Family therapy for all recovering families is not a realistic goal. Some families may not need it, while others, for a variety of reasons, may be unable to participate in family therapy (for example, because of motivational deficits, financial resources, and unavailability of services). In contrast, family-centered nursing services are necessary for all families during recovery. The nurse can expect to assume multiple roles: counselor, guide, role model, teacher, crisis intervener, and resource person, with nursing process providing the framework for intervention.

Assessment

In assessing the family, the nurse focuses on individual members and how members interact with and impact on each other. Interest is on how the alcoholism has affected each member and the family as a unit, individual recovery concerns, and recovery issues shared by the entire family. In the initial assessment the nurse seeks to gather as much information as possible to gain an understanding of family recovery needs amenable to nursing intervention and those needs that may best be met through referral to other support services. This information includes demographic data, physical and emotional health, family background, recovery concerns, current family structure, family roles, communication patterns, member relationships, current family stressors, resources, available familial and community supports, coping behaviors, and family expectations for recovery. Given the broad range of information required to conduct a comprehensive assessment, the nurse may choose to have families complete standardized self-report family assessment instruments. One outcome of the recent advances in family theory and research has been the development of several reliable and valid family questionnaires. The interested reader is referred to *Family Assessment Inventories for Research and Practice*.[23]

Nursing Diagnoses

Having completed the initial assessment, the nurse analyzes the data according to the theoretical frameworks and formulates family-specific nursing diagnoses. A list of potential diagnoses are presented as suggestions. The diagnoses derive from the document *Standards of Addictions Nursing Practice with Selected Diagnosis and Criteria*.[3] No attempt has been made to prioritize the diagnoses, since the needs of recovering families are quite diverse. The information in parentheses represents defining characteristics that have been documented in the family and alcoholism literature.

- *knowledge deficit* (disease concept, noncompliance, denial, inaccurate perceptions of health status)
- *noncompliance* (informed choice, psychosocial stress, progression of the disease)
- *sexual dysfunction* (alcohol-induced physiologic alterations, marital relationship issues)
- *alteration in thought process* (irritability, impairment in memory resulting from past blackouts or current stress, irrational beliefs about alcoholism and recovery)
- *impaired communication* (verbal-nonverbal incongruencies, inability to express feelings, inadequate listening skills)
- *alteration in self-concept* (self-esteem issues, faulty role performance, personal identity concerns)
- *fear* (recovery stressors, lack of control over alcohol, unexplained anxiety)
- *social isolation* (disease stigma, deviant past behavior, rejection)

- *dysfunctional family process* (interaction and relationship issues, inability to access social support and resources, faulty problem-solving and decision-making, disturbances in family functioning, dependency issues, alterations in role performance)
- *altered parenting* (inappropriate parenting behaviors, child neglect or abuse)
- *spiritual distress* (questioning relationship with a higher power)
- *powerlessness* (loss of control, reluctance to participate in recovery program, passive coping responses, dependency)
- *hopelessness* (passivity, depression, suicidal ideation, negative expectations for recovery)
- *grief* (loss experienced in giving up alcohol and associated lifestyle, guilt, depression, shame)

Planning and Implementation

When planning interventions, the nurse should be aware that families with an alcoholic member may not see themselves as clients; therefore, they are reluctant to become involved in family-centered treatment. Family members are willing to do what they can to help the alcoholic maintain sobriety but may not realize that they too have developed symptoms of alcoholism and need professional assistance. By helping families understand that alcoholism is a family disease, the nurse refocuses the problem from the alcoholic and presents it as a shared concern. Exploring and clarifying this issue should be addressed in the initial assessment session. Recommending that family members attend an Al-Anon/Al-Ateen support group or community educational programs will facilitate their understanding and enhance future nursing interventions. Learning about the disease is essential to recovery.

Goal setting is a joint activity between the nurse and family members. Short-term goals center around stabilizing the family system. Long-term goals address making family-level changes and establishing patterns for maintaining changes.

Stabilizing the Family System

Upon entering an alcoholic family system during early recovery, the nurse soon realizes the family is both optimistic and relieved by the sobriety of the alcoholic member and skeptical and concerned about recovery. Postcrisis the family is in transition and highly vulnerable. This is a difficult period; adjustment to life without alcohol may be more problematic for some families than others. The nurse will want to identify those families considered at high risk. These families should be linked to additional supportive services early in recovery. Based on the research literature, alerting family factors include low cohesion, high conflict, few shared interests and activities, multiple stressors, inadequate resources, passive coping behaviors, a history of relapse and marital dissatisfaction, and alcohol abuse serving an adaptive function in family system maintenance. A referral for marital or family therapy is often necessary when family discord dominates member interactions. Because the decision to go into therapy may be a difficult one, the nurse can help families to make this commitment by providing information, encouragement, and support.

Strategies for stabilizing less dysfunctional families should focus on decreasing family stressors and augmenting resources. Counseling families about the negative impact of life change events and assisting family members in working through resentments about past alcohol-related hardships represent two important areas that decrease family system demands. Expectations for recovery need to be explored, as these may be unrealistic. Families want to believe that current abstinence means the alcoholic has been cured. Whether this belief represents family denial of alcoholism or lack of knowledge about recovery, the nurse can provide accurate information, as well as refer them to educational programs in the community.

Limited access to resources is, in part, related to an alcoholic family lifestyle. The stigma of alcoholism, reinforced by disruptive, embarrassing behaviors by the alcoholic, results in varying degrees of social isolation. Recovery adjustment problems are intensified by the family's lack of social contacts and shared pleasures.[42] Support groups such as Alcoholics Anonymous and Al-Anon facilitate re-entry into the community and serve as a contact for developing new relationships. The nurse can use contracting techniques or homework assignments to encourage participation in family recreational activities. Families need to have fun together. Building positive experiences in their lives fosters family cohesion, a critical factor in lasting recovery.

Making Changes and Establishing Patterns for Maintaining Change

Based on systems theory concepts, strategies for making changes should be directed at the family's structure and function. Realigning family members according to parental and children hierarchical subsystems will facilitate reinstating the alcoholic member into the family and foster role-appropriate behaviors. Issues around trust and responsibility will surface and should be addressed by the nurse in counseling sessions. Confronting family myths represents another sensitive topic. Family members believe alcohol has been the primary cause of their conflicts. The nurse explores with the family how each member both has been affected by the alcoholism and has contributed to it. Understanding this dynamic can help restore family control over alcoholism and the recovery process.

Improving family interactions is an important condition for maintaining change. Interventions should be directed at improving communication skills, developing problem-solving abilities, identifying and expressing feelings, and learning negotiating strategies. Conducting skills training programs using a couples group format is one option. This approach is cost effective, efficient, and enjoyable for the nurse. It offers a number of benefits for couples: learning valuable skills, feedback from other couples, and an opportunity to focus on healthy behaviors rather than on alcoholism, which has previously dominated their relationship and activities. Recovery can be a positive experience for the family and the nurse.

Evaluation

The nurse uses the nursing diagnoses and treatment goals to determine the effectiveness of selected interventions. In evaluating the family's current level of interacting and functioning, it is important to recognize that progress may be slow. Setbacks are inevitable. The nature of a family system is to maintain established patterns; therefore, intellectual understanding will exceed attitudinal and behavioral change. Involving the family in self-evaluation allows the nurse to point out subtle improvements members may not readily recognize, reinforce identified gains, and provide support when discouragement is experienced. This is a time to reassess the needs and determine the future direction of additional services.

SUMMARY

The problems families face during recovery from alcoholism are complex and pervasive. Sobriety for the alcoholic without concurrent alterations in family member relationships and improved family functioning too often leads to relapse and the demise of the family unit. The degree to which a family is able to modulate demands, use resources, implement effective coping strategies, and make necessary relationship adjustments may determine the extent to which treatment effects will be maintained. For those families who have successfuly worked together to overcome the negative effects of alcoholism, the experience becomes a major catalyst to continued growth, maturity, and a healthier lifestyle. The nurse has a significant role in assisting the family with early recovery needs and in developing new behaviors for maintaining therapeutic gains.

REFERENCES

1. Ablon, J. Family structure and behavior in alcoholism. A review of the literature. In Kissin, B., & Begleiter, H. (eds), *Biology of alcoholism,* vol 4. *Social biology.* New York: Plenum, 1976, pp. 4–29.
2. Ablon, J. The significance of cultural patterning for the alcoholic family. *Family Process 19:*127–144, 1980.
3. American Nurses' Association. Standards of addictions nursing practice with selected diagnosis on criteria. Kansas City, MO:, American Nurses' Association, 1988.
4. Billings, A., & Moos, R. Psychosocial processes of recovery among alcoholics and their families: Implications for clinicians and program evaluators. *Addict Behav 8:*205–218, 1983.
5. Burr, W. *Theory construction and the sociology of the family.* New York: John Wiley and Sons, 1973.
6. Captain, C. Marital adaptation during recovery from alcoholism. Doctoral dissertation, University of Wisconsin, 1987.
7. Codogan, D. Marital group therapy in the treatment of alcoholism. *Q J Stud Alcohol 34:*1187–1194, 1973.
8. Davis, D., Berenson, D., Steinglass, P., & Davis, J. The adaptive consequences of drinking. *Psychiatry 37:*209–215, 1974.
9. Ewing, J., Long, V., & Wenzel, G. Concurrent group psychotherapy of alcohol patients and their wives. *Int J Group Psychother 11:*329–338, 1961.
10. Ewing, J., & Fox, R. Family therapy of alcoholism. In Masserman, J. (ed), *Current psychiatric therapies.* New York: Grune & Stratton, 1968, pp. 86–91.
11. Finkelhor, D. *Sexuality victimized children.* New York: The Free Press, 1979.

12. Gallup, C. *Alcohol abuse: A problem in one of three American families.* Princeton, NJ: The Gallup Poll, November 15, 1982.
13. Gelles, R., & Straus, M. Determinants of violence in the family: Toward a theoretical integration. In Burr, W., Nye, F., & Reiss, I. (eds), *Contemporary theories about the family.* New York: The Free Press, 1979, pp. 549–581.
14. Hill, R. *Families under stress.* New York: Harper & Row, 1949.
15. Hill, R. Generic features of families under stress. *Soc Casework 39*:139–150, 1958.
16. Jackson, J. The adjustment of the family to the crisis of alcoholism. *Q J Stud Alcohol 15*:562–574, 1954.
17. Jacobs, T., Dunn, N., & Leonard, K. Patterns of alcohol abuse and family stability. *Alcohol Clin Exp Res 7*:382–385, 1983.
18. Knight, J. The family in the crises of alcoholism. In Gitlow, S., & Peyser, H. (eds), *Alcoholism. A practical treatment guide.* New York: Grune & Stratton, 1980, pp 205–226.
19. Kogan, K., & Jackson, J. Stress, personality, and emotional disturbances in wives of alcoholics. *Q J Stud Alcohol 26*:468–495, 1964.
20. Lisansky-Gomberg, E. Women, sex roles, and alcohol problems. *Professional Psychology 12*:146–155, 1981.
21. McCubbin, H., & Patterson, J. Family stress and adaptation to crisis: A double ABCX model of family behavior. *Family Studies Review Yearbook.* Beverly Hills, CA: Sage Publications, 1981.
22. McCubbin, H., & Patterson, J. The family stress process: The double ABCX model of adjustment and adaptation. In McCubbin, H., Sussman, M., & Patterson, J. (eds), *Social stress and family: Advances and developments in family stress theory and research.* Marriage and Family Review, vol 6. New York: Haworth Press, 1983, pp. 7–38.
23. McCubbin, H., & Thompson, A. Family Assessment Inventories for Research and Practice. Madison, Wisconsin, University of Wisconsin-Madison Family Stress and Coping Project, 1987.
24. Meeks, D., & Kelly, C. Family therapy with the families of recovering alcoholics. *Q J Stud Alcohol 31*:399–413, 1970.
25. Miller, P., & Barlow, D. Behavioral approaches to the treatment of alcoholism. *J Nerv Ment Dis 157*:10–20, 1973.
26. Moos, R., & Moos, B. The process of recovery from alcoholism: III. Comparing functioning families of alcoholics and matched control families. *J Stud Alcohol 45(2)*:111–116, 1984.
27. Mulford, A. Stages in the alcoholic process: Toward a cumulative, nonsequential index. *J Stud Alcohol 38*:63–583, 1977.
28. Olson, D., McCubbin, H., Barnes, H., et al. *Families: What makes them work.* Los Angeles, CA: Sage Publishing, 1983.
29. Orford, J., Guthrie, S., Nicholls, P., et al. Self-reported coping behavior of wives of alcoholics and its association with drinking outcome. *J Stud Alcohol 36*:1254–1267, 1975.
30. Orme, T., & Rimmer, J. Alcoholism and child abuse. *J Stud Alcohol 42(3)*:273–287, 1981.
31. Paolind, T., & McCrady, B. *Marriage and marital therapy: Psychoanalytic, behavioral and systems theory.* New York: Brunner/Mazel, 1977.
32. Reiss, D., & Oliveri, M. Family paradigm and family coping: A proposal for linking the family's intrinsic adaptive capacities to its responses to stress. *Fam Relations 29*:443–552, 1980.
33. Schutkit, M., & Morrissey, E. Psychiatric problems in women admitted to an alcohol detoxification center. *Am J Psych 136*:611–617, 1979.
34. Smith, C. Alcoholics: Their treatment and their wives. *Br J Psychiatry 115*:1039–1042, 1969.
35. Speer, D. Family systems: Morphostasis and morphogenesis, or is homeostasis enough? *Fam Process 9*:259–278, 1970.
36. Steinglass, P., Tislenko, L., & Reiss, D. Stability/instability in the alcoholic marriage: The interrelationships between cause of alcoholism, family process, and marital outcome. *Fam Process 25*:365–376, 1985.
37. Steinglass, P., Weiner, S., & Mendelson, J. A systems approach to alcoholism: A model and its clinical application. *Arch Gen Psychiatry 24*:401–408, 1971.

38. Steinglass, P. Experimenting with family treatment approaches to alcoholism, 1950–1975: A review. *Fam Process* 15:97–123, 1976.
39. Ward, F., & Faillace, L. The alcoholic and his helpers. *Q J Stud Alcohol* 31:684–691, 1970.
40. *Webster's ninth new collegiate dictionary.* Springfield, MA: Merriam Webster, Inc., 1987, p. 603.
41. Woodruff, R., Guge, S., & Clayton, P. Divorce among outpatients. *Br J Psychiatry* 121:289–292, 1972.
42. Zackon, F., McAuliffe, W., & Chien, J. Issues of the recovering family. Treatment Research Monograph Series. Addict Aftercare: Recovering Training and Self-Help. Washington DC, US Government Printing Office, Publication #(ADM) 86–1341, 1985.
43. Zweben, A. Problem drinking and marital adjustment. *J Stud Alcohol* 47:167–172, 1986.

UNIT 4

FAMILY HEALTH NURSING EDUCATION

Nursing education must perpetuate an environment that is favorable for preparing competent practitioners as well as generate new knowledge and refine current knowledge. One way to increase the promotion of family health, then, is to educate nurses and nursing students in the concepts and interventions revolving around family health. The articles in this section serve as a general overview of the body of knowledge currently available in the literature. However, very little in the literature describes this process in the academic or clinical practice settings. This is surprising, considering the value placed on education as an intervention strategy for all nursing.

CHAPTER **36**

Helping Nursing Students Communicate with High-Risk Families: An Educator's Challenge

Helen Lerner, Mary Woods Byrne

Helping students have a positive experience in the clinical laboratory is a goal of all nursing educators. In the field of parent–child nursing, students encounter families who are at increased health risk because of a complicated pregnancy, delivery, or chronic illness, and at increased social risk because of such factors as poverty, illiteracy, and drug addiction. Families with these risk factors often have histories of poor personal support systems and negative experiences with health care providers.

Difficulties can arise when nursing students meet these families and try to establish communication. Because nursing educators want to give students the best possible preparation for beginning practice, the question arises whether it is appropriate to involve students with families at high risk. Decisions can be made to avoid having students care for these families and to avoid contracting for student experiences in the kinds of institutions most likely to be utilized by multiproblem families. In our view, however, this deprives students of an essential learning opportunity and sends the message that the care of certain populations is beyond the scope and interest of the average nurse.

In reality, it is increasingly impossible to avoid multiproblem clients. The student who has carefully guided experiences caring for high-risk families is better prepared for entry level practice.

To provide a positive experience, the faculty must consider student awareness and ability to cope in three areas. First, nursing students are novices when it comes to the

Reprinted from *Nursing and Health Care, Vol. 12* (No. 2), February 1991, pp. 98–101. Used by permission of National League for Nursing.

ability to communicate professionally. Second, it is difficult to communicate with many people at high risk because their absorption with multiple problems leaves little energy for building helping relationships. Third, even though students feel empathy for young families who are in a similar age group, students can become discouraged if their efforts to communicate are not well received. Students need help to preserve these caring feelings despite factors that threaten students' self-esteem.

STUDENTS AS
NOVICE PROFESSIONALS

Nursing students' range of interpersonal skills begins with the social ability to make introductions and simple explanations and must quickly proceed in clinical situations to far more sophisticated therapeutic techniques. These essential and complex communications skills are not easy for students to master. This process is compounded by the stressful environment of the clinical setting as well as the need to integrate novice interpersonal skills with equally new psychomotor skills.

In one exploratory study of nursing students' perceptions of their education, the difficulties they experienced in talking to patients emerged as a major problem category of their clinical experiences. So baffled were the students at times that the researchers labeled this category "nursing in the dark" (Melia, 1982).

The challenge of communicating with high-risk, multiproblem families is more difficult because the student professional has limited experience on which to rely. Students tend to critique negatively the communication skills of many of the staff with whom they are closely associated in their clinical experiences (Byrne, 1988). Lacking experience and perspective, students fail to see positive aspects of staff interaction. Staff who work in facilities that deal with high-risk families do so because they are committed to caring for these families. It is important for the instructor to help both staff and student benefit from this experience. Staff need to know that their nursing care is a positive feature for the students. Students can grow in their communication abilities by emulating successful staff–client interaction.

SECOND ISSUES:
NEGATIVE FEEDBACK

It is well known that nursing students are most gratified by working with patients and families who respond well to them (Baer & Lowery, 1987). Many high-risk families most in need of nursing care are the ones that respond less well to students and to other health care providers. When the students receive negative feedback, they become less eager to be in a situation where they must care for high-risk families. In addition, many families at social risk are cared for in settings that are chronically under-funded and are heavily burdened with problems that reflect the social and economic ills of the particular area where they are located. These factors contribute to the student's perceptions of negative feedback and hopelessness. Despite factors that faculty cannot modify, they can be alert to opportunities to help the students understand and depersonalize hostile or distant client behavior.

A student was rebuffed in her first attempts to care for a mother hospitalized with antepartal bleeding. "I don't want to eat. I don't want to take my medicine and *I don't want to talk to you.*" The mother continually rebuffed the student's efforts to provide any kind of care. With the help of the instructor, necessary care was delivered. The situation was discussed in postconference, and the student received group support and several interpretations of the mother's behavior. The following week, the student was assigned to a different client purposely. The mother she had cared for previously came up to her and said, "Where have you been? How come you aren't my nurse anymore? I have been looking for you." The student and instructor were both surprised. Perhaps the instructor had misinterpreted the mother's real cues?

Often, high-risk families have difficulty seeking help. Many are isolated from their neighbors and families and lack the social skills to develop a relationship with a health care provider (McElmurry, et al., 1987). Many families have not had helping relationships with others, and, thus, they take a long time to develop trust in a health care provider. Many are defensive and withdrawn during short-term relationships. The apathy that these families exhibit is often a symptom of an underlying depression (Spietz, 1988). The resulting avoidance of relationships and negative feedback fails to produce for these families the kind of support that they need and reinforces the negative perceptions they have of the health care system and providers.

Negative experiences with sporadic health care encounters reinforces the devaluing of established health care services. When neighbors and acquaintances have also had negative encounters, this social network validates the pattern of resistance to engagement with health service providers. The resulting situation is characterized by mistrust of health professionals and the sending out of negative signals. Nursing students are very vulnerable to negative signals, can misread their complex origins, and perceive only personal rejection and negative feedback.

EMPATHETIC STUDENTS
BECOME DISCOURAGED

Trying to understand the concerns of high-risk families may be very difficult for those who have not had similar life experiences. Students need the help of the nursing instructor and the staff to understand the concerns of the family.

Empathy comes easily to nursing students. We have observed the deep sense of caring that students typically bring with them to their clinical learning experiences. Because the students are still bridging the transition from lay person to professional, they perceive the realities of the clinical scene from a point of view close to the patient's perspective. Not yet comfortable with technological gadgetry, students empathize with young mothers on the intrapartum unit who are intimidated by fetal monitors, intravenous lines, and such. Students still respond to the sense of shame and embarrassment that patients feel whose unclothed bodies are observed by a crowd of strangers. Students bristle with the anger laboring patients feel when they are accosted without introductions, asked to repeat histories and identifying data, while pain is seemingly taken for granted.

Students often come with a sense of helpfulness and caring. They are ready and eager to provide the bridge to social support that has been chronically absent in the lives of many high-risk families. Students have impressed us with their humanity and caring in their approaches to even the most difficult patients. Yet often it is because of their caring attitudes that hostile remarks and rejection are most upsetting.

STRATEGIES FOR IMPROVING COMMUNICATION WITH HIGH-RISK FAMILIES

Foster continuity in care. In order to assist mothers in learning to care for a new infant and to develop parenting skills, students need to realize that they must first gain the mother's trust. This is often difficult even for seasoned nurses. Barnard and colleagues (1985) have reported that contrary to expectations, the newborn period is not an optimum time to establish a relationship with a mother and actually a poor time to begin intervention.

Initiating the helping process for these mothers is very time-consuming (Barnard et al., 1985). It takes many contacts with the parent before the parent is ready to work with the nurse. This time lag can cause dissatisfaction for the nursing student.

Nursing students on the postpartum unit may have only one or two contacts with a parent and no follow-up of the situation. Mothers may not see the need for a nurse, since they require minimal physical care, and the nursing student may be unsure of her role and assume that the instructor wants students to "teach" the mother no matter what!

Providing experiences where more than one contact with the mother is possible is beneficial to both the mother and the student. Many nursing schools do this when they have a student follow a mother from the labor and delivery unit to the postpartum unit. We try to increase the number of contacts by providing the student with opportunities to make home visits when the mother goes home from the hospital.

Through the experience of continuity of care, a nursing student helped a client cope with a tragic situation. Ms. R. was in labor and presenting many difficulties for the staff when the instructor and the students arrived on the labor and delivery unit. In addition to yelling and cursing at those who cared for her, she refused to be examined, even though the fetal heart tracing showed late decelerations. She began demanding, "let me have may pocketbook" and became abusive when the staff, fearing drug ingestion, refused to give it to her. The student stayed with her and supported her through labor with assistance from the instructor and the staff nurses. She ignored the abusive comments and kept telling the mother of her progress. The student accompanied the mother to the delivery room and stayed with her, coaching her and supporting her. After the infant was born, the mother appeared to be in a heavily drugged state and refused to look at the infant. The student held the infant and spoke to the mother softly, pointing out his positive features.

The following day, the student cared for the mother in the postpartum unit. The mother was more amenable to communication and appeared very frightened about caring for the infant. The student supported the mother when caring for the infant and praised her efforts pointing out how well the infant responded. Ms. R. thanked the student for being there yesterday with her when she was "so crazy!" The mother requested that the student visit her at home to help her learn how to care for the infant. The mother left after 3 days, but the infant stayed an additional day because of appearance of drugs in his urine. The evening before the infant was due to go home, he expired.

The student contacted the mother by telephone and spoke with her, giving condolences. The student made arrangements to visit with the mother at her boyfriend's home where she was staying. The visit occurred 3 days later. The mother spoke with the student at length about the experience and the guilt that she felt. She showed evidence of enrollment in a drug treatment program, and both she and her partner expressed gratitude to the student for the support that they had been given. Obviously, this is not the end of this unfortunate story, but it is reasonable to expect that the mother and her partner will be more able to seek and accept help in the future.

It is essential for the instructor to stress that the most important need of the mother at this point in time is to feel that she is accepted and valued. Nursing students should be encouraged to look for positive aspects of the mother's behavior and family strengths that can provide a basis for intervention. Examples of this are a positive parent–child relationship, concern for other children, or seeking information about health or child care. It is only after the mother can feel this acceptance on the part of the nurse that effective and continuing intervention is possible.

Instructors need to speak with the student before the student goes in to care for the mother in the postpartum unit. The charts of many patients report so many overwhelming problems that it is often difficult for the student to focus on any specific goals for providing nursing care.

Identifying social problems or psychological problems is a very important part of nursing education. Vincent and Davis (1987) noted in their study of public health nurses that baccalaureate-educated nurses identified more social problems than nurses without a baccalaureate degree. On the postpartum unit, however, it is important for the instructor to make the distinction among what problems are in need of referral and what problems are beyond the scope of the health care facility at that time.

PRESERVE STUDENT EMPATHY

The following page is an excerpt from a clinical process recording that was submitted by a student in a parent-child nursing course to describe a difficult interaction.

Student empathy needs to be reinforced and rewarded. This responsibility falls primarily to the clinical faculty person. Students are expressing themselves sincerely but tentatively, always seeking affirmation of their becoming professional selves (Byrne, 1988). They need to know that empathy is an appropriate positive component of professionalism. Faculty can reinforce empathy by commending it. They must also demonstrate how it can be incorporated with the skills needed for comfort, assessment, and

TABLE 1

Nursing Student	Client	Evaluation
"...sounds like you didn't sleep well last night."	"Yeah, it was too G...d... hot last night. I was jumping up turning the f...fan on and off. My f...nose is all stopped up." (Client looking toward the window.)	Neutral response to show interest and involvement without attaching a value to it. Ms. S.'s use of profanity caught me off guard. I only hoped that my expression had not changed.
"May I sit here?" (indicating the chair at the end of the bed)	"I have to go make a phone call."	I felt like I was being tested. First she wanted to go back to sleep and now she wanted to make a phone call.
"If your call isn't urgent, I'd like to do a postpartum check, which includes checking your breasts, your bleeding, and blood pressure, temperature, and pulse." (Eye contact made.)	"Okay, just don't take too long." (Eye contact brief)	

teaching. One student was frustrated in the recovery room of the delivery suite because her soft-spoken, compassionate statements were being rebuffed by the rising anger of her newly delivered patient. The instructor joined the student, and while continuing the empathic statements, implemented perineal care, and positioning of the patient for comfort. The patient became more relaxed, and the student learned how to combine compassion with essential physical care.

Be patient—don't expect instant solutions. The problems generated by poverty, poor health, addiction, and other societal ills affect our whole society and require a multisystem approach. These problems sometimes seem insurmountable.

A student cared for a mother in labor who was 31 weeks pregnant. The mother had no prenatal care and delivered twins unexpectedly. The father was unemployed, and the family was homeless. The parents were very angry at the staff for not knowing that there were twins. When the student cared for the mother on the following day in the postpartum unit, the mother still appeared angry and hostile. The students brought the mother to the neonatal intensive care unit to see the babies and touch them in the incubators. The patient continued to be angry and hostile with staff and the student. The student explained why staff members needed to ask the questions that they did and pointed out the good care that the babies were getting. The student also explained to the entire family what was going on. In addition, the student recommended resources for the family such as WIC, which could help extend the family's meager resources. She included information about possible drug treatment programs. At the end of the day, the mother appeared less hostile and expressed her gratitude to the student. It was pointed out to the student in postconference by her peers and the instructor just how significant that achievement was.

We need to communicate to our students that they are making significant contributions to the health care of socially high-risk families and that they are doing this as part of a joint effort of health professionals and institutionalized programs. They need to combine their knowledge as professionals with their responsibility as citizens to make needed changes in the lives of high-risk families. This requires communication of hope, support, inspiration, and commitment to students. We are most fortunate in having staff nurses who do this on a continuing basis. We must let the students know that together it is possible to move beyond the daily frustrations and make significant changes in families' lives.

REFERENCES

Baer, E. D., & Lowery, B. J. (1987). Patient and situational factors that affect nursing students' like or dislike of caring for patients. *Nursing Research, 36*(5), 298–302.

Barnard, K., Hammond, M., Mitchell, S., Booth, C. , Spietz, A., Snyder, C., & Elsas, T. (1985). Caring for high risk infants and their families. In M. Green (Ed.), *The psychosocial aspects of the family*, Lexington, MA: D. C. Heath.

Byrne, M. W. (1988). *An ethnography of undergraduate nursing student's clinical learning field*. Doctoral dissertation. Adelphi University, New York (University Microfilms No. 8814972).

McElmurry, B., Swider, S., Grimes, M., Dan, A., Irvin, Y., & Lourenco, S. (1987). Health advocacy for young, low income, inner city women. *Advances in Nursing Science, 9*(4), 62–75.

Melia, K. (1982). 'Tell it as it is'—qualitative methodology and nursing research: Understanding the student nurse's world. *Journal of Advanced Nursing, 7*, 327–335.

Spietz, A. (1988). Working with depressed moms. *NCAST National News, IV* (1), 1–2 & 5.

Vincent, P. & Davis, J. (1987). Social problems encountered by public health nurses: Identification and response differences according to education and experience. *Journal of Nursing Education, 26* (4), 144–149.

CHAPTER 37

Flaws in Family Nursing Education

Janice M. Bell, Lorraine M. Wright

Canadian nurses pay lip service to family-centered care, but can't always put it into practice. Does the fault lie in our nursing programs?

The family plays a vital role in promoting and maintaining health. We've all come to recognize this role, and knowledge in family nursing has grown dramatically over the past decade. But how is family nursing being taught? What are nursing students learning about caring for the family?

We asked those questions of Canada's 27 undergraduate nursing programs and 10 graduate programs. All but one program (undergraduate) responded. Their replies sketched a picture of family nursing education in Canadian universities, highlighting six major flaws. Based on those flaws, we developed recommendations for nurse clinicians and educators.

Flaw 1: Family nursing education is well integrated in undergraduate programs, but is not emphasized in graduate nursing programs.

Undergraduate programs make a concerted effort to implement and teach two areas of family nursing in particular: family assessment and families in health and illness. Although few programs offered specific courses with the family as the primary focus, teaching about family nursing occurred in other courses.

Graduate programs compared poorly. We were most concerned by the finding that graduate programs without a family-related specialty had no other family content. On

Reproduced with permission from *The Canadian Nurse. L'infirmière canadienne*, Volume 86, Number 6.

the average, less than one specific course title directly related to the family was reported by Canadian graduate nursing programs.

Flaw 2: Definitions of the family are becoming broader, but models and theories are many, varied and often inappropriate for understanding family dynamics.

Increasingly, university nurse educators are accepting nontraditional definitions of "family." With today's wide variety of family types and structures, the most advanced definition of family may be "the family is who the client says it is."

A plethora of assessment frameworks and family theories are being used to teach family nursing. Nursing models/theories most often identified were Roy's adaptation model, Orem's self-care model and Neuman's system model. Other programs taught developmental, systems, structural/functional, social support, communication, role, crisis, or stress and coping theory. Interestingly, few of the university programs use cybernetics theory.

Nurse educators are caught in a dilemma. They strive to educate within a nursing theory and they recognize the importance of caring for families. Yet few nursing theories include any aspect of family nursing. Trying to modify the frameworks to include the family is unsatisfactory.

One possible solution is to marry some of the more established nursing theories to such mid-range theories as cybernetics, systems theory and communication theory. This newly-wed framework of family nursing would not focus on the number of people being cared for (individual, family and community), but rather would look at responses to health problems from a systemic viewpoint. Nursing care would focus on the interactions between family members and the reciprocal effect of these interactions on the etiology, maintenance and impact of health and illness.

Although systems theory seems to be making its way into family nursing, cybernetics has not. Using cybernetics could dramatically enhance the nurse's ability to consider the reciprocal connections between illness, individuals and families.

Flaw 3: Nursing programs do not make enough use of textbooks and journals related to family nursing.

Each university was asked to identify the three textbooks and three journals most commonly used in nursing courses related to the family. Friedman's *Family Nursing: Theory and Assessment* and Wright and Leahey's *Nurses and Families: A Guide to Family Assessment and Intervention* headed the list. But 23 other textbooks—ranging from community health to maternity nursing—were also identified. Such a tremendous diversity shows the lack of national consensus in how family nursing should be taught and what students should learn. Family science or family therapy textbooks and journals were rarely mentioned. Notably, such journals as *Family Process, Family Relations and Family Systems Medicine* were missing.

We offer two recommendations. First, nurse educators must become more familiar with existing interdisciplinary family journals such as *Family Relations, Journal of Marital and Family Therapy* and *Family Process*. Secondly, Canada needs a journal of family nursing. Currently, information about family nursing is scattered haphazardly throughout many journals. A journal of family nursing would give nurse educators, clinicians, researchers and theorists a common forum to discuss families and family nursing.

Flaw 4: Few Canadian nursing programs teach advanced family intervention skills.
Family intervention strategies are taught by 21 of the undergraduate programs. Specific interventions, ranked in order of frequency, include praising the strength of the family or an individual; educating family members; validating affect; assigning behavioral tasks; and normalization. All interventions are taught at a level appropriate to undergraduate nurses. They seem to be the usual family-as-context interventions suggested in the nursing literature. Graduate programs reported a similar list of the beginning-level interventions, but seldom mentioned advanced interventions based on family relationships, interactions and beliefs, such as reframing, systemic reframing, ritual, metaphor and externalizing the symptom.

The survey shows that family assessment takes priority over family intervention. Nursing programs place little emphasis on designing or implementing interventions that would bring about positive changes. The existing family nursing literature, which is focused on description, offers few solutions to this over-emphasis on assessment. Although advanced knowledge about interaction, reciprocity and family interventions is available from the disciplines of family science and family therapy, our nurse educators apparently do not use it, even at the graduate level.

The lack of focus on interventions may be a direct reflection of the lack of strong clinical skills among nurse educators. We recommend that nurse educators become strong family clinicians. They will then focus more and more on developing and testing sophisticated family nursing interventions and reporting these new strategies in the literature.

Flaw 5: Not enough programs use live or videotaped interviews to demonstrate and supervise clinical work with families.
Family assessment, family interviewing skills and family intervention are usually taught through lectures or seminars. Only half the programs use videotape demonstrations or live interview demonstrations. Role playing is used by half the programs, but our experience and the literature indicate that skills practiced in role-playing are seldom transferable. In other words, nursing students have little opportunity to view skilled demonstrations of family assessment, family intervention and family interviewing. No wonder nurses pay lip service to family-centered care but have difficulty putting it into practice. Those programs without live or videotaped demonstrations could use the series of videotapes written and produced by Dr. Wendy Watson for family nursing education (see bibliography).

Programs use a wide variety of methods for supervising and evaluating students. Ranked in order of common use, the methods include case consultation, process recording, live clinical supervision, group supervision, audiotape supervision and videotape supervision. The predominant methods, case consultation and process recording, do not give direct observational data to nurse educators. Live or videotaped supervision leaves little to speculation and provides the most certain means of monitoring a student's skill development in family nursing.

Frequently, three main reasons are offered for the limited use of live or videotaped supervision: workload, lack of equipment and logistical problems. Our concern is that nurse educators may not be providing this necessary type of supervision and evaluation because they themselves lack clinical competence in family nursing.

Flaw 6: Canadian programs make no distinction between family nursing, family systems nursing and family therapy.

We asked our respondents which approach they use when working with families: family nursing, family systems nursing or family therapy, or some combination of the three. We defined family nursing as a focus on the individual in the context of the family; family systems nursing as a focus on the family system as the unit of care; and family therapy as a focus on emotional or behavioral problems.

Undergraduate nursing programs reported the following ranking: 23 use a family systems nursing approach, 20 also use a family nursing approach and four use a family therapy approach. All six of the 10 graduate programs offering a family-related specialty use a family systems nursing approach; four also use a family nursing approach; and two use a family therapy approach.

The reported frequency of a family systems nursing approach (family as the unit of care) seems inconsistent with the reported lack of teaching about reciprocity and complex interactions of families in assessment, intervention and interviewing. Perhaps the distinction between family-as-context (family nursing) and family-as-target (family systems nursing) was not clearly understood or described. Programs should make distinctions among family nursing, family systems nursing and family therapy. In turn, the theory and clinical skills that accompany each approach need to be taught at appropriate levels, from beginning to advanced competency. A focus on the complex interactions of the family is appropriate for advanced nursing practice at the graduate level. Undergraduate theoretical and clinical competence should focus on the family as context.

ABRÉGÉ

Formation boîteuse en soins infirmiers à la famille. Une étude portant sur tous les programmes de sciences infirmières au Canada a trouvé que la formation en soins infirmiers à la famille se concentre sur l'évaluation de la famille, et sur les familles et la maladie. Des lacunes graves ont été décelées vis-à-vis des interventions et des techniques de'entrevue, tout particulièrement au plan de l'exercice de pointe de ces soins. Des méthodes d'enseignement et d'évaluation plus efficaces sont nécessaires. Les chercheurs s'inquiètent du fait que ces faiblesses découlent du manque de compétences cliniques des enseignantes.

At the heart of the flaws in family nursing education is the lack of nurse educators who are also expert family clinicians. Strong clinical skills emphasizing family interaction and reciprocity would enable nurse educators to model family nursing skills, develop and test advanced interventions and fully use the existing interdisciplinary knowledge about families. Nurse educators must become committed to clinical scholarship and clinical supervision, as well as clinical teaching.

BIBLIOGRAPHY

Friedman, M. *Family nursing: Theory and assessment.* 2d ed. Norwalk, CT: Appleton-Century-Crofts, 1986.

Watson, W. L. A *family with chronic illness: A "tough" family copes well.* Videotape. The University of Calgary, 1988.

Watson, W.L. *Aging families and Alzheimer's disease.* Videotape. The University of Calgary, 1988.

Watson, W.L. *Fundamentals of family systems nursing.* Videotape. The University of Calgary, 1988.

Watson, W.L. *Families with psychosocial problems.* Videotape. The University of Calgary, 1989.

Watson, W. L. *Family systems nursing interventions.* Videotape. The University of Calgary, 1989.

Wright, L.M. and Leahey, M. *Nurses and families: A guide to family assessment and intervention.* Philadelphia: F.A. Davis, 1984.

CHAPTER 38

Prenatal Education and Family Centered Health Promotion at the Worksite

Donna J. MacLachlan, Shelby F. Merkel

The purpose of occupational health programs is to protect and enhance the health and well being of the worker. More and more of the U.S. work force includes women with young children. A recent study (Zylke, 1988) showed that more than 50% of mothers with children under 6 years of age were employed outside the home. Women often work up to the time of their delivery and return to work at the conclusion of their postpartum period or following a leave of absence. Calculated from *A Current Population Survey, Marital and Family Package*, 15% of all families with children have working single parents (Bureau of Labor Statistics, 1988).

Occupational health nurses play an important role in promoting healthy family functioning (deChesnay, 1988). More specifically, the National Commission to Prevent Infant Mortality (1988) states that whenever possible, companies should provide prenatal health promotion educational programs as part of comprehensive health benefit policies. Many people live away from their extended families and may need to learn their wellness and parenting skills in the workplace, or to have work serve as a channel of information for appropriate community resources.

Corporate America is faced with escalating health insurance premiums; expenditures for health care rank second only to payroll. Healthy babies make good business sense. Infants with low birth weight (less than 5½ lbs.) have a significantly higher

Reprinted by permission of the American Association of Occupational Health Nurses, *AAOHN Journal*, Vol. 38, No. 3 March 1990.

mortality rate during the neonatal period than normal birth weight infants (Shapero, 1980). These infants also have an increased rate of morbidity. Behrens (1987) makes the point that "babies born with birth defects, low birth weight, or other health problems also affect businesses directly:

- Physician and hospital costs for initial hospitalization of a low birth weight baby average $14,616, compared with $2,378 for a normal weight baby.
- Almost 19% of low birth weight babies are rehospitalized for an average of 12 days each.
- Sick babies may delay mothers' return to work and cause increased absences among concerned parents."

An Office of Technology Assessment report estimated that every low birth weight birth avoided by prenatal care saves the U.S. health care system between $14,000 and $30,000 in initial hospitalization and long term costs ("Bradley Introduces Infant Mortality and Children's Health Legislation." Washington, D.C.: News release, February 1, 1989). Education for workers about proper prenatal health care and enhanced coping skills should lower absenteeism and increase work efficiency. Employer disability and insurance costs should also decrease, demonstrating that the occupational health nurse supports not only the family but also the employer.

Petschek (1987) identified a need for occupational health nurses to receive a clear definition of the scope and purpose of prenatal education. This article also stated that the occupational health nurse should be encouraged to initiate prenatal education programs when the staff perceives that such a program is needed.

The purpose of this article is to address those issues. The nursing process, which includes assessment, planning, implementation, and evaluation, provides the format. Two comprehensive prenatal education programs are presented, as well as the activities and factors related to their success. Occupational health nurses may be more eager to present prenatal education programs at their worksites when they see how this program dynamically extended by networking into other family centered health promotion activities.

ASSESSMENT

The work setting in which these programs were developed and are currently taught is the research and development arm of AT&T, with about 30,000 employees in facilities in the Midwest and East. A significant number of pregnant employees are in the high risk category due to age (third decade). Delivery is one of the primary causes of benefit absence in this company. Work hours may be very irregular with evening and night laboratory times, making attendance at community prenatal classes difficult. Although the population is very wellness oriented, the need for a prenatal education program in the workplace became apparent.

PLANNING

The purpose of the prenatal education programs is to provide information that will contribute to safe, healthy, and productive pregnancies, deliveries, and family functioning. Goals include:

- Teaching the prevention of birth defects and premature births, and proper health habits, anatomy, and physiology of pregnancy/labor/delivery, comprehensive prenatal care, infant care, and parenting.
- Encouraging women to work during their pregnancies, since pregnancy is a normal healthy state, and to return to work after delivery.
- Referring employees to community resources for additional education and/or care.
- Supporting father and mother as a team.

Contact was also made with the March of Dimes, a certified nurse lactation consultant, nurse childbirth educators, and nurse midwives. Input from surrounding hospitals and obstetricians was sought.

With the support of the company medical director, a two hour pilot class was presented to assess employee interest. The test lecture on prenatal nutrition generated a large employee response. A comprehensive course outline and student class evaluation questionnaire for a 12-week prenatal lecture series was then developed. Guest speakers were contacted for availability, and course handouts and visual aids were obtained from pharmaceutical firms, government agencies, and educational companies. Monetary outlay was minimal, since the majority of the literature was free.

The initial planning stage encompassed approximately 4 months. Ongoing planning and course modification continue as new materials and information become available.

IMPLEMENTATION

The initial prenatal series, designed and presented in the Chicago area work location in 1983, has been ongoing since. Four series are taught each year. Employees, spouses, and single parents-to-be, which include women who are in their second and third trimesters, enroll in the free, 12-week, lunch hour classes held in the employee health department conference room. Class size is limited to 30 to facilitate discussion and networking. The content includes information about anatomy and physiology of late pregnancy, nutrition, exercise, prenatal tests, health care provider visits, the labor and delivery process, types of deliveries, the role of the father, postpartum care, newborn characteristics and illnesses, infant safety and care, breast and bottle feeding, child care issues, company benefits and parenting.

The occupational health nurse is the primary instructor. This identifies the nurse as a resource and support person throughout the pregnancy and early parenting period. The company physician, a benefit representative, and an employee counselor also present information. Class "alumni" enthusiatically offer experiential knowledge on a caesarean section delivery, infant supplies, and selection of alternative child care. The new babies are always an attraction. Community speakers may include hospital nutritionists and child care specialists.

Comprehensive handouts and visual aids are provided by pharmaceutical and educational firms, local health departments, hospitals, and other community agencies. Videos, slides, and films graphically portray vaginal and caesarean section deliveries and many aspects of child care. The caesarean section class is well received in the health care community and, as a result, is approved by the surrounding hospitals for admission of the father to the caesarean section delivery room. At the completion of the series, certificates are awarded.

A separate 3-week preregistered lunch hour program addresses the health education needs of those in their first trimester of pregnancy and those couples contemplating pregnancy.

The prenatal education class presented in a New Jersey work location is similar in course content, but different in design. The occupational health nurse who developed this course chose to keep each presentation autonomous. Each lunch hour program is advertised with posters and company mail. Preregistration is not required, and walk-ins are welcome. Twenty to 50 employees, spouses, singles, parents-to-be, and children attend programs in a worksite conference room separate from the employee health department.

This 12-week series encompasses all three trimesters of pregnancy, infant care, and preconceptual counseling information. In addition to the occupational health nurse, many outside community health professionals make presentations with varied formats. This series has been taught once a year for the past 3 years at two New Jersey locations. The community networking in and out of the company has generated cooperation for additional programs and has added strength and breadth to the prenatal program.

Both program formats incorporate assessment of family functioning into this health promotion activity. The class content considers specific potential problem areas for the population served, capitalizes on this population's strengths, and promotes health rather than focusing on the negative. Information is presented in a manner commensurate with the students' education and lifestyle. Throughout the class, open communication in all areas of the couple relationship is stressed, shared problem solving is encouraged, and role flexibility is introduced. Many appropriate community resources are identified for individual use.

EVALUATION

The prenatal programs are well attended at all locations, with waiting lists for the preregistered program. Evaluation questionnaires are obtained from all class participants (see Figure 1). One comment that appears routinely is the appreciation for the course being taught in the work environment. Convenience, the perception of

EXPECTANT PARENT CLASS EVALUATION FORM

Your answers to the following questions will help me evaluate my current classes as well as plan for the future. Thank you for your cooperation.

1. Please circle:
   A. Father   Mother   First Baby?   Yes   No
2. What prompted you to attend these classes? (circle)
   Doctor   Friend   Newsletter Article   Personal Interest
   Other _____
3. Are you attending/will attend any other classes: (circle)
   Hospital Expectant Parent   Lamaze   Health Dept.
   Other _____
4. Did these classes meet your expectations?
   Very well _____   Fairly well _____   Not at all _____
5. What part did you find most beneficial? _____
   _____
6. Do you feel you have made any changes as a result of this course? _____
   Could you please mention at least one?
   _____
7. Describe how you feel about the classes now that you have completed the series. Recommendations and comments are encouraged! _____
   _____
   _____
8. What advantages are there to having these classes presented in your work environment? _____
   _____
   _____
9. Do you have any personal concerns? _____
   _____
   _____

For Statistical Purposes:
Age _____
Hospital _____
OB _____
Requesting analgesia/anesthesia? _____
Preference? _____
Planning on breast feeding? _____
Use of formula? _____
Presently using/practicing relaxation techniques? _____
_____

FIGURE 1.

corporate support for pregnant employees, and the work support group are often the reasons given. Information on work policies, benefits, and alternative child care resources is well received

Many attendees believe this program familiarizes them with the occupational health nurse as a resource person for their questions and concerns during the child bearing and parenting phases of their lives. They appreciate having this resource person conveniently located at the worksite. For some employees, the prenatal class is the initial interaction with the company employee health department. This program acts as an introduction to other services available.

The guest speakers/new parents are often referred to in the evaluations as "special treats" and "favorite program." The emotional/experiential aspect of childbirth appears to be very important to pregnant women. The written materials distributed at every session are identified on many evaluations as being of great importance for references, resources, and supporting information.

A significant number of attendees are able to identify behavior changes they have made after completing the prenatal series. Men and women believe they take a more active role in their prenatal care by questioning and communicating more assertively with their health care providers. Pregnant women identify an improvement in their nutrition and/or exercise habits.

Both parents-to-be believe they have more realistic expectations of the labor and delivery processes. Many express the perception of an improved level of confidence in their ability to be a good parent—better prepared for childbirth and parenthood, more positive about breast feeding, more comfortable with the father and coach roles, better able to make decisions, calm and reassured.

Evaluation questionnaires from the lectures have provided much positive feedback and insight on new programs desired. As a result, spin-off family centered health promotion programs have been planned and initiated with other committees using networking. Networking performs three basic functions:

- Reduces costs by not competing with other groups' programs.
- Opens access to information by sharing people, background information, data, and resources.
- Promotes good feelings and communication between groups.

SPIN-OFF PROGRAMS

A noontime lecture series on parenting was cosponsored by employee health departments at three company locations and by several child care committees. Rotating through five company locations in New Jersey, these free, 15-week lectures addressed all phases of parenting and considered many different age levels. This annual series continues to increase in variety—from "medical savvy," to child/school liaison, raising street-wise kids, and preparing creative meals.

Parents Fairs were held at four company locations, with booths staffed by company and community representatives. A 5-week, noontime child growth and development lecture series was sponsored by the employee health department and presented by a community child development specialist. A formal noon hour presentation on ultrasound and the prevention/identification of birth defects was delivered by a well known radiologist. Grandparents To Be and Parenting the Parent classes were also offered.

Programs on "how to find child care" are presented regularly at several locations. Working mothers' and working parents' support groups are active and thriving, with regular input from occupational health nurses.

Electric breast pumps are now being utilized at six company locations. In the cleanliness and privacy of an employee health department room, new mothers find a support system as they provide nourishment for their infants. This service also encourages mothers to return to work sooner than they might otherwise do.

Child growth and development libraries are continuing to grow. Networking has allowed company occupational health nurses to serve on Child Care Committees and the Women's Networking Planning Board, and to speak at forums about various women's health issues involving subcommittees of nurses from in-house medical departments.

Also, the occupational health nurses serve as a community resources for PTAs, outside women's networks, outside medical departments; as role models and teachers of nutrition for minority grade schoolers who tour the worksite; and as coordinators of the AT&T Pioneer Indian Children's Clothing Drive at the worksite.

The networking, cooperation, and teamwork demonstrated within the work community and among the company employee health departments are very rewarding to the nurses. The prenatal programs and associated activities combine community and company resources in a dynamic way to help improve the health and future of AT&T Bell Laboratories families.

The workplace prenatal program

- Teaches employees to understand how to stay healthy on their own.
- Helps combat increasing health benefits costs.
- Provides health education, the impetus for lifestyle changes.

REFERENCES

Behrens, R.A. (1987). Healthy pregnancies, healthy babies make healthier workforce. *Worksite wellness media report*. Washington, D.C.: Washington Business Group on Health Office of Disease Prevention and Health Promotion.

Bureau of Labor Statistics. (1988, March). *A current population survey, marital and family package*. Washington, D.C.: Bureau of Labor Statistics, Table 39.

deChesnay, M., & Magnuson, J. (1988). How healthy families cope with stress. *AAOHN Journal, 36*(9), 361-365.

National Commission to Prevent Infant Mortality. (1988, April). *The private sector's role in reducing infant mortality*. Washington, D.C.: author.

Petschek, M.A. (1987). Prenatal education—should it be part of your worksite health program? *AAOHN Journal, 35*(11), 485-486.

Shapero, S., McCormick, M.C., Starfield, B.H., Krischer, J.P., & Bross, D. (1980). Relevance of corre-lates of infant deaths for significant morbidity at one year of age. *American Journal of Obstetrics and Gynecology, 136,* 363-373.

Zylke, J.W. (1988). Day-care quality and quantity becomes challenges for parents, politicians and medical researchers. *Journal of the American Medical Association, 260*(22), 3247–3249.

CHAPTER **39**

Innovations in Family and Community Health

Angeline Bushy, Rebecca Graner

PRECONCEPTION EDUCATION: A PROGRAM FOR COMMUNITY HEALTH NURSES

The cause and effect relationship of life-style behaviors on pregnancy outcomes is well documented. The early reproductive years are a preparatory time for prospective parents, especially women, to become aware of, evaluate, and alter at-risk life-style behaviors. Consequently, anticipatory guidance prior to conception is important for all. Particularly in need of health-promoting information are young women who are at risk for poor pregnancy outcomes, such as adolescents, those who smoke or live in households where others smoke, those who have poor nutritional status, and those in low socioeconomic minority groups. Preconceptional education also is critical for men of reproductive age, since a man's life style can directly influence his partner's pregnancy outcome.[1-3]

Prenatal classes target those who already are pregnant; their content does not address those individuals who are contemplating becoming pregnant in the future. Stemming from this information deficit, a Planning Pregnancy Class (see Table 1) was developed by one of the authors (RG). Its purpose is to augment—ideally, to preempt—participation in prenatal classes.

The anticipated outcomes of the Planning Pregnancy Class are threefold:

1. reduce the infant mortality rate by improving pregnancy outcomes,

Reprinted from *Family & Community Health*, Vol. 13, No. 3, pp. 82–84, with permission of Aspen Publishers, Inc., © 1990.

TABLE 1
Planning Pregnancy Class Goal, Objectives, and Content

Goal: To improve pregnancy outcomes within the market area

Objectives: The purpose of this class is to
1. promote awareness of individual responsibility in pregnancy outcomes and infant mortality rates,
2. discuss the anticipated role changes that accompany childbearing and childrearing,
3. describe the manner in which pregnancy affects family dynamics,
4. identify childbirth options available to consumers in the health care delivery system,
5. list formal and informal community resources for support during childbearing and childrearing, and
6. facilitate informal networking among program participants.

Topic	Content
Life-style patterns	Health-promoting versus high-risk life-style activities
	Marital transitions
	Parental expectations
	Optimal pregnancy outcome
	Costs, demands, rewards of parenting
Employment issues	The super mom syndrome
	Dynamics associated with life/family transitions
Developmental issues	Becoming pregnant
	Genetics
	Health of the parents
	Maintaining the pregnancy
	In-utero risk factors
	The new baby
	Childcare skills
Planning for pregnancy	Primary considerations: Why? When?
	Mapping ovulation
	Gender selection
	Calculating the estimated date of conception
	Birthing options
Social support	Natural versus formal systems
	Community resources
Obstetrical unit	Optional tour; meet staff
Evaluation	

2. enhance participants' parenting skills after they have children, and
3. reduce obstetrical malpractice litigations and thereby affect esclating health care costs.[4]

The topics addressed in the 4-hour, consumer-oriented class include information about nutrition; healthy versus at risk life-style behaviors; social and environmental factors that influence pregnancy outcomes; the role of genetics; selecting an "ideal time" to have a baby; issues related to fetal rights; information on birth control; techniques for determining a child's gender; an overview of informal and formal maternal, child, and family support services in the community; and an optional tour of an obstetrical unit in a hospital that cosponsors the class. The target audience is anyone contemplating pregnancy in the near future, both men and women. No arbitrary time constraints delineate "near future" so as to not restrict participation.

Community health nurses' primary role is to provide meaningful, cost effective primary health care to groups of clients. Preconceptional counseling has the potential of being one of the most cost effective methods of improving the health of future generations. To be effective, though, the programs must be accessible to vulnerable populations that are identified as at risk for poor pregnancy outcomes.[5]

Benefits of such counseling may be difficult to quantify, however, because the full ramifications of the class may not be realized for several generations. In essence, the class attempts to expose participants to the notion of individual responsibility for having healthy offspring. It is hoped that awareness will motivate participants to modify or replace at-risk behaviors with healthy practices *before* becoming pregnant. Ultimately, healthy life styles also should increase opportunities for improved pregnancy outcomes.

The Planning Pregnancy Class is an initial effort to address a major, national health concern: high maternal-infant mortality rates. The greatest challenge to community health nurses will be delivering the program to vulnerable populations who are most in need of the information.

REFERENCES

1. Briggs, S. A vision for America's future agenda for the 1990s: A children's defense budget. *NAACOG Newletter.* 1989; 16 (5):5.
2. Chez, R., Cefalo, R., & Jmerkatz, I. Why it's important to help patients prepare for pregnancy. *Contemp Ob/Gyn.* 1989; 33(6):64–85.
3. Davis, M., & Akridge, K. The effects of promoting intrauterine attachment in primiparas on post delivery attachment. *JOGNN.* 1987; 16(6):430–437.
4. Moos, M., & Cefalo R. Preconceptional health promotion: A focus for obstetric cre. *Am J Perinatol.* 1987; 4(1):63–69.
5. Bushy, A. Body image and self-esteem: A comparison of rural and urban pregnant women. Austin, TX: University of Texas at Austin; 1988. Dissertation.

Index

Numbers followed by an *f* indicate a figure; *t* following a page number indicates tabular material.

/